UNUSUAL PRODUCTIONS IN PHONOLOGY

The universalist view that acquisition of phonology is guided by universal principles has been the dominant position for decades. More recently, an alternative view has brought into focus the relationship between developmental markedness and language-specific input frequencies. With entirely original chapters on non-ambient-like productions by typically and atypically developing children and second language learners, *Unusual Productions in Phonology* delves deeply into these competing explanations to show that the patterns observed do not uniquely lend themselves to one or the other explanation. Rather, they point toward the need for both universal markedness and statistical input considerations in any attempted explanation.

Containing contributions from leading researchers from around the world, this impressive collection is a must-have resource for any researcher, practitioner, or advanced student specializing in phonology, cognitive psychology, applied linguistics, and communication disorders.

Mehmet Yavaş is a Professor of Linguistics at Florida International University. He has published numerous articles on applied phonology and is the principal author of *Avaliação Fonologica da Criança* (1990), a phonological assessment procedure for Brazilian Portuguese. His other publications include *Phonological Disorders in Children* (1991), *First and Second Language Phonology* (1994), *Phonology: Development and Disorders* (1998), and *Applied English Phonology* (3rd edition forthcoming).

LANGUAGE AND SPEECH DISORDERS BOOK SERIES

Series Editors:

Martin J. Ball, Linköping University, Sweden
Jack S. Damico, University of Louisiana at Lafayette

This new series brings together course material and new research for students, practitioners, and researchers in the various areas of language and speech disorders. Textbooks covering the basics of the discipline will be designed for courses within communication disorders programs in the English-speaking world, and monographs and edited collections will present cutting-edge research from leading scholars in the field.

PUBLISHED

Recovery from Stuttering, Howell

Handbook of Vowels and Vowel Disorders, Ball & Gibbon (Eds.)

Handbook of Qualitative Research in Communication Disorders, Ball, Müller & Nelson (Eds.)

Dialogue and Dementia, Schrauf & Müller (Eds.)

Understanding Individual Differences in Language Development Across the School Years, Tomblin & Nippold (Eds.)

Unusual Productions in Phonology: Universals and Language-Specific Considerations, Yavaş (Ed.)

For continually updated information about published and forthcoming titles in the *Language and Speech Disorders* book series, please visit **www.psypress.com/language-and-speech-disorders**

UNUSUAL PRODUCTIONS IN PHONOLOGY

Universals and Language-Specific Considerations

Edited by
Mehmet Yavaş

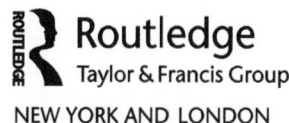

Routledge
Taylor & Francis Group
NEW YORK AND LONDON

First published 2015
by Psychology Press

Published 2023 by Routledge
605 Third Avenue, New York, NY 10017
4 Park Square, Milton Park, Abingdon, Oxon OX14 4RN

*Routledge is an imprint of the Taylor & Francis Group,
an informa business*

Library of Congress Cataloging-in-Publication Data
Unusual productions in phonology : universals and language-specific considerations /
    edited by Mehmet Yavas.
        pages cm
    Includes bibliographical references and index.
  1. Articulation disorders.   2. Articulation disorders in children.   3. Language acquisition.
I. Yavas, Mehmet S. editor.
    RC424.7.U58 2014
    618.92'855—dc23
    2014021182

ISBN: 978-1-848-72670-3 (hbk)
ISBN: 978-1-138-80980-2 (pbk)
ISBN: 978-1-315-74282-3 (ebk)

Typeset in Times New Roman
by Apex CoVantage, LLC

CONTENTS

CONTRIBUTORS

Rachel Aghara—University of Houston, Houston, Texas

B. May Bernhardt—University of British Columbia, Vancouver, Canada

Natasha Bouchat-Laird—Western University, Ontario, Canada

Françoise Brosseau-Lapré—McGill University, Montreal, Canada

Katherine M. Brown—Indiana University, Bloomington, Indiana

Ferenc Bunta—University of Houston, Houston, Texas

Emily Byers—Indiana University, Bloomington, Indiana

Robert S. Carlisle—California State University, Bakersfield, California

Mario E. Chávez-Peón—Centro de Investigaciones y Estudios Superiores en Antropologia Social, Mexico, DF

Juan Antonio Cutillas Espinosa—Universidad de Murcia, Murcia, Spain

Daniel A. Dinnsen—Indiana University, Bloomington, Indiana

Judith A. Gierut—Indiana University, Bloomington, Indiana

Jette G. Hansen Edwards—The Chinese University of Hong Kong, Shatin, Hong Kong

Margaret Kehoe—University of Geneva, Geneva, Switzerland

Elizabeth Morin-Lessard—Concordia University, Montreal, Canada

Michele L. Morrisette—Indiana University, Bloomington, Indiana

Amanda L. Procter—University of Houston, Houston, Texas

Paula M. Reimers—University of Essex, Colchester, Essex, United Kingdom

Roswitha Romonath—University of Cologne, Cologne, Germany

Susan Rvachew—McGill University, Montreal, Canada

Joseph Paul Stemberger—University of British Columbia, Vancouver, Canada

Mehmet Yavaş—Florida International University, Miami, Florida

Tania S. Zamuner—University of Ottawa, Ottawa, Canada

ACKNOWLEDGMENTS

I would like to express my gratitude to the authors who have contributed to this book. Their enthusiastic response with original contributions made it possible for me to set the goals of this volume. I am extremely grateful for their cooperation.

My deep thanks also go to the following scholars who gave their help in the review of the chapters:

Martin Ball, Linköping University, Sweden
Jessica Barlow, San Diego State University, United States
B. May Bernhardt, University of British Columbia, Canada
Walcir Cardoso, Concordia University, Canada
Andrea MacLeod, University of Montreal, Canada
Roy Major, Arizona State University, United States
Cliffton Pye, University of Kansas, United States
Keren Rice, University of Toronto, Canada
Yvan Rose, Memorial University, Canada
Carol Stoel-Gammon, University of Washington, United States
Tania Zamuner, University of Ottawa, Canada

I am very appreciative of their generosity.

Finally, I would like to thank Paul Dukes of Taylor & Francis for his constant support, and my students Jake Guyton and Yaobin Liu for their assistance in the preparation of the manuscript.

INTRODUCTION

Mehmet Yavaş

The universalist view of acquisition, which espouses the idea that children's acquisition of phonology is guided by universal principles, has been the dominant position for decades. However, a growing body of literature during the last two decades on children's early use of words in various languages has brought into focus the relationship between developmental patterns and language-specific input frequencies. The works in this volume look at these two competing explanations—universal markedness and statistical input conditions—with data from three populations that reveal non-ambient-like productions: typically and atypically developing children, and second language learners.

While the acquisition of first language phonology—typical and atypical—has long been viewed as a legitimate area of inquiry for phonological theory, investigations on second language/interlanguage phonologies have not had the same status. The basic reason for this was the thinking that the non-ambient-like productions of an L2 speaker could be explained with reference to his/her first language. The recognition of L2 phonology as relevant to phonological acquisition and to phonological theory has been a result of a multitude of studies in the last two to three decades; these investigations have revealed that several aspects of non-ambient-like productions in L2 phonologies need to be explained through universal markedness. Although the influence of the learners' L1 cannot be completely shut out in the explanation of the non-ambient-like productions, increasingly the attention has turned to markedness, especially for speakers with intermediate levels of L2. Thus, the dynamism regarding the effects of universals in

1

L2 phonology has been very visible. As for statistical input frequencies, however, interest in L2 phonological acquisition studies has only been relatively recent (Cardoso 2008; Cardoso & Liakin 2009; Piske & Young-Scholten 2009).

Simply stated, frequency is the rate of a phonological unit. Two types of frequency that are discussed are 'type' and 'token' frequencies. Token frequency refers to the frequency of occurrence of a given word (e.g. *the*, *big*), while type frequency refers to a specific sound or sequences of sounds (/ð/, /tr/). For example, an initial /st/ cluster has high 'type' frequency, whereas /ʒ/ and the onset cluster /fj/ rank low. Sometimes, there is a clash between the two frequencies. For example, word-initial /ð/ has low type frequency (not found in many different words) but high token frequency (e.g. very frequently used grammatical morphemes *the*, *that*).

Another concept that is relevant here is 'neighborhood density' (hereafter ND), which combines frequency and similarity. Typically, this is defined through the number of words that differ from the target word by a single phoneme substitution, insertion, or deletion. Generally, words from dense neighborhoods (i.e. words with many phonetically similar counterparts), such as *bit*, which has several neighbors (e.g. *bet*, *but*, *bat*, *beat*, *bill*, *bitch*, *bid*, *bought*, *big*, *pit*, *sit*, *wit*, *knit*, *built*, *it*, etc.), are produced faster and more accurately than words from sparse neighborhoods, such as *giant*, with no neighbors, or *jeans*, with very few neighbors.

The significance of input frequencies in phonological development has been reported for several languages. For example, the palato-alveolar affricate /ʧ/ is acquired earlier in Spanish than in English due to its high frequency in the former (Macken 1995). Similarly, post-alveolar retroflex fricatives and affricates are among the earliest acquired sounds in Potunghua (Hua & Dodd 2000), whereas similar palato-alveolar sounds in English (/ʃ/, /ʧ/, /ʤ/) are acquired later. /d/ provides another example; it is one of the early acquired sounds in English but is acquired later in Finnish, due to its low frequency (Macken 1995). /v/ seems to be mastered earlier in Swedish, Estonian, and Bulgarian than it is in English, because of its higher frequencies in those languages (Ingram 1988). /l/ is mastered earlier by French-speaking children compared to English-speaking children due to its greater token frequency in the former (Chevrie-Muller & Lebreton 1973). Some reports on the development of CVC structures also lend support to the influence of the ambient language; the development is earlier in English than in Spanish. This seems to be due to the differences in the percentages of codas in child-directed speech, which is 60% in English and only 25%

in Spanish (Roark & Demuth 2000). Interestingly, Spanish final coda consonants are acquired earlier by Spanish-German bilingual children than by Spanish monolinguals (Lleó 2006). This suggests that the high frequency of coda consonants in children's German has an effect on their Spanish.

Although in many instances there is an overlap between the unmarked and the frequent and thus early-learned phonological units, there are obvious clashes between the two. For example, while sonorant consonants are less marked in coda position than obstruents, Stites, Demuth, and Kirk (2004) showed that alveolar stops, which are the most frequent coda consonants in English, were the first-acquired coda consonants in English. This is interpreted as showing that robust frequency effects override markedness tendencies.

Zamuner, Gerken, and Hammond (2004), however, suggest that frequency effects within the syllable rhyme, rather than the coda alone, are better at predicting order of acquisition. This raises the question of what units need to be considered for statistical computing. Similarly, the interaction of prosodic factors with frequency may add further variables. Kirk and Demuth (2006) suggest that English-speaking 2-year-olds are more likely to produce coda consonants when they occur in either stressed or final syllables, where their duration is longer.

There are also reports, however, that reveal conflicting results for the same target(s). In the examination of the acquisition of English initial /s/ clusters in typically developing monolingual children, Yavaş and Core (2006) state that /st/, which is most frequent in English, has the highest correct realization, and /sn/, which has the lowest frequency in these clusters, has the lowest percentage correct. The higher percentage of correct realizations of /st/ has also been reported in Haitian Creole-English-speaking bilingual children (Yavaş & Beaubrun 2006). While these results seem supportive of frequency, /st/ is found with no special status in Spanish-English bilingual children—either in typical development (Yavaş & Barlow 2006) or in atypical development (Yavaş 2010). Moreover, data from atypically developing monolingual English-speaking children (Yavaş & McLeod 2010) show that markedness based on the sonority distance between /s/ and C2 is a much better explanation of the patterns; low frequency /s + nasal/ clusters had much greater accuracy than the most frequent but sonority-reversing /st/.

Moreover, there are also instances where frequency-based predictions have been challenged. For example, Levelt, Schiller, and Levelt (2000) argue that Dutch-speaking children's order of acquisition of syllable types can be predicted through the frequency of syllable structure in child-directed speech. However, Rose (2009), looking at the Dutch data, states that the findings cannot be explained by frequency-based explanations and that approaches based on representational complexity offer better explanations for the observed phenomena. Rose and Inkelas (2011), looking at some other patterns discussed in the literature—consonant harmony, velar fronting, and cluster reduction, among others—state that, due to their emerging nature, these cannot be predicted from statistical tendencies. To explain children's productions, they call for a multi-faceted approach, where frequency may be only one of the factors. As can be seen from all these, there are unsettled issues. In order to contribute further to the discussion of the effects of frequency and markedness with additional new data from various languages, this volume brings together studies on three different populations.

The first four chapters in this volume address data from typical development of first language phonology. In chapter 1, Gierut, Morrisette, and Brown explore the link between language-specific input statistics and universal principles in acquisition. Language-specific probabilistic phonotactics and universal syllable well-formedness are examined through two computational studies, with the aim of determining which principle would best align with the distribution of words in the child lexicon of English. Findings indicate that the distribution of words in child lexicons was not in agreement with either model; neither language-specific input statistics nor universal principles were sufficient in capturing the composition of the child lexicon. The authors suggest an integrated approach whereby language-specific input statistics contribute to the refinement of language universals. They also stress the need for cross-linguistic studies, as input statistics vary from language to language.

NDs have been shown to be a factor in lexical development for several languages. At the same time, these studies demonstrated that the effects of ND vary, and this is likely due to the language-specific structures and lexical patterns of individual languages. In chapter 2, Zamuner, Morin-Lessard, and Bouchart-Laird investigate the role of ND in Québec French-speaking children's lexicons. Results indicate that NDs in children's vocabularies are similar to adult French in that both have many rhyme neighborhoods (lexical items distinguished by a change in the initial consonant) and different from adult French in that they have a greater number of consonant neighborhoods (lexical items distinguished by changes in vowels). The authors suggest language-specific input patterns (children first learn words with open syllables) as the likely explanation for these discrepancies.

Before children acquire clusters, reduction to a single member is a common process in languages. Data from European languages are generally supportive of an explanation in terms of sonority sequencing of the clusters: the consonant with the lowest sonority in the cluster is generally the retained member. In chapter 3, Stemberger and Chávez-Peón investigate this topic by looking at a language, Valley Zapotec, which has unusual complex onsets that are not rising in sonority. Their findings suggest different explanations for different cluster types. Such facts lead to a conclusion that while there are some shared universals reported for European languages, there are also language-specific factors at play.

While the studies in the above chapters are concerned with segments and phonotactic restrictions, in chapter 4 Reimers takes a different route to evaluate markedness in first language acquisition. Assuming that markedness guides the infant in language development from birth, Reimers suggests that the initial state has to be taken as far back as possible towards infant perceptual studies. Since this state does not contain any segments, the unit to be considered is the rhythm-bearing unit, the syllable. Looking at evidence from Japanese infants, Reimers questions the CV syllable as the basic type and suggests that a coda constituent needs to be included when ambient language influence is taken into account.

The next four chapters, chapters 5–8, feature analyses of data from children with phonological disorders. The first two examine data from groups, and the last two are longitudinal single case studies. In chapter 5, Bernhardt, Romonath, and Stemberger examine the patterns of singleton fricative development in German and English through data from 30 children in each language. Their findings, mirroring several others in the volume, give support to universal patterns (e.g. /f/ was the most advanced in both languages, despite being less frequent than /v/ in German and less frequent than /s/ in English) and also to language-specific considerations (e.g. /v/ in German is more advanced than in English because it is more frequent in German). The effects of frequency are also present in German data through more affricate substitutions in mismatches.

In chapter 6, Rvachew and Brosseau-Lapré provide an analysis of pre- and post-treatment productions of syllable-initial /ʁ/-clusters by Québec French-speaking children. Their focus is on patterns related to syllable stress, co-articulatory challenges, and the sonority profile within the onset. Their findings indicate greater accuracy of clusters in stressed syllables (universal perceptual salience), possible co-articulatory factors (correct tokens observed most frequently for dorsal targets; i.e. dorsal stop + [ʁ]), and phonological factors (partial support for 'sonority' (Jongstra 2003)). Also noteworthy, however, is the language-specific influence regarding some surprising productions, which might be due to the ambiguous status of Québec French [ʁ] (children may have classified this target as a fricative or an approximant).

In chapter 7, Dinnsen, Gierut, and Morrisette examine the error pattern 's > θ > f chain shift', whereby grooved coronal fricatives are replaced by interdental fricatives and interdental fricatives are replaced by labial fricatives. The conspiracy to avoid coronal fricatives is driven by two universal markedness constraints. The authors suggest that the optimality theoretic account they provide, which relies on both language-specific and universal properties, also offers some insight into why this chain shift has been so problematic in clinical treatment studies.

Another case study, chapter 8 by Kehoe, is an analysis of data from a trilingual (English, German, and French) child, Max, who shows protracted phonological development. The focus is on Max's acquisition of CV forms and velar consonants and the production of consonant clusters with respect to place of articulation. Max's early speech is characterized by a U-shaped pattern of development, in which, after a period of producing codas and velar consonants, his production of these structures declines. These changes cannot be accounted for by frequency but are consistent with the emergence of unmarked forms. The obstruent + liquid cluster reductions, however, are consistent with place-determined onset reduction; Max selects 'labial', produces [wʌk] for *truck* (closely tied to his analysis of English /r/ as labial), and applies this to his English but not to his German and French words because in French and German /r/ is 'dorsal', not 'labial'. Thus, the findings lend support to both universals and language-specific features.

The last four chapters introduce data from second language acquisition and/or from bilingual productions. Chapters 9 and 10 focus on the acquisition by speakers from various L1 language backgrounds of specific English #sC onset clusters, where the C is an alveolar (i.e. /st/, /sn/, /sl/). The objective is to see if input frequency and/or sonority-based markedness can explain the patterns observed. In chapter 9, Carlisle and Cutillas Espinosa examine longitudinal data from Spanish L1 speakers under Major's (2001) Ontogeny Phylogeny Model, which suggests different degrees of influence from L1 interference and the universals at different stages of interlanguage phonology. The study compares the correct productions of the above-cited #sC clusters at two time points, one year apart, in intermediate-level learners. The results reveal that the influence of markedness remains as strong at time 2 as it is at time 1. The fact that there is a greater increase in the correct productions of more marked onsets supports the Ontogeny

Phylogeny Model's claims that the influence of markedness declines in later stages of acquisition. In chapter 10, Hansen Edwards looks at the acquisition of the same clusters by L1 speakers of Mandarin Chinese, Cantonese, and Vietnamese. The explanations for the findings point in three different directions for the three languages examined: markedness for Vietnamese, L1 transfer for Cantonese, and input frequency for Mandarin Chinese. Hansen Edwards attributes the differences between her findings and those of previous studies to the type of data collected (naturalistic versus word lists or sentence reading) and to the language type; that is, it depends whether the learners' L1 allows complex onsets other than #sC clusters.

The last two chapters concentrate on productions in bilingual populations. In chapter 11, Procter, Bunta, and Aghara examine the voice onset time (hereafter VOT) productions of Spanish-English bilingual children and their monolingual peers in each language. They find that the VOTs of the English /p/ and /b/ are significantly shorter in the productions of bilingual children than in their monolingual peers; however, the tendency is the reverse for /g/. Overall, their findings indicate that although their performance is not identical to the VOTs from their monolingual peers in relation to VOTs, bilingual children have autonomous systems for their two languages. The language that is more significantly affected is English (L2); the authors explain this in terms of language dominance and greater language use, which favor Spanish (L1).

Yavaş and Byers, in chapter 12, look at the productions of adult Spanish-English bilinguals, examining the VOTs of voiceless stops in monolingual utterances in the two languages as well as in code-switched utterances in either direction. Similar to the findings of Procter et al., the results show that bilinguals' VOTs for /p, t, k/, although not identical to those found in monolinguals, are clearly separated for the two languages. In those cases in which the direction of code-switching has a significant effect, we see the effects of the precursor language. Overall, Spanish (L1) VOTs are influenced more than those of English (L2). Although this may seem contrary to expectations, because it shows a movement from less marked (short-lag) to more marked (long-lag) productions, the best explanation seems to reside in language (L2 English) dominance and greater use of the L2.

As is obvious from the findings of these chapters, the patterns observed do not uniquely lend themselves to one or the other explanation. Rather, they point towards the need for both universal markedness and statistical input considerations in any attempted explanation. The data presented here provide clear evidence for this and should stimulate further discussion.

REFERENCES

Cardoso, W. (2008). The development of sC onset clusters in interlanguage: Markedness vs frequency effects. In R. Slabakova (Ed.) *Proceedings of the 9th Generative Approaches to Second Language Acquisition Conference*, 15–29. Somerville, MA: Cascadilla.

Cardoso, W. & Liakin, D. (2009). When input frequency patterns fail to drive learning: Evidence from Brazilian Portuguese English. In B. Baptista, A. Rauber & M. Watkins (Eds.) *Recent Research in Second Language Phonetics/Phonology: Perception and Production*, 174–202. Newcastle upon Tyne: Cambridge Scholars.

Chevrie-Muller, C. & Lebreton, M.T. (1973). Etude de la realization des consonnes au cours d'une epreuve de mots, sur des groupes d'enfants de 3 ans et 5 ans ½ [Study of the pronunciation of consonants during a word repetition test in groups of children aged 3 and 5 and one-half years]. *Revue de laryngologie*, 94, 109–152.

Hua, Z. & Dodd, B. (2000). The phonological acquisition of Putonghua. *Journal of Child Language*, 27, 3–42.

Ingram, D. (1988). The acquisition of word-initial [v]. *Language and Speech*, 31, 77–85.

Jongstra, W. (2003). Variable and stable clusters: Variation in the realization of consonant clusters. *Canadian Journal of Linguistics,* 48, 265–288.

Kirk, C. & Demuth, K. (2006). Accounting for variability in 2-year-olds' production of coda consonants. *Language Learning and Development*, 2, 97–118.

Levelt, C. C., Schiller, N. O. & Levelt, W. J. (2000). The acquisition of syllable types. *Language Acquisition*, 8, 237–264.

Lleó, C. (2006). The acquisition of prosodic word structures in Spanish by monolingual and Spanish-German bilingual children. *Language and Speech*, 49, 207–231.

Macken, M. (1995). Phonological acquisition. In J. Goldsmith (Ed.) *The Handbook of Phonological Theory*, 671–696. Oxford: Basil Blackwell.

Major, R. (2001). *Foreign Accent: The Ontogeny and Phylogeny of Second Language Phonology.* Mahwah, NJ; Lawrence Erlbaum Associates.

Piske, T. & Young-Scholten, M. (Eds.) (2009). *Input Matters in SLA*. Bristol: Multilingual Matters.

Roark, B. & Demuth, K. (2000). Prosodic constraints and the learner's environment: A corpus study. In C. Howell, S. A. Fish & T. Keith-Lucas (Eds.) *Proceedings of the 24th Annual Boston University Conference on Language Development*, 597–608. Somerville, MA: Cascadilla.

Rose, Y. (2009). Internal and external influences on child language productions. In F. Pellegrino, E. Marsico, I. Chitoran & C. Coupe (Eds.) *Approaches to Phonological Complexity*, 329–351. Berlin: Mouton de Gruyter.

Rose, Y. & Inkelas, S. (2011). The interpretation of phonological patterns in first language acquisition. In C.J. Ewen, E. Hume, M. van Oosterdorp & K. Rice (Eds.) *The Blackwell Companion to Phonology*, 2414–2438. Malden, MA: Wiley-Blackwell.

Stites, J., Demuth, K. & Kirk, C. (2004). Markedness versus frequency effects in coda acquisition. In A. Brugos, L. Micciulla & C.E. Smith (Eds.) *Proceedings of the 28th Annual Boston University Conference on Language Development*, 565–576. Somerville, MA: Cascadilla.

Yavaş, M. (2010). Acquisition of /s/-clusters in Spanish-English bilingual children with phonological disorders. *Clinical Linguistics and Phonetics*, 24:3, 188–198.

Yavaş, M. & Barlow, J.A. (2006). Acquisition of #sC clusters in Spanish-English bilingual children. *Journal of Multilingual Communication Disorders,* 4:3, 182–193.

Yavaş, M. & Beaubrun, C. (2006). Acquisition of #sC clusters in Haitian Creole-English bilingual children. *Journal of Multilingual Communication Disorders*, 4:3, 194–204.

Yavaş, M. & Core, C. (2006). Acquisition of #sC clusters in English-speaking children. *Journal of Multilingual Communication Disorders*, 4:3, 169–181.

Yavaş, M. & McLeod, S. (2010). Acquisition of /s/ clusters in English-speaking children with phonological disorders. *Clinical Linguistics and Phonetics*, 24:3, 177–187.

Zamuner, T., Gerken, L. & Hammond, M. (2004). Phonotactic probabilities in young children's speech production. *Journal of Child Language*, 31, 515–536.

1

SONORITY PRINCIPLES MEET PROBABILISTIC PHONOTACTICS IN LEXICAL DEVELOPMENT

**Judith A. Gierut, Michele L. Morrisette,
and Katherine M. Brown**

Contemporary research on language acquisition has been dominated by models that appeal to statistical regularities of the input to guide children's learning (Aslin, Saffran, & Newport, 1999; Jusczyk, 1997; Kelly & Martin, 1994). These models make use of the probabilistic occurrence of language-specific structures to predict the developmental course, speed, and accuracy of learning. Evidence in support of probabilistic proposals has come primarily from experimental psycholinguistic studies of English (Edwards, Beckman, & Munson, 2004; Jusczyk, Luce, & Charles-Luce, 1994; Storkel, 2001).

This theoretical perspective stands in sharp contrast to early foundational research on language acquisition, which was dominated by universalist models (Chomsky, 1999; Ferguson, 1977; Jakobson, 1941/ 1968). The intent was to instantiate formal principles of language in the context of acquisition to gain insight into the range and variation of possible grammars and their change over time. Supporting evidence came largely from longitudinal cross-linguistic descriptions (de Boysson-Bardies & Vihman, 1991; Ingram, 1988; Locke, 1983).

This chapter aims to unite psycholinguistic and linguistic perspectives by exploring the link between language-specific input statistics and universal principles in acquisition. The focus was on phonotactic probability as the language-specific variable and syllable well-formedness as the universal principle. Two computational studies of the developing mental lexicon of English are reported. The purpose was to determine whether the distribution of words in the child lexicon best aligns with phonotactic probability, principles of well-formedness, or some combination of the two. A brief overview of the variables of interest, framed within the context of acquisition, provides the background and motivation for the hypotheses to be tested.

PROBABILISTIC PHONOTACTICS

The developing mental lexicon is said to be organized into neighborhoods, which consist of phonetically similar forms defined by one-phoneme substitutions, deletions, or additions (Luce, 1986). Words with many phonetically similar counterparts make dense neighborhoods—e.g., 'cat' has neighbors 'mat, hat, sat, cot, kit, cut, cap, can, catch' among others (as retrieved from http://neighborhoodsearch.wustl.edu)—whereas words with few similar counterparts make sparse neighborhoods—e.g., 'push' has just three neighbors, 'bush, pull, put' (as retrieved from http://neighborhoodsearch.wustl.edu). One hypothesis is that children initiate the language acquisition process by building dense neighborhoods (Jusczyk et al., 1994). They acquire and add new words to their developing lexicon that overlap in phonological form (Walley, 1993). Support for this idea comes from computational studies, which show that children's early words are phonologically more similar than the words they learn later (Storkel, 2004a). The neighborhoods of children also tend to be denser than those of adults (Coady & Aslin, 2003; cf. Charles-Luce & Luce, 1990, 1995). Behavioral evidence from perception shows too that infants encode words from dense neighborhoods with enough phonetic detail to detect mispronunciations (Swingley & Aslin, 2002). Moreover, in production, toddlers readily acquire new words that are comprised of IN sounds, which occur in the phonetic inventory, as opposed to OUT sounds, which do not (Schwartz & Leonard, 1982). Likewise, toddlers produce the sounds that occur in words from dense neighborhoods more accurately than those from sparse neighborhoods (Sosa & Stoel-Gammon, 2012). This pattern of performance continues through mid-childhood and beyond because preschoolers—with and without language learning disorders—benefit from dense neighborhoods for purposes of word learning (Demke, Graham, & Siakaluk, 2002), phonological learning (Gierut & Morrisette, 2012), syntactic learning (Hoover & Storkel, 2013), and metalinguistic awareness (De Cara & Goswami, 2003). Thus, the organization of phonetically similar words into dense neighborhoods appears to have multifaceted consequences for language acquisition (Stoel-Gammon, 2011).

A related observation is that the developing mental lexicon of English is largely comprised of Consonant-Vowel-Consonant (CVC) words (Charles-Luce & Luce, 1990). The CVC words in dense neighborhoods are further made up of the most commonly occurring sounds of English (Coady & Aslin, 2003; Storkel, 2013). More precisely, neighborhood density is positively correlated with phonotactic probability (Vitevitch & Luce, 1999). *Phonotactic probability* is the statistical likelihood of sounds and sound sequences in a given language (Vitevitch & Luce, 2004 for English; http://www.people.ku.edu/~mvitevit/PhonoProbHome.html) and is computed as the sum of segment frequency (SSF) and/or the sum of biphone frequency (SBF). SSF reflects the likelihood of a given sound occurring in a given position relative to all other possible segments in the language, whereas SBF reflects the likelihood of the occurrence of pairs of sounds relative to all other pairs in that language. The greater the SSF or SBF value, the more common the phonological form.

As with neighborhood density, studies have shown that phonotactic probability affects language acquisition. In perception, Jusczyk et al. (1994) showed that infants listen longer to words that consist of common as opposed to rare phonotactic patterns. In production, Beckman and Edwards (2000) found that preschoolers imitate nonwords composed of common sound sequences more accurately than rare sequences. Storkel (2001) likewise found that phonotactic probability influences children's acquisition and retention of novel words. It is important to clarify that phonotactic probability is independent of normative age of sound mastery (Storkel, 2013). Phonotactic probability is based on the statistical regularity of sounds in the target language input, whereas normative age of sound mastery is based on the cross-sectional order of acquisition of sounds in children's outputs.

The relevance of these data is that they offer a testable prediction about the composition of the developing lexicon of English from the vantage of language-specific input statistics. Specifically, it is predicted that the developing lexicon will contain a greater proportion of CVC words with common as opposed to rare phonotactic patterns; this is one hypothesis to be tested herein.

SYLLABLE WELL-FORMEDNESS

It has long been thought that the syllable is a prosodic bootstrap to language acquisition (Gleitman & Wanner, 1982). The syllable has been described as the 'frame' from which the lexical and phonological 'content' emerge (MacNeilage & Davis, 1990). Numerous studies have described the range of syllable types produced by children and their corresponding orders of emergence (Ingram, 1978; Levelt, Schiller, & Levelt, 2000; Lleó & Prinz, 1997; Vihman, 1992). The data are rich, capturing the use of syllables beginning in the earliest stages of babbling. The data are also detailed, highlighting cross-linguistic similarities and differences.

Complementary experimental work has further demonstrated that children are sensitive to the internal structure of syllables. In perception, infants detect commonalities among syllables based on properties of the onset (Juscyzk, Goodman, & Baumann, 1999). In production, children's erred outputs implicate the syllable, such that simplifications and reductions affect unstressed units (Gerken & McGregor, 1998). Other production studies have found that children's learning is differentially affected by exposure to different types of syllable structure (Gierut, 1999; Gierut & Champion, 2001). Syllables with branching onsets (i.e., clusters), for example, induce greater phonological learning than syllables comprised of adjuncts /sp-/, /st-/, /sk-/. Finally, metalinguistic research has demonstrated that preliterate children are able to accurately judge and manipulate words based on syllables (Treiman & Breaux, 1982). This ability emerges well before children have explicit knowledge of the syllable as a linguistic unit.

The function of the syllable in acquisition takes on added interest in light of known universal principles that dictate syllable well-formedness. The *Sonority Sequencing Principle* posits that onsets rise in sonority to the nucleus and remain level (or fall) to the coda (Sievers, 1881), where sonority is defined by intensity and intraoral air pressure (Parker, 2002). This principle dictates permissible sequences of segments within the onset or within the coda. In complement, the *margin hierarchy* further identifies low sonority onsets as better formed than high sonority onsets and, conversely, high sonority codas as better formed than low sonority codas (Prince & Smolensky, 1993/2004; Vennemann, 1988). Obstruents (stops, fricatives, affricates) are low sonority segments, and sonorants (nasals, liquids, glides) are high sonority segments. For example, the CVC 'dear' has optimal structure given its obstruent|sonorant margins (hereafter OBS|SON). By comparison, the CVC 'rid' is not as well-formed due to its sonorant|obstruent margins (hereafter SON|OBS). This is not to say that the latter is precluded from occurring, but only that it does not follow basic cross-linguistic preferences for margin sonority.

Of special interest are CVCs that have exclusively low sonority margins or exclusively high sonority margins. A word like 'did' has obstruents in both the onset and coda (OBS|OBS), whereas 'rear' has sonorants in both the onset and coda (SON|SON). In each case, the sonority of the segment at one edge of the word is preferred and at the other edge dispreferred. The well-formedness of such sequences is unclear based on the linguistics literature. Many studies support the perceptual salience of the onset (Cutler & Norris, 1988; Marslen-Wilson & Zwitserlood, 1989). Yet, other studies report a scarcity of codas and coda combinations in English (Kessler & Treiman, 1997). The limited range of segmental occurrences in coda position makes this context more predictable and thus more reliable as a linguistic cue. Cross-linguistic studies further note that segments which occur in onset and coda positions are not uniformly distributed (Parker, 2001). Permissible segments in the onset are not necessarily the same sounds or subset of sounds that are permissible in the coda, and vice versa. The literature on language acquisition also leaves open the indeterminacy of OBS|OBS and SON|SON sequences. One body of research supports the onset as crucial to early acquisition (Ferguson & Farwell, 1975; Jusczyk et al., 1999; Storkel, 2002). Yet, other work posits the coda as a prominent context early on, with a shift to the onset only later in development (Aitchison & Straf, 1981; Brooks & MacWhinney, 2000; Dinnsen & Farris-Trimble, 2008).

This notwithstanding, the relevance of these observations is that they again give rise to a testable hypothesis about the composition of the developing lexicon of English but from the vantage of universal principles of syllable well-formedness. The prediction is that the developing lexicon will contain a greater proportion of CVCs with OBS|SON margins because this is the universally preferred structure.

STUDY 1

The purpose was to document the distribution of words in an idealized child lexicon of English to establish conformity to predictions that follow from probabilistic phonotactics versus syllable well-formedness. A computational approach was adopted as a first step toward establishing possible relationships between input statistics and universals.

Procedures

Corpus

Following established procedures (e.g., Charles-Luce & Luce, 1990), a corpus of CVCs was first identified as representative of the child lexicon. CVCs were the focus given their importance to phonological acquisition and the developing lexicon. CVCs also permit control of word length, which is a known confound in the computation of phonotactic probability (Storkel, 2004b).

An adult database was consulted to identify all legal CVCs of English. The Hoosier Mental Lexicon (HML; Nusbaum, Pisoni, & Davis, 1984) was used for consistency with the existing literature. The HML is an online database consisting of 20,000 words of the 1967 *Merriam-Webster Pocket Dictionary*, accessed at http://neighborhoodsearch.wustl.edu/Neighborhood/Home.asp. A search of the HML identified 961 legal CVCs in English (Jusczyk et al., 1994; Luce & Large, 2001; Vitevitch, personal communication, December 17, 1999; see Storkel, 2013, for revised estimates). These were unambiguous CVCs, with elimination of the stressed rhotic vowel because it yields a coda cluster. The legal CVCs were then trimmed to best match the words of the child lexicon. To determine which CVCs might be in the child lexicon, a second database—the Child Mental Lexicon Calculator (CMLC; Storkel & Hoover, 2010)—was consulted. This is an online database accessed at http://www.bncdnet.ku.edu/cgi-bin/DEEC/post_ccc.vi. The CMLC consists of 10,000+ words spoken by children in kindergarten and first grade based on the combined resources of Kolson (1960) and Moe, Hopkins, and Rush (1982). The 961 legal CVCs retrieved from the HML were compared against the CMLC. Any CVC of the HML that was not also in the CMLC was eliminated. The result was a corpus of 656 CVCs that defined the child lexicon evaluated herein.

Coding and Calculations

The 656 CVCs of the child lexicon were coded and sorted for syllable well-formedness based on margin sonority. There were four logically possible groupings as defined above: OBS|SON, OBS|OBS, SON|SON, SON|OBS. The number of words in a given group was tallied for the 656-word child lexicon.

Phonotactic probability was also computed for words of the child lexicon. SSF values were retrieved because we were specifically interested in the quality of the segments in onset and coda positions. Recall that SSF reflects the statistical likelihood of a given sound in a given word position relative to all other sounds of the English language. SSF values were obtained from the CMLC for each word of the child lexicon. Mean SSF values were then computed for words grouped by margin sonority.

The reliability of coding and computing SSF was determined for 10% of the data (inclusive of Studies 1 and 2). An independent examiner checked the accuracy of the child corpus as derived from the HML, the coding of CVC well-formedness, and the computation of SSF. Reliability of these procedures was 99.8% agreement.

Results and Discussion

Table 1.1 reports the number of words in the child lexicon grouped by margin sonority. Of 656 words, 154 had universally preferred OBS|SON margins, and 171 had dispreferred SON|OBS margins. For completeness, 258 words had OBS|OBS and 73 had SON|SON edges.

These data were evaluated against predictions that derived from universal principles of well-formedness, as in (1). Recall that the child lexicon of English was expected to have the most words with OBS|SON margins and the fewest with SON|OBS margins. It can be seen that the predictions did not match the observations; instead, most words had OBS|OBS margins.

(1) Predicted: OBS|SON > SON|OBS
     Observed: OBS|OBS > SON|OBS > OBS|SON > SON|SON

Table 1.2 reports the mean SSF values of words in the child lexicon grouped by margin sonority. These were statistically

Table 1.1 Number and distribution of words in the child lexicon and its neighborhoods grouped by margin sonority

	Lexicon	Neighborhoods				
		OBS|SON	OBS|OBS	SON|SON	SON|OBS	Total
OBS|SON	154	1271	360	318	—	1949
OBS|OBS	258	385	2066	—	516	2967
SON|SON	73	324	—	414	209	947
SON|OBS	171	—	521	230	1290	2041
Total	656	1980	2947	962	2015	7904

Table 1.2 Mean sum of segment frequency values of words in the child lexicon and its neighborhoods grouped by margin sonority

	Lexicon	Neighborhoods			
		OBS|SON	OBS|OBS	SON|SON	SON|OBS
OBS|SON	0.1956	0.2047	0.1714	0.1844	—
OBS|OBS	0.1617	0.2078	0.1741	—	0.1570
SON|SON	0.1761	0.2040	—	0.1828	0.1503
SON|OBS	0.1422	—	0.1727	0.1802	0.1529

distinct and nonoverlapping categories based on a one-way ANOVA, $F(3, 652) = 51.15$, $p = .00$. It can be seen that the greatest SSF was associated with OBS|SON margins, and the least with SON|OBS margins. Words with OBS|OBS and SON|SON edges fell in between. This means that, for English, words in the child lexicon with OBS|SON margins were the most common in phonological form, whereas words with SON|OBS edges were rarest in phonological form.

SSF data were evaluated against the predictions stemming from language-specific input statistics, as ranked in (2) from most to least common segment frequencies. It was expected that words with OBS|OBS edges, which constituted the greatest proportion of the child lexicon, would be one of the most common phonological patterns in the input following from SSF values. Once again, the predictions did not align with the observations.

(2) Predicted: OBS|OBS > SON|OBS > OBS|SON > SON|SON
     Observed: OBS|SON > SON|SON > OBS|OBS > SON|OBS

Thus, it appeared that the distribution of words in the child lexicon of English did not align either with universal principles or with language-specific input statistics. Neither was sufficient in and of itself in capturing the composition of the child lexicon. This notwithstanding, there is a striking observation to be made. Notice, in (1), that universal principles of well-formedness support OBS|SON and SON|OBS margins as optimal and nonoptimal, respectively. In (2), language-specific input statistics showed that words with OBS|SON and SON|OBS margins consist of the most common and rare phonological patterns of English, respectively. The insight to be gained is that the *predictions* of the universal principles in (1) agree precisely with *observed* language-specific probabilities in (2). The implication is that the two may be isomorphic, at least as reflected by the distribution of words in the child lexicon of English.

STUDY 2

The purpose was to test the apparent isomorphism between universal and language-specific predictions through a finer grained analysis of neighborhoods of the child lexicon of English. Recall that a neighborhood is a pocket of the lexicon comprised of phonetically similar words, as defined by one-phoneme substitutions, deletions, or additions. If there were a 1:1 correspondence between syllable well-formedness and phonotactic probability as predicted, this should be borne out within neighborhoods as well as across the lexicon at large. The evaluation of neighborhoods afforded a further methodological advantage by increasing the sample size of the child lexicon.

Procedures

Neighborhood corpora were developed using the child lexicon of Study 1. There were four corpora, corresponding to the four groupings of words by sonority margins identified in Study 1. Each grouping of words coded in Study 1 as OBS|SON, OBS|OBS, SON|SON, and SON|OBS was re-entered into the CMLC. Then, a neighbor search was completed to yield each neighborhood corpus. To illustrate the procedure, consider that 154 words of the child lexicon had been coded as having OBS|SON margins in Study 1; one of these words was 'sign'. 'Sign' was re-entered into the CMLC, and 15 words were retrieved as its neighbors, including 'sun, side, mine' among others. Each of these neighbors was then coded and grouped based on margin sonority. To continue the example, the neighbors 'sun, side, mine' were coded respectively as OBS|SON, OBS|OBS, and SON|SON. Additionally, SSF values of the neighbors were retrieved. This process was then repeated for all words coded as OBS|SON in the child lexicon. Moreover, it was repeated again for all remaining groupings by margin sonority. This thereby allowed for the analysis of well-formedness and phonotactic probability in four neighborhoods to parallel Study 1.

Results and Discussion

Table 1.1 reports the distribution of words in the four neighborhoods based on margin sonority. Notice that, for any given neighborhood, three of four logically possible margins were represented. This is due to the definition of a neighbor as a one-phoneme substitution, deletion, or addition. In each neighborhood, the margin that was missing entailed a two-phoneme difference. To illustrate, the OBS|SON neighborhood was comprised of words with OBS|SON, OBS|OBS, and SON|SON margins, consistent with the prior example of 'sign' having neighbors 'sun, side, mine'. Words with SON|OBS margins were precluded in this case because these would have involved phonetic differences in both the onset *and* the coda. For example, 'nice' is not a neighbor of 'sign' because there are two segmental substitutions, which is at odds with the definition of a neighbor.

A second point to be gleaned from Table 1.1 was that the majority of words in a neighborhood mimicked the margin sonority that defined that corpus. Specifically, the OBS|SON neighborhood was comprised of 1949 words; of these, 1271 likewise had OBS|SON margins. There were

2967 words in the OBS|OBS neighborhood, and 2066 had OBS|OBS margins. The SON|SON neighborhood was comprised of 947 words, 414 of which had SON|SON margins. Finally, the SON|OBS neighborhood contained 2041 words, 1290 of which followed the SON|SON pattern. From these data, it seems that words in a neighborhood tend to mirror each other in margin sonority. This is consistent with the view that children build dense neighborhoods by adding words to the lexicon which are phonologically similar and overlapping in phonological form (Walley, 1993). Here, the novel extension is that phonological similarity is likely based on syllabic as well as segmental structure.

Neighborhood corpora were also evaluated for phonotactic probability, with mean SSF values reported in Table 1.2 for each corpus. One-way ANOVAs with Bonferroni post hoc comparisons showed that the SSFs of each neighborhood were statistically distinct, where $F(2, 944–2964) = 100.24–173.04$, $p = .00$. These values are ranked in (3) from common to rare phonotactic patterns for each corpus.

(3) OBS|SON corpus: OBS|SON > SON|SON > OBS|OBS
   OBS|OBS corpus: OBS|SON > OBS|OBS > SON|OBS
   SON|SON corpus: OBS|SON > SON|SON > SON|OBS
   SON|OBS corpus: SON|SON > OBS|OBS > SON|OBS

Two observations emerge from the rankings. One is that, for every corpus, neighbors with OBS|SON margins have the greatest SSF values and therefore reflect the most common phonotactic patterns of English. Keep in mind, too, that OBS|SON margins are universally preferred. A second observation is that, for every corpus, neighbors with SON|OBS margins have the lowest SSF values and, accordingly, reflect the least common phonotactics of English. Notably, SON|OBS margins are universally dispreferred. These observations confirm the hypothesis being tested, namely, that phonotactic probability and syllable well-formedness appear to be isomorphic in the lexical neighborhoods of children acquiring English.

There is a third observation that can be gleaned from the rankings in (3). Recall that universal principles are unable to differentiate the well-formedness of words with OBS|OBS or SON|SON margins. In such cases, one margin has a preferred structure and the other a dispreferred structure: obstruents are ideal onsets, but sonorants are ideal codas. If universal principles align 1:1 with language-specific input statistics as proposed, then it may be possible to discern syllable well-formedness from probabilistic phonotactics in these ambiguous cases. The rankings in (3) inform this issue. Notice that, for every corpus, neighbors with SON|SON margins contained the more commonly occurring phonotactic patterns of English than neighbors with OBS|OBS margins. The implication is that the sonority of the coda takes priority over the onset in determining well-formedness in these cases. The significance is that language-specific input statistics revealed new insights which were previously unavailable from universal principles.

GENERAL DISCUSSION

The collective results of two computational studies contribute to ongoing debates about the effects of language universals and language-specific input statistics on acquisition. This research highlighted, in particular, the mutual benefits that arise from an integrated approach to the puzzle. This is best illustrated by the findings of Study 1, which showed that universal principles of syllable well-formedness were insufficient in capturing the composition of words in the child lexicon. Likewise, Study 1 showed that language-specific input statistics associated with probabilistic phonotactics were equally inadequate in accounting for the data. However, when principled and statistical data were examined in tandem, the perspectives converged. Specifically, words of the child lexicon with universally preferred low sonority onsets and high sonority codas were also statistically the most likely phonological patterns of English. This symmetry hinted that universals and language-specific statistics might be one and the same, at least as evidenced computationally for the developing lexicon of English.

This research demonstrated too that language-specific input statistics have a central purpose in refinement and clarification of language universals. This was best exemplified by the findings of Study 2, where the predicted isomorphism between principles of syllable well-formedness and phonotactic probabilities was borne out in fine-grained analyses of lexical neighborhoods. More important, language-specific input statistics directly addressed known ambiguities in syllable well-formedness. Based on probabilistic patterns of the child lexicon, it was established that SON|SON margins were better formed than OBS|OBS margins. When phonotactic probability was taken into account, the sonority of the coda emerged as more important to syllable well-formedness than the onset. In this way, language-specific input statistics illuminated that which was obscured from the vantage of language universals. In strong form, it might be said that language-specific input statistics 'trumped' universals because the latter were wholly derivable from probabilistic data.

The consequence of these findings for theory and application are multifaceted in light of the opportunities that are afforded for continued research. On the side of theory, it will be essential to capitalize on the insights of language-specific input statistics to aid the precision of language universals. This tack would likewise address some of the limitations of the present set of studies. For example, the focus herein was on syllable structure, but there are numerous other universals that could be explored. Studies of segmental markedness come to mind given their extensive coverage in the developmental literature (Bernhardt & Stoel-Gammon, 1996; Demuth, 1995; Dinnsen & Elbert, 1984; Gnanadesikan, 2004; Ingram, 1988; Rice & Avery, 1995). While developing grammars are conventionally characterized by unmarked structure, it remains to be established whether unmarked structure also occurs most frequently in the input language (Levelt et al., 2000 for Dutch).

The present work focused exclusively on CVC words of an idealized child lexicon of English. Our narrow examination of CVC words afforded distinct methodological advantages because margin sonority could be unambiguously determined and the calculation of phonotactic probability was not confounded by word length (Storkel, 2004b). Yet, the words of a child's lexicon vary in canonical shape and include forms with no onsets, no codas, and multisyllabicity. It will be important to take into account the full range of syllable types in future studies. Our approach was also computational in nature and would benefit from complementary behavioral studies. These might include descriptive, experimental, longitudinal, or cross-sectional alternatives.

The work herein on English needs to be expanded to include cross-linguistic research. This is relevant because input statistics vary from language to language. It would be an especially powerful demonstration if statistical and universal patterns were to align uniformly in cross-linguistic studies, despite the known statistical variation across languages.

Finally, our interpretation was purposefully theory-neutral given the paucity of research of this type. In the spirit of the Stanford Universals Project (Greenberg, 1978), our aim was to first identify relationships between universals and statistical regularities of English. As evidence accrues, it will be incumbent on linguistic theory to incorporate language-specific regularities in explanatory models of language structure. Similarly, psycholinguistic theory will need to accommodate universals in explanatory models of language function. In all, a convergence of evidence across principles, languages, methodologies, and theories holds promise for firmly establishing the boundaries and workings of language universals and input-specific properties in acquisition.

On the side of application, the present findings have the potential to bear on clinical populations with language learning disorders. The clinical literature is rich with data showing the relevance of language universals to the goals of treatment (for reviews, see Gierut, 2001, 2007, 2008; Thompson, 2007). Specifically, treatment of complex (marked) structure facilitates greater learning than treatment of simpler (unmarked) structure. Likewise, language-specific input statistics have informed the design of treatment by specifying the words to be taught. For example, treatment of high frequency words from dense neighborhoods facilitates greater phonological learning (Gierut & Morrisette, 2012). Thus, language universals and language-specific input statistics have each contributed independently to clinical treatment.

To our knowledge, there have been no attempts to integrate the treatment recommendations that derive from universals with those that derive from input statistics so as to maximize the benefits. An example lies in a possible extension of the present findings to treatment of children with phonological disorders. Consider a child who is taught a sound produced in error using CVC words in treatment. To boost learning, the CVC words chosen for treatment might have optimal OBS|SON margins and, further, common probabilistic phonotactics. The learning to result under this scenario is likely to differ from that of another child, who might be treated using words with optimal OBS|SON margins but rare phonotactics. It is easy to see that the full complement of logically possible treatment scenarios obtains in the orthogonal manipulation of sonority margins and phonotactic probability. The various manipulations are likely to trigger differential learning, with the results being traceable to the unique contribution of universals versus language-specific input statistics. The practical advantage of an integrated approach of this type is obvious. More important, applied research along these lines has the potential to disentangle the effects of universals from input statistics in language acquisition. As data continue to amass from theoretical and applied research of the sort suggested, it is conceivable that we will come closer to understanding how the formal study of linguistic structure interfaces with language-specific regularities in the input to inform the acquisition process.

ACKNOWLEDGMENTS

This research was supported in part by the National Institute on Deafness and Other Communication Disorders of the National Institutes of Health under Award Number R01DC001694. The content is solely the responsibility of the authors and does not necessarily represent the official views of the National Institutes of Health. Portions of the research were reported at the 2011 American Speech-Language Hearing Association Convention, San Diego.

REFERENCES

Aitchison, J., & Straf, M. (1981). Lexical storage and retrieval: A developing skill? *Linguistics, 19,* 751–795.

Aslin, R. N., Saffran, J. R., & Newport, E. L. (1999). Statistical learning in linguistic and nonlinguistic domains. In B. MacWhinney (Ed.), *The emergence of language* (pp. 359–380). Mahwah, NJ: Erlbaum.

Beckman, M. E., & Edwards, J. (2000). Lexical frequency effects on young children's imitative productions. In M. Broe & J. Pierrehumbert (Eds.), *Papers in laboratory phonology V* (pp. 207–217). Cambridge, UK: Cambridge University Press.

Bernhardt, B., & Stoel-Gammon, C. (1996). Underspecification and markedness in normal and disordered phonological development. In C. E. Johnson & J. H. V. Gilbert (Eds.), *Children's language* (Vol. 9, pp. 33–53). Mahwah, NJ: Erlbaum.

Brooks, P. J., & MacWhinney, B. (2000). Phonological priming in children's picture naming. *Journal of Child Language, 27,* 335–366.

Charles-Luce, J., & Luce, P. A. (1990). Similarity neighbourhoods of words in young children's lexicons. *Journal of Child Language, 17,* 205–215.

Charles-Luce, J., & Luce, P. A. (1995). An examination of similarity neighbourhoods in young children's receptive vocabularies. *Journal of Child Language, 22,* 727–735.

Chomsky, N. (1999). On the nature, use, and acquisition of child language. In W. C. Ritchie & T. K. Bhatia (Eds.), *Handbook of child language acquisition* (pp. 33–54). New York: Academic Press.

Coady, J. A., & Aslin, R. N. (2003). Phonological neighbourhoods in the developing lexicon. *Journal of Child Language, 30,* 441–469.

Cutler, A., & Norris, D. G. (1988). The role of strong syllables in segmentation for lexical access. *Journal of Experimental Psychology: Human Perception & Performance, 14,* 113–121.

de Boysson-Bardies, B., & Vihman, M. M. (1991). Adaptation to language: Evidence from babbling and first words in four languages. *Language, 67,* 297–319.

De Cara, B., & Goswami, U. (2003). Phonological neighborhood density effects in a rhyme awareness task in 5-year-old children. *Journal of Child Language, 30,* 695–710.

Demke, T. L., Graham, S. A., & Siakaluk, P. D. (2002). The influence of exposure to phonological neighbours on pre-schoolers' novel word production. *Journal of Child Language, 29,* 379–392.

Demuth, K. (1995). Markedness and the development of prosodic structure. *North East Linguistic Society, 25*, 13–25.

Dinnsen, D. A., & Elbert, M. (1984). On the relationship between phonology and learning. In M. Elbert, D. A. Dinnsen, & G. Weismer (Eds.), *Phonological theory and the misarticulating child (ASHA Monographs No. 22)* (pp. 59–68). Rockville, MD: ASHA.

Dinnsen, D. A., & Farris-Trimble, A. W. (2008). The prominence paradox. In D. A. Dinnsen & J. A. Gierut (Eds.), *Optimality theory, phonological acquisition and disorders* (pp. 277–308). London: Equinox.

Edwards, J., Beckman, M., & Munson, B. (2004). The interaction between vocabulary size and phonotactic probability effects on children's production accuracy and fluency in nonword repetition. *Journal of Speech, Language, and Hearing Research, 47*, 421–436.

Ferguson, C. A. (1977). New directions in phonological theory: Language acquisition and universals research. In R. W. Cole (Ed.), *Current issues in linguistic theory* (pp. 247–299). Bloomington: Indiana University Press.

Ferguson, C. A., & Farwell, C. B. (1975). Words and sounds in early language acquisition: English initial consonants in the first fifty words. *Language, 51*, 419–439.

Gerken, L., & McGregor, K. (1998). An overview of prosody and its role in normal and disordered child language. *American Journal of Speech-Language Pathology, 7*, 38–48.

Gierut, J. A. (1999). Syllable onsets: Clusters and adjuncts in acquisition. *Journal of Speech, Language, and Hearing Research, 42*, 708–726.

Gierut, J. A. (2001). Complexity in phonological treatment: Clinical factors. *Language, Speech and Hearing Services in Schools, 32*, 229–241.

Gierut, J. A. (2007). Phonological complexity and language learnability. *American Journal of Speech-Language Pathology, 16*, 1–12.

Gierut, J. A. (2008). Fundamentals of experimental design and treatment. In D. A. Dinnsen & J. A. Gierut (Eds.), *Optimality theory, phonological acquisition and disorders* (pp. 93–118). London: Equinox.

Gierut, J. A., & Champion, A. H. (2001). Syllable onsets II: Three-element clusters in phonological treatment. *Journal of Speech, Language, and Hearing Research, 44*, 886–904.

Gierut, J. A., & Morrisette, M. L. (2012). Density, frequency and the expressive phonology of children with phonological delay. *Journal of Child Language, 39*, 804–834.

Gleitman, L., & Wanner, E. (1982). Language acquisition: The state of the state of the art. In E. Wanner & L. R. Gleitman (Eds.), *Language acquisition: The state of the art* (pp. 3–48). Cambridge, UK: Cambridge University Press.

Gnanadesikan, A. (2004). Markedness and faithfulness constraints in child phonology. In R. Kager, J. Pater, & W. Zonneveld (Eds.), *Constraints in phonological acquisition* (pp. 73–108). Cambridge, UK: Cambridge University Press.

Greenberg, J. H. (1978). *Universals of human language: Volume 2: Phonology*. Stanford, CA: Stanford University Press.

Hoover, J. R. & Storkel, H. L. (2013). Grammatical treatment and specific language impairment: Neighborhood density and third person singular -s. *Clinical Linguistics & Phonetics, 27*, 661–680.

Ingram, D. (1978). The role of the syllable in phonological development. In A. Bell & J. B. Hooper (Eds.), *Syllables and segments* (pp. 143–155). Amsterdam: North-Holland.

Ingram, D. (1988). Jakobson revisited: Some evidence from the acquisition of Polish. *Lingua, 75*, 55–82.

Jakobson, R. (1941/1968). *Child language, aphasia, and phonological universals* (A. R. Keiler, Trans.). The Hague: Mouton.

Jusczyk, P. W. (1997). *The discovery of spoken language*. Cambridge, MA: MIT Press.

Jusczyk, P. W., Goodman, M. B., & Baumann, A. (1999). Nine-month-olds' attention to sound similarities in syllables. *Journal of Memory and Language, 40*, 62–82.

Jusczyk, P. W., Luce, P. A., & Charles-Luce, J. (1994). Infants' sensitivity to phonotactic patterns in the native language. *Journal of Memory and Language, 33*, 630–645.

Kelly, M. H., & Martin, S. (1994). Domain-general abilities applied to domain-specific tasks: Sensitivities to probabilities in perception, cognition, and language. In L. Gleitman & B. Landau (Eds.), *The acquisition of the lexicon* (pp. 105–140). Cambridge, MA: MIT Press.

Kessler, B., & Treiman, R. (1997). Syllable structure and the distribution of phonemes in English syllables. *Journal of Memory and Language, 37*, 295–311.

Kolson, C. J. (1960). *The vocabulary of kindergarten children*. (Unpublished doctoral dissertation.) University of Pittsburgh, Pittsburgh.

Levelt, C. C., Schiller, N. O., & Levelt, W. J. M. (2000). The acquisition of syllable types. *Language Acquisition, 8*, 237–264.

Lleó, C., & Prinz, M. (1997). Syllable structure parameters and the acquisition of affricates. In S. J. Hannahs & M. Young-Scholten (Eds.), *Focus on phonological acquisition* (pp. 143–164). Amsterdam: John Benjamins.

Locke, J. L. (1983). *Phonological acquisition and change*. New York: Academic Press.

Luce, P. A. (1986). *Neighborhoods of words in the mental lexicon (Technical report no. 6)*. Bloomington: Indiana University, Speech Research Laboratory.

Luce, P. A., & Large, N. R. (2001). Phonotactics, density, and entropy in spoken word recognition. *Language and Cognitive Processes, 16*, 565–581.

MacNeilage, P. F., & Davis, B. (1990). Acquisition of speech production: Frames, then content. In M. Jeannerod (Ed.), *Attention and performance XIII: Motor representation and control* (pp. 453–475). Hillsdale, NJ: Erlbaum.

Marslen-Wilson, W., & Zwitserlood, P. (1989). Accessing spoken words: The importance of word onsets. *Journal of Experimental Psychology: Human Perception and Performance, 15*, 576–585.

Moe, A. J., Hopkins, C. J., & Rush, R. T. (1982). *The vocabulary of first-grade children*. Springfield, IL: Charles C. Thomas.

Nusbaum, H. C., Pisoni, D. B., & Davis, C. K. (1984). *Sizing up the Hoosier mental lexicon* (Research on spoken language processing progress report no. 10, pp. 357–376). Bloomington: Indiana University, Speech Research Laboratory.

Parker, S. (2001). Non-optimal onsets in Chamicuro: An inventory maximized in coda position. *Phonology, 18*, 361–386.

Parker, S. (2002). *Qualifying the sonority hierarchy.* (Unpublished doctoral dissertation.) University of Massachusetts, Amherst.

Prince, A., & Smolensky, P. (1993/2004). *Optimality theory: Constraint interaction in generative grammar*. Malden, MA: Blackwell.

Rice, K., & Avery, P. (1995). Variability in a deterministic model of language acquisition: A theory of segmental elaboration. In J. Archibald (Ed.), *Phonological acquisition and phonological theory* (pp. 23–42). Hillsdale, NJ: Erlbaum.

Schwartz, R. G., & Leonard, L. B. (1982). Do children pick and choose? An examination of phonological selection and avoidance in early lexical acquisition. *Journal of Child Language, 9*, 319–336.

Sievers, E. (1881). *Grundzüge der Phonetik*. Leipzig, Germany: Breitkopf & Hartel.

Sosa, A. V., & Stoel-Gammon, C. (2012). Lexical and phonological effects in early word production. *Journal of Speech, Language, and Hearing Research, 55*, 596–608.

Stoel-Gammon, C. (2011). Relationships between lexical and phonological development in young children. *Journal of Child Language, 38*, 1–34.

Storkel, H. L. (2001). Learning new words: Phonotactic probability in language development. *Journal of Speech, Language, and Hearing Research, 44*, 1321–1337.

Storkel, H. L. (2002). Restructuring of similarity neighborhoods in the developing mental lexicon. *Journal of Child Language, 29*, 251–274.

Storkel, H. L. (2004a). Do children acquire dense neighborhoods? An investigation of similarity neighborhoods in lexical acquisition. *Applied Psycholinguistics, 25*, 201–221.

Storkel, H. L. (2004b). Methods for minimizing the confounding effects of word length in the analysis of phonotactic probability and neighborhood density. *Journal of Speech, Language, and Hearing Research, 47*, 1454–1468.

Storkel, H. L. (2013). A corpus of consonant-vowel-consonant real words and nonwords: Comparison of phonotactic probability, neighborhood density, and consonant age of acquisition. *Behavior Research Methods, 45*, 1159–1167.

Storkel, H. L., & Hoover, J. R. (2010). An online calculator to compute phonotactic probability and neighborhood density on the basis of child corpora of spoken American English. *Behavior Research Methods, 42*, 497–506.

Swingley, D., & Aslin, R. N. (2002). Lexical neighborhoods and the word-form representations of 14-month-olds. *Psychological Science, 13*, 480–484.

Thompson, C. K. (2007). Complexity in language learning and treatment. *American Journal of Speech-Language Pathology, 16*, 3–5.

Treiman, R., & Breaux, M. (1982). Common phoneme and overall similarity relations among spoken syllables: Their use by children and adults. *Journal of Psycholinguistic Research, 11*, 569–598.

Vennemann, T. (1988). *Preference laws for syllable structure and the explanation of sound change: With special reference to German, Germanic, Italian and Latin.* New York: Mouton de Gruyter.

Vihman, M. M. (1992). Early syllables and the construction of phonology. In C. A. Ferguson, L. Menn, & C. Stoel-Gammon (Eds.), *Phonological development: Models, research, implications* (pp. 393–422). Timonium, MD: York Press.

Vitevitch, M. S., & Luce, P. A. (1999). Probabilistic phonotactics and neighborhood activation in spoken word recognition. *Journal of Memory and Language, 40*, 374–408.

Vitevitch, M. S., & Luce, P. A. (2004). A web-based interface to calculate phonotactic probability for words and nonwords in English. *Behavior Research Methods, Instruments, & Computers, 36*, 481–487.

Walley, A. C. (1993). The role of vocabulary development in children's spoken word recognition and segmentation ability. *Developmental Review, 13*, 286–350.

2

PHONOLOGICAL PATTERNS IN THE LEXICAL DEVELOPMENT OF FRENCH

Tania S. Zamuner, Elizabeth Morin-Lessard and Natasha Bouchat-Laird

Systematic patterns have been found in adult and child language across the traditional areas of linguistic analyses: phonetics, phonology, morphology, syntax and semantics. While a great deal of research has focused on the acquisition of English, more cross-linguistic research is needed which incorporates languages with different structures and, specifically for the focus in this work, languages with different phonological and lexical patterns. This is essential in understanding the potential universal and language-specific aspects of development, as recently emphasized by Stoel-Gammon (2011). This task is made even more difficult because the predictions from universal and input accounts often converge (Zamuner, 2003; Zamuner, Gerken & Hammond, 2005). Our focus is to explore the development of neighbourhood densities in a less examined language: French. Based on previous findings from English, it was predicted that the developmental data would pattern like adult French such that the patterns of neighbourhood densities in child French would be similar to those in the input language. While we found that child French differed in some ways from adult French, we suggest that this reflects properties of the input language, namely the distribution of syllable shapes in frequent French words.

NEIGHBOURHOOD DENSITIES

Lexical items vary in the degree of phonological overlap they have with other words. The degree of sound similarity is measured by a word's (phonological) neighbours, which are created by the addition, deletion or substitution of a phoneme (Luce & Pisoni, 1998). The French word *balle* /bal/ (Eng. 'ball') has the neighbours *salle* /sal/ (Eng. 'room'), *mal* /mal/ (Eng. 'wrong' or 'pain'), *belle* /bɛl/ (Eng. 'pretty'), *bulle* /byl/ (Eng. 'bubble') and *bas* /ba/ (Eng. 'socks' or 'low'), among others. Neighbourhoods are further differentiated between dense and sparse neighbourhoods. These concepts capture the degree to which words vary in their phonological similarity and the way that words are thought to be stored in the lexicon. Words with a large degree of sound similarity to other words are said to reside in dense neighbourhoods, and words with a small degree of sound similarity to other words are said to reside in sparse neighbourhoods. The French word *balle* has many neighbours and resides in a dense neighbourhood, whereas the word *boeuf* (Eng. 'beef') has few neighbours and resides in a sparse neighbourhood. The degree of sound similarity measured by neighbourhood densities (NDs) has been shown to be a factor in how lexical information is processed, retrieved and produced (Luce & Pisoni, 1998; Vitevitch, Luce, Pisoni & Auer, 1999). In adult word recognition tasks, words from dense neighbourhoods are retrieved more slowly than words from sparse neighbourhoods, described by competition effects during word recognition (Luce & Pisoni, 1998). Speech production tasks, on the other hand, yield different patterns: words from dense neighbourhoods are produced faster and more accurately than words from sparse neighbourhoods (Garlock, Walley & Metsala, 2001; Vitevitch, 2002).

One growing area of research interest has been to examine patterns across children's emerging lexicons as defined by ND. These types of studies have a variety of aims. For example, they attempt to provide insight into how children represent and organize phonological and lexical representations, how existing representations can influence children's phonological and lexical acquisition and how new representations are integrated with existing representations. The influence of phonological and lexical development is most likely bidirectional, but how they develop and interact is not fully understood (see Stoel-Gammon, 2011 for a discussion of these issues). ND has been shown to be a factor in development, with many studies simultaneously considering multiple cues, such as phonotactic probability and word frequency (e.g. Storkel, 2009; Stokes, 2010; Stokes, Kern & dos Santos, 2012). For the purposes of the discussion here, we will focus on previous findings on NDs alone. Different methodologies have been employed to look at NDs. For example, work has examined the effects of NDs in children's word recognition, word production and lexical acquisition, where the finding is that words with high NDs are acquired earlier compared to words with low NDs (Storkel, 2009). Sosa and Stoel-Gammon (2012) found that 2-year-olds produce dense ND words more accurately and with less variability than sparse ND words. Other constructs such as prosodic NDs have also been proposed (Gladfelter & Goffman, 2013).

The role that NDs play in children's early phonological and lexical development has yet to be fully understood and as such is of great empirical interest, especially cross-linguistically. Beyond English, a handful of studies have looked at NDs in language development, using a variety of experimental methodologies. For example, Freedman and Barlow (2012) examined the effects of NDs on spoken word production with English-speaking, Spanish-speaking and English-Spanish bilingual children aged 2–8 years and found differences in how words with low NDs were produced in English and Spanish. As compared to English, Spanish has few monosyllabic words, and the majority of words are disyllabic (Vitevitch & Rodríguez, 2005). Work on spoken word recognition has been done with Mandarin-speaking children aged 4–7 years. Mandarin has a high proportion of monosyllabic words as well as many multisyllabic words (Wang, Wu & Kirk, 2010). Wang et al. (2010) found effects of lexical frequency and ND in children's spoken word recognition of disyllables but not with monosyllabic stimuli. They argued that one possibility is that this is due to the high number of homophones in Mandarin. Research has also looked at NDs in the development of German (Zaba & Schmidt, 2011) and Finnish (Kirjavainen, Nikolaev & Kidd, 2012), as well as at the effects of orthographic NDs in reading in a variety of languages, such as Italian (Marinelli, Traficante, Zoccolotti & Burani, 2013). These cross-linguistic studies demonstrate that the effects of ND vary, likely due to the influence of the sound structure and lexical patterns of individual languages.

NDS AND LEXICAL ACQUISITION

Another line of research has looked at NDs in lexical acquisition. Rather than experimentally manipulating NDs as a factor in an experimental design, these studies have looked at patterns of ND in children's emerging vocabularies. The original studies were driven by the question of how children store early lexical information. One proposal argued that the initial encoding of lexical information is more holistic (Charles-Luce & Luce, 1990; Metsala & Walley, 1998). The other proposal was that although children's lexicons are smaller than adults' lexicons, children nevertheless encode lexical information with the same amount of detail (Coady & Aslin, 2004). These studies have been based both on children's spontaneous productions and on lexical norm data from the MacArthur-Bates Communicative Development Inventory (MB-CDI). For example, in an analysis of children's vocabularies from ages 1;4 to 2;6, Storkel (2009) found that children acquire shorter words with a higher ND earlier than longer words with a lower ND (also see Storkel, 2004). However, in a study using naturalistic, longitudinal data from three children, Maekawa and Storkel (2006) did not find consistent effects of ND in children's expressive vocabulary development and in fact found the opposite effect for one child, who acquired words from sparse neighbourhoods before those from dense neighbourhoods. In other work based on young children's vocabularies measured from parental responses to the MB-CDI for English (Stokes, 2010), the Inventaire Français du Développement Communicatif (IFDC) for European French (Stokes, Kern, et al., 2012) and the Danish Communicative Development Inventory (DCDI) for Danish (Stokes, Bleses, Basbøll, & Lambertsen, 2012), Stokes and colleagues found that across these languages ND has an inverse relationship with vocabulary size. Children with smaller vocabularies have more words from dense neighbourhoods than sparse neighbourhoods. This is perhaps surprising given the differences in the lexical and phonological structures of the languages.

NDS AND POSITIONAL STUDIES

ND is a very broad definition of sound similarity in the lexicon. Recall that the definition of neighbours is words that differ by the addition, deletion or substitution of a phoneme (Luce & Pisoni, 1998). This distinction fails to capture acoustic similarities between words, treating neighbours which differ in manner, place and voicing features (*pit* ~ *nit*) the same as pairs which differ only in voicing (*pit* ~ *bit*). It also fails to capture positional differences between neighbours, for example, treating words that differ in word-initial position (*pit* ~ *bit*) the same as pairs that differ in word-final position (*pit* ~ *pin*). Among the set of neighbours a word has, they can be classified by where in the word the substitution, deletion or addition takes place. Rhyme neighbours (RNs) are distinguished by changes in the initial consonant (*peur* ~ *coeur*), consonant neighbours (CNs) are distinguished by changes in the vowel (*beurre* ~ *bar*), and lead neighbours (LNs) are distinguished by changes in the final consonant (*douche* ~ *douce*) (De Cara & Goswami, 2002).

Research has found similar and different patterns of positional neighbours depending on which language is being investigated. Ziegler and Goswami (2005) provided a comparison of neighbour types in monosyllabic words for English, Dutch, German and French and found that in all four languages, RNs are the most frequent, but language differences were found in the proportion of CNs and LNs. This type of cross-linguistic comparison suggests that there are both language-universal effects of ND, in the high proportion of RNs, but also language-specific effects, in the proportions of CNs and LNs. Presumably, these differences arise from the phonological structures in the various languages. In other words, the phonological patterns of a given language, such as syllable structure or phonotactic patterns, will influence the language's distribution of NDs. For example, languages differ in the ratio of vowels and consonants in their phonemic inventories, which may result in differences in neighbourhood types (Stokes, Bleses, et al., 2012, p. 1268). Languages such as Hua, which permits only CV syllables, will by default not have any neighbours distinguished in final position. Languages also differ in their phonotactics, such as restricting certain segments in syllable-final position to only sonorants, as in Manam (Lichtenberk, 1983). In these languages, one would predict fewer LNs because fewer lexical distinctions can be made in final position.

In addition to cross-linguistic comparisons, research has also contrasted NDs in children's early lexicons to the target language. English-speaking children's NDs pattern closely to those of English-speaking adults (De Cara & Goswami, 2002; Zamuner, 2009). Moreover, at the earliest stages, there are even more RNs in CVC words in child English compared to English-speaking adults (Zamuner, 2009). These differences may reflect learners' early speech perception sensitivities, driven by the language input of high RNs or based on other factors such as the acoustic saliency of word-initial position over other word positions. This is characterized as a reciprocal relationship between phonological representations and the lexicon (Stoel-Gammon, 2011), where phonological sensitivities influence lexical acquisition at the early stages of language development. Another possibility is that at the earliest stages, learners rely on a statistical learning cue from high ND as a cue for lexical development (Stokes, Bleses, et al., 2012). As this is driven by patterns across words in the lexicon, it raises the possibility that the distributions of neighbour types may differ across languages. For example, Danish has a low ratio of consonants to vowels (Bleses, Basbøll, Lum, & Vach, 2011). This may lead to increased difficulty for Danish-learning infants to segment words from the speech stream and may impact the rate of lexical acquisition. Stokes, Bleses, et al. (2012) further hypothesize that this might impact Danish children's sensitivity to different neighbour types, relying more on CNs compared to RNs or LNs.

CURRENT RESEARCH

Despite the steps taken in our understanding of how children structure and organize their early lexicons, there remain issues that need further investigation. The majority of research has been conducted on English, which tends to have many monosyllabic and CVC words compared to other languages (Fikkert, 2007; Stoel-Gammon, 2011). An examination of languages with different syllable and prosodic patterns may yield cross-linguistic similarities and/or differences in how children acquire their phonology and build their lexicons. French has diverse sound structures compared to English, such as having a different rhythm and different syllable patterns. French is a syllable-timed language (Abercrombie, 1967), stress tends to fall on the final syllable of a phrase (Dell, 1984; Walker, 1984; Hayes, 1995; Hirst & Di Cristo, 1998), and French has a high frequency of open syllables (Demuth & Johnson, 2003). See Demuth and Johnson (2003) and Stokes, Kern, et al. (2012) for further discussion of phonological differences between English and French.

This research investigates the phonological patterns of NDs in the early vocabularies of French-speaking children using the Québec French version of the MB-CDI (henceforth QF-CDI) (Trudeau, Frank & Poulin-Dubois, 1997, 1999). As previously discussed, similarities and differences have been found across distributions of RNs, CNs and LNs for adults and children in English (De Cara & Goswami, 2002; Zamuner, 2009). Comparisons between adult and child French might yield similar relationships. First, early child French may pattern like child English (Zamuner, 2009) and may have a greater proportion of RNs at the early stages of lexical acquisition. The distribution of RNs will more closely approximate the target language as vocabulary size grows. To illustrate, at the early stages of lexical development, one might expect more distinctions in children's vocabularies to occur at the beginnings of words. With time, lexical distinctions will occur at all positions in the word. Alternatively, given the larger proportion of open syllables in French, there may be more CNs in the early lexicons of French, as hypothesized by Stokes, Bleses, et al. (2012) for the development of Danish. For instance, one might expect at the earliest stages of development that most lexical distinctions in children's vocabularies would occur in the vowel position.

To test these scenarios, the first objective was to establish patterns of phonological NDs in French to allow for comparative analyses between adult and child language. The first analysis was on the lexicon of French and will be referred to as adult French (Analysis I). The second analysis examined the early lexicons of children acquiring French (Analysis II).

We then present longitudinal analyses of the QF-CDI, providing a breakdown of neighbour types between 1;7 to 2;6 (Analyses III and IV). Last, as Maekawa and Storkel (2006) found varying results for NDs when looking at children's expressive vocabularies compared to lexical norm data, we also examined naturalistic data from one child learning French (Rose, 2000) (Analysis V).

Researchers have varied the types of words included in their analyses, such as all nouns (Storkel, 2009), monosyllables (Stokes, 2010) or CVC words (Zamuner, 2009). We present both monosyllabic and CVC analyses and note differences between the analyses below. The standard definition for phonological neighbours was used. A word was considered a phonological neighbour if it differed from another word through the substitution, deletion or addition of a single phoneme. Each neighbour was coded for whether it was an RN (*faire* /fɛr/ (Eng. 'to do') vs. *verre* /vɛr/ (Eng. 'glass')), CN (*bulle* /byl/ (Eng. 'bubbles') vs. *balle* /bal/ (Eng. 'bullet' or 'ball')) or LN (*langue* /lɑ̃g/ (Eng. 'language') vs. *lampe* /lɑ̃p/ (Eng. 'lamp')).

ANALYSIS I: ADULT FRENCH ND

NDs for French were based on the Lexop database and served as the baseline from which to compare child data. Lexop (Peereman & Content, 1999) contains the subset of all monosyllabic words ($n = 2249$) extracted from the BRULEX database (Content, Mousty, & Radeau, 1990) and provides phonetic transcriptions, as well as a number of measures, such as word frequency. Bisyllabic words were included if they ended in a consonant cluster + schwa, because schwa is never phonetically realized word-finally (Charette, 2006, p. 29). Therefore, words such as *triste* (Eng. 'sad') were included. To test whether this had an effect on the results, Analyses I through IV were redone with the exclusion of these words, with similar results to when the words were included. Masculine and feminine forms of nouns and adjectives have separate entries. Although Ziegler and Goswami (2005) provide a summary of NDs in French, analyses of ND in adult French were done to ensure that the coding and analyses were held constant across both child and adult French.

NDs were calculated based on the words' phonetic transcriptions. Note that the adult French corpus is based on European French. Although there are some differences between European French and Canadian French, it was assumed that the dialects are similar enough to compare for the purposes of the study. Canadian French differs from European French in the realization of vowels in certain contexts. Open CV syllables are typically realized the same in Canadian French as in

European French, but the following changes take place in closed syllables: [a] → [ɑ] (e.g. *ça* /sa/ (Eng. 'this') and *sale* /sɑl/ (Eng. 'dirty')), [i] → [ɪ] (*vie* /vi/ (Eng. 'life') and *vite* /vɪt/ (Eng. 'fast')), [y] → [ʏ] (*lu* /ly/ (Eng. 'read') and *lune* /lʏn/ (Eng. 'moon')), [u] → [ʊ] (*doux* /du/ (Eng. 'soft', masc.) and *douce* /dʊs/ (Eng. 'soft', fem.)). In some varieties of Canadian French, vowel laxing of /i/ and /y/ does not typically take place before lengthened consonants (voiced fricatives). Also, the change [a] → [ɑ] (e.g. *ça* /sa/ (Eng. 'this') and *sale* /sɑl/ (Eng. 'dirty')) takes place in closed syllables, but it is most often attested at the end of words in open syllables (Rose & Wauquier-Gravelines, 2007). To test whether these differences had an effect on the results, these vowel changes were encoded and Analyses I through IV were redone, with no impact on the results.

Each monosyllabic word in the database was analyzed for the number and proportion of RNs, CNs and LNs, and the same analyses were done on the subset of CVC words. For monosyllables, adult French yields the greatest proportion of RNs (8679 (.42)), followed by CNs (5924 (.29)) and LNs (5984 (.29)). These results are similar to those reported for adult French in Ziegler and Goswami (2005). Similar results are found for RNs when the analyses are restricted to CVC words: RNs (3669 (.40)), followed by CNs (1890 (.21)) and LNs (3561 (.39)). What differs in the monosyllabic and CVC analyses is the proportion of CNs and LNs. Results are presented in Figure 2.1.

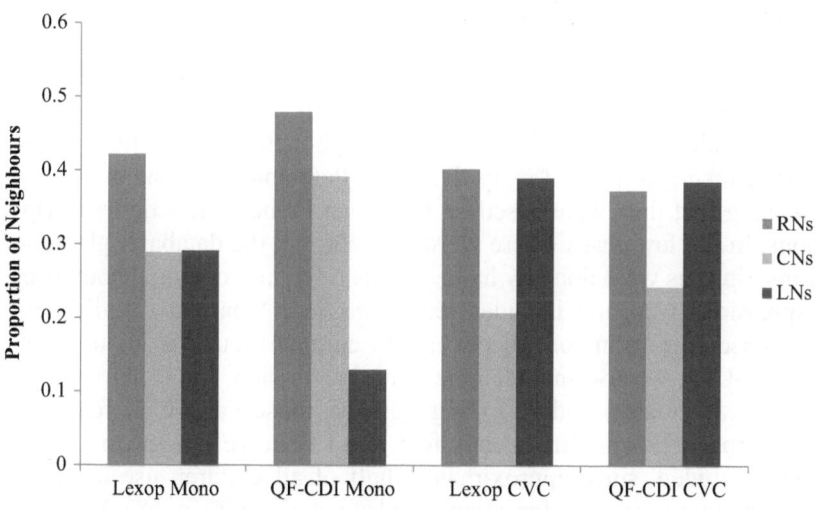

Figure 2.1 Overall proportions of RNs, CNs and LNs in monosyllabic and CVC words in Lexop and QF-CDI.

ANALYSIS II: CHILD FRENCH ND

Analyses of child French were based on the lexical norm data of all monosyllabic and CVC words from the QF-CDI (Trudeau et al., 1997), for expressive vocabularies of children between 1;3 and 2;6 years of age. The lexical norms are divided into two acquisition rates: 50% and 90% acquisition. This criterion describes which words were produced by 50% and 90% of the children at any given month, as measured by parental questionnaire (Trudeau et al., 1997). The lexical norm data provide a breakdown of how many new words are acquired from month to month, for expressive vocabularies.

Various criteria have been used to establish which words to include in analyses. Storkel (2004) used a 50% acquisition rate as a cut-off point, whereas the cut-off rate of 25% was used in Zamuner (2009). For the QF-CDI, the lexical norms are divided into two broad categories: 50% and 90% acquisition rates. As a result, the lexical norm data for the QF-CDI are not as fine-grained as the English normative data. To make the results as parallel as possible to previous studies, acquisition was defined as 50%; thus, at any given month, only words that were reported to have been typically produced by 50% of children were analyzed. Additional monosyllabic words are found on the QF-CDI questionnaire but are not reported to have been acquired by 50% of children by 30 months of age. For example, the word *thon* (Eng. 'tuna') is on the QF-CDI form but is not reported in the lexical norm data as being acquired by 50% of children by 30 months of age and therefore was not included.

Following Peereman and Content (1999), bisyllabic words ending in a consonant cluster + schwa were included in the set of monosyllabic words. Calculations of ND were based on phonetic transcriptions of the words, taken from the Lexop database (Peereman & Content, 1999), meaning that they were based on European French phonetic transcriptions. In the few cases where words were not in the database, phonetic transcriptions were done by hand. Words referring to animal sounds or expressions were not included, e.g. *bêêê bêêê* 'baa baa'. While only the masculine form for adjectives and animate nouns is included on the QF-CDI, we also included the feminine version. For example, *chat* (Eng. 'cat', masc.) and *vert* (Eng. 'green', masc.) and their feminine counterparts *chatte* (Eng. 'cat', fem.) and *verte* (Eng. 'green', fem.) were included, since approximately half of all children use forms in both the masculine and feminine (Trudeau et al., 1999, p. 68). Verbs on the QF-CDI are listed in the infinitive. Approximately 85% of children use the form of the future tense which is constructed with the verb *aller*

(Eng. 'to go') + the infinitive. A decision was made not to use common forms of conjugated verbs. One potential issue is that the Lexop database includes verb forms, making the adult and child French analyses not comparable. However, to test whether this decision made any difference in the distribution of NDs, Analyses I through IV were redone with all verbs excluded, with the same results.

A total of 211 phonologically unique monosyllabic words are reported for the lexical norm data for the QF-MCI. The number and proportion of neighbour types based on monosyllabic words on the QF-CDI was RN (n = 316, Proportion .48), CN (n = 259, Proportion .39) and LN (n = 85, Proportion .13). There were 70 phonologically unique CVC words. The number and proportion of CVC words in the QF-CDI was RN (n = 60, Proportion .37), CN (n = 39, Proportion .24) and LN (n = 62, Proportion .39). These distributions are presented in Figure 2.1. For both analyses, RNs were the most represented, but the difference between CNs and LNs varied between the monosyllabic and CVC analyses.

COMPARISONS OF NDS IN CHILD FRENCH AND ADULT FRENCH

A comparison between child French and adult French in Figure 2.1 indicates that the distribution of neighbour types is both similar and different. They are similar in that they have a high proportion of RNs. In the monosyllabic analyses, it is striking that the proportion of CNs is much greater in child French than in adult French. These differences were unexpected since it was predicted that NDs in child French would mimic those of adult French. One possible account for the differences may be that children initially acquire words with less complex syllable structures, such that French children have a higher proportion of words with open syllables in their vocabulary. Therefore, French-speaking children have yet to acquire the more complex structures that allow for LNs to arise. Support for this possibility is seen when one compares the results from the monosyllabic versus CVC analyses. When words are restricted to CVCs, NDs in child French pattern like those in adult French.

Another account for the differences between adult and child French comes from the nature of the adult French data. Recall that adult French data were taken from the Lexop database (Peereman & Content, 1999), which includes all possible monosyllabic words in French. This means the analysis includes very low frequency words which children are unlikely to have acquired. If these low frequency words have a different

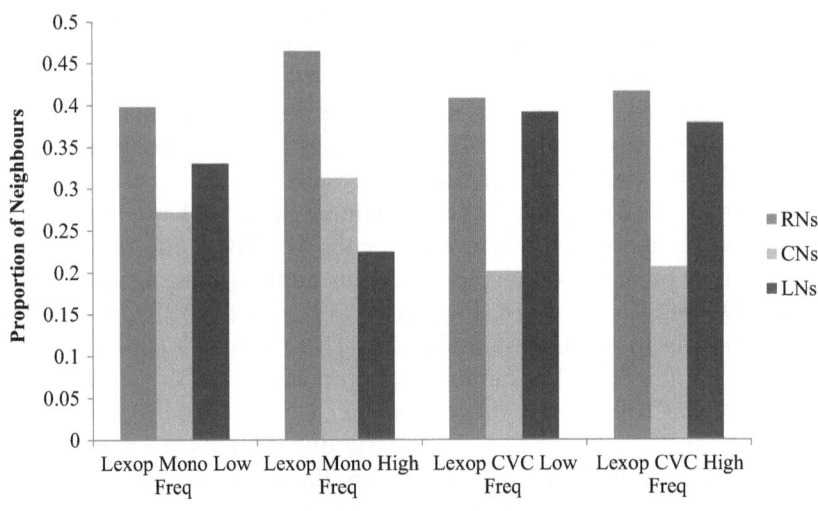

Figure 2.2 Overall proportions of RNs, CNs and LNs in monosyllabic and CVC words in Lexop, by lower half and upper half of word frequency estimates.

distribution of NDs, this might provide a reason for why the adult and child language data differ. The Lexop database provides word frequency estimates, and NDs were recalculated based on a medium split of these frequency estimates (lower half and upper half), provided in Figure 2.2. When examining NDs in infrequent and frequent monosyllabic words, varying patterns of NDs are found. When words are restricted to lower frequencies, there are more LNs than CNs, similar to the analyses based on all monosyllabic words in adult French and similar to the results for adult French in Ziegler and Goswami (2005). However, if words are restricted to the subset of words with higher frequencies, the distribution of NDs in monosyllabic words is similar to the patterns found for child French: RNs > CNs > LNs. Therefore, there are differences in the distribution of syllable and/or word shapes in infrequent vs. frequent French words. It might be that children have yet to acquire the structures of infrequent lexical items, which is why they have fewer LNs. For CVC words, the frequency analyses are similar to the analyses collapsed across all CVC words (also see Figure 2.2).

ANALYSIS III: CHILD FRENCH LONGITUDINAL ANALYSES OF MONOSYLLABIC WORDS

Recall that in previous analyses of English, it was found that early vocabularies have a greater proportion of RNs than expected. To look

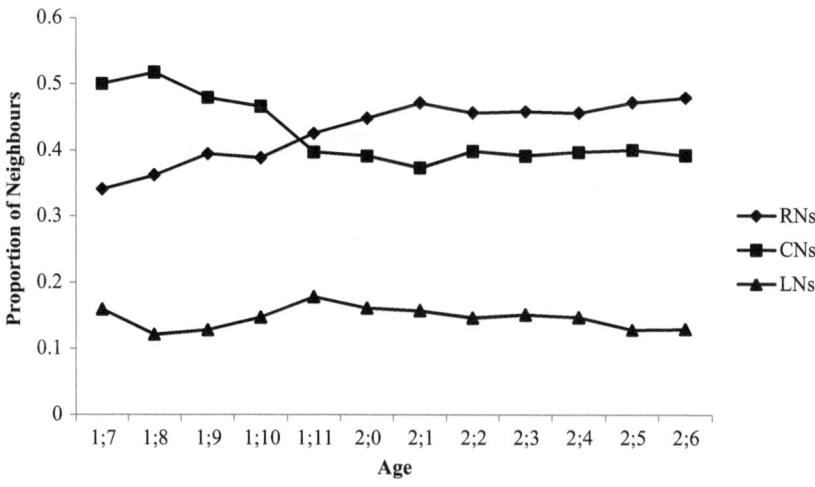

Figure 2.3 Overall proportions of RNs, CNs and LNs in French-speaking children's early lexicons (QF-CDI)—monosyllables.

at whether parallel results were found in French, longitudinal analyses were carried out on the lexical norm data from the QF-CDI. To ensure that lexicons were large enough to provide meaningful results, analyses were restricted to months where children acquired a minimum of 25 monosyllabic words. The size of the lexicons varied across 1;7–2;6 (range: 30–211 words, $M = 118.83$ words). For each month, NDs were calculated for the set of monosyllabic words that were scored as having a 50% rate of acquisition or higher, as seen in Figure 2.3.

To examine whether there were statistical differences in the distribution of neighbour types at the different months, a repeated measures ANOVA was used with position as the between subjects factor (RN, CN, LN). The condition of sphericity was violated and corrected using Greenhouse-Geisser values. There was a statistically significant effect of position: $F(1.17, 12.94) = 127.01$, $p < 0.001$, $\eta^2_p = 0.92$, with the average proportions: RNs (.43), CNs (.42), LNs (.15). Follow-up comparisons on position using Bonferroni-corrected alpha found that both RNs and CNs differed statistically from LNs but that RNs and CNs were not appreciably different from each other. Thus, the ranking of the three positions was RN, CN > LN.

ANALYSIS IV: CHILD FRENCH LONGITUDINAL ANALYSES OF CVC WORDS

The next analysis looked at the subset of CVC words, restricted to months where a minimum of 25 CVC words were acquired by children:

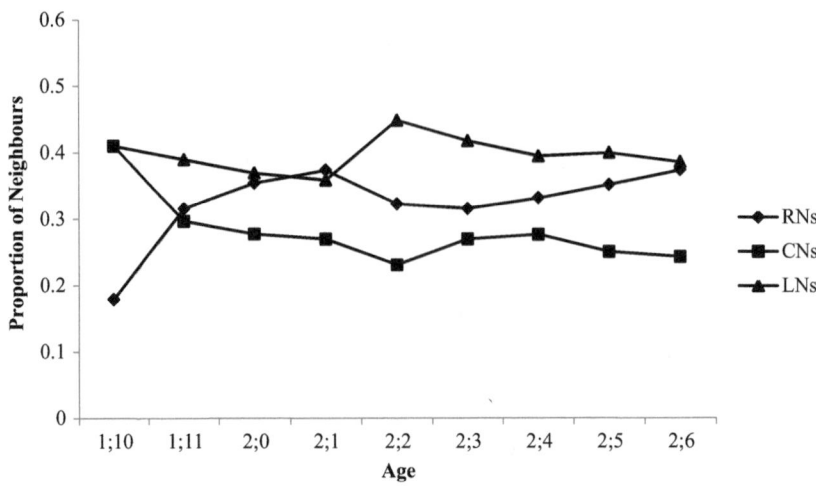

Figure 2.4 Overall proportions of RNs, CNs and LNs in French-speaking children's early lexicons (QF-CDI)—CVC.

1;10–2;6, range: 27–70 words, $M = 49.88$ words. Similar to the analysis with monosyllabic words, an analysis with CVC words was done to determine whether there were statistical differences in the distribution of neighbour types across the months. A repeated measures ANOVA was used with position as the between subjects factor (RN, CN, LN). There was a statistically significant effect of position: $F(2, 16) = 8.99$, $p < 0.01$. $\eta^2_p = 0.53$, with the average proportions: RNs (.32), CNs (.28), LNs (.40). Again, follow-up comparisons on position, corrected using Bonferroni adjusted alpha levels, found that only CNs and LNs statistically differed from each other. Regarding the distribution of neighbour types, Figures 2.3 and 2.4 show that the results from the CVC analyses look more like the results from monosyllables at the later ages. Unlike in the analyses with monosyllables, the CVC analyses do not consistently have higher CNs at the younger months.

ANALYSIS V: CHILD FRENCH SPONTANEOUS PRODUCTION DATA

The analyses conducted on the lexical norm data from the QF-CDI were based on parental responses to checklists rather than naturalistic data. We attempted to address this limitation and examined the spontaneous speech of a Canadian French-speaking child. The child's productions were analyzed for phonological neighbours (RNs, CNs, LNs), with

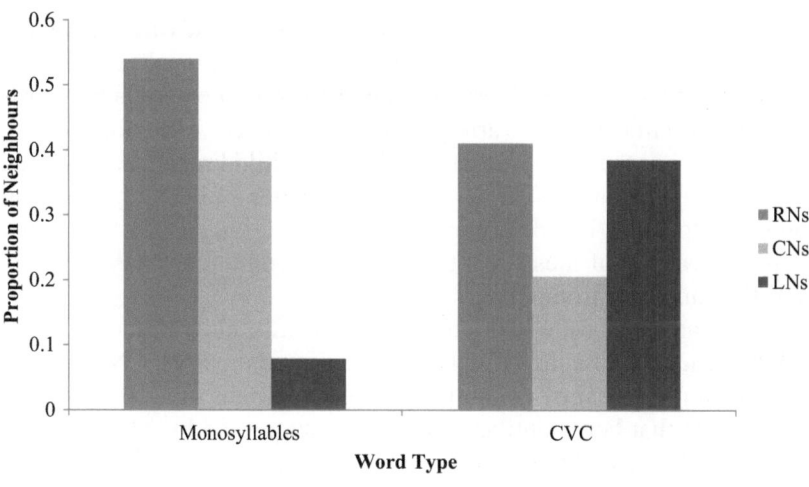

Figure 2.5 Overall proportions of RNs, CNs and LNs in monosyllabic and CVC words in Clara's vocabulary between 2;6 and 2;7 years of age.

the expectation that the same distributions would be found in spontaneous speech as with the lexical norm data. Spontaneous production data from Clara were taken from the French Goad-Rose corpus (Rose, 2000), taken from CHILDES/PhonBank database (Rose et al., 2006; Rose & MacWhinney, to appear). These are naturalistic data, recorded bi-monthly in the child's home. Clara's data were collapsed across three sessions, from ages 2;6.5 to 2;7.19. The ND analyses were based on idealized transcriptions of Clara's expressive speech. Analyses identified all the unique monosyllable words (57) and CVC words (17) in Clara's vocabulary which also occurred on the QF-CDI. NDs for these words were then taken from the calculations based on the QF-CDI. As seen in Figure 2.5, Clara's proportions of RNs, followed by CNs and LNs, are similar to patterns in the QF-CDI for monosyllables (RNs ($n = 312$, Proportion .48), CNs ($n = 259$, Proportion .40) and LNs ($n = 73$, Proportion .13)) and for CVC words (RNs ($n = 60$, Proportion .38), CNs ($n = 39$, Proportion .25) and LNs ($n = 58$, Proportion .37)).

DISCUSSION AND CONCLUSION

This study examined NDs in the development of French with the aim of expanding our understanding of phonological and lexical factors in language development. In comparing French data, it was found that the patterns of ND were both similar and different. What was similar was the high proportion of RNs in both child and adult French. Differences were seen when we considered CNs and LNs. In monosyllabic words, patterns in child French varied from adult French. The most striking difference was the high proportion of CNs in child French, and even the highest proportion of CNs at the earliest stages of development from ages 1;7 to 1;10. The disproportionate distribution of CNs was found across a variety of measures: the QF-CDI, longitudinal data from the QF-CDI and data from Clara.

When analyses were restricted to CVC words, child French was like adult French. Across the QF-CDI lexical norm data, RNs, CNs and LNs showed a great deal of variability between the ages of 1;10 and 2;6. It is possible that here, similar to what was suggested by Maekawa and Storkel (2006), children have not yet mastered cues of ND in CVC words for lexical development, potentially because CVC words are less frequent in French. Rather, they have picked up on the most frequent syllable shape patterns in French: open syllables.

These findings, although not in the expected direction, nevertheless help to establish the phonological and lexical structures of French-speaking children. It was initially predicted that child French would mirror adult French, based on previous research showing that NDs in child English were similar to adult English, though more exaggerated (De Cara & Goswami, 2003; Zamuner, 2009). The fact that NDs are different across child and adult French monosyllables is somewhat perplexing if the overall frequency of NDs in the language alone drives language development (see Demuth, 2007; Rose & Inkelas, 2011 for a discussion on some of the limitations of frequency-based explanations in language development). Although further research is needed to explain why these differences are found, the first hypothesis was that this reflects differences in the syllable structure across English and French. When children are acquiring French, they are likely to first learn words with the most frequent syllable structure: open syllables. As such, francophone children have a greater proportion of CNs and have yet to acquire the more complex syllable structures that allow for LNs to arise in the first place. This illustrates how the structure of the target language may lead to different patterns of acquisition cross-linguistically, as predicted by Stokes, Bleses, et al. (2012). Another possible explanation comes from the analyses which restricted NDs to low and high frequency words. NDs in adult French across these two measures were quite different (Figure 2.2). When NDs in monosyllabic words were restricted to the higher frequencies, parallels were found between adult and child French. NDs within adult French vary by frequency, with infrequent words having different syllable and/or word shapes which allow for more lexical distinctions to be made in final position. Children first acquire the frequent words of French and are subsequently less likely to acquire words with the structures of infrequent lexical items.

Studies of lexical development have often examined corpora that are based on idealized transcription of children's productions. While it is informative to use idealized data as a baseline for what to expect in child language, it is also informative to consider children's production accuracy. In other words, idealized data do not take into account any production errors. For example, the current analyses do not take into account whether children produced the target word *parc* (Eng. 'park') as /paʁ/ or /paʁk/. While analyses from Clara consisted of spontaneous speech, there was not enough data to make any meaningful comparisons between NDs and production accuracy. NDs and production were recently examined by Sosa and Stoel-Gammon (2012) (also see Freedman & Barlow, 2012). They found that children produce words with high NDs more accurately and with less variability compared to words with low NDs. This is compatible with a theory in which children's phonological representations develop based on distributions of NDs in their lexicon. One could also consider different types of neighbours (RNs, CNs and LNs) combined with ND (dense or sparse neighbourhoods) and compare this to children's production accuracy. Thus, a possible avenue for future research is to examine whether children make fewer production errors in initial position with words that have many RNs compared to fewer RNs. If such a relationship is found, this would suggest that phonological representations are also dependent on patterns of ND across different positions. Alternatively, one might compare the structures in children's outputs to see whether this has an effect on the words children acquire, for example, to see whether children who delete final segments and produce CV syllables are less likely to acquire CVC words compared to children who can produce final segments. These analyses can be compared across languages and may reveal cross-linguistic similarities and differences.

Another approach would be to compare the tendencies in individual children's lexical development to milestones in their phonological development. Rose (2000) proposes distinct stages of syllable structure acquisition for Québec French, beginning with the unmarked CV syllable. This pattern was observed in Clara's data and also in Theo's data, a child speaking a dialect of Québec French characteristic of Montreal. Rose notes, however, that children may have different structural representations. Differences emerged between Clara and Theo in when they acquired word-final [ʁ], and Rose argues that this is due to different representations of the phonological structure of French words: Clara's representation of [ʁ] was a placeless word-final coda and was thus acquired at a later stage, while Theo's was a word-final onset acquired in the first stages. If children's phonological structures impact their lexical tendencies, one would predict that children like Clara would have a greater proportion of RNs and CNs in their lexicons than children like Theo, who would have both RNs and CNs, as well as LNs.

One limitation to the current study is that the analyses were limited to monosyllabic words, yet French has many multisyllabic words. In an examination of data from CHILDES, Demuth and Johnson (2003) found that there was a large percentage of monosyllabic (45%) and disyllabic words (47%) in French. The fact that the current analyses focused solely on monosyllabic words may limit the generalizability of the current findings. Another limitation is that the analyses presented here have focused strictly on ND; there are other factors that may interact with ND, however, such as word frequency (Stokes, 2010). To tease apart these relationships, access to a larger database with child frequency counts is needed.

The challenge of understanding the universal versus language-specific aspect of development is especially demanding if we consider the variety of languages that children learn. Our focus was to explore the patterns of ND in French to determine whether child language reflected universals or the language-specific input. The differences between child French and adult French varied from previous work on English. This suggests that there are language-specific ways in which patterns of ND emerge across languages. Although child French showed a unique distribution of NDs, particularly in monosyllabic words, we suggest that this reflects the syllable structure of frequent French words. This points to a complex relationship between the input and patterns of phonological and lexical development. Previous research has shown that many different factors can interact in development, such as the production and perception capabilities of learners, morphological patterns, word stress and word length, just to name a few (Fikkert, 2007; Sosa & Bybee, 2008; Demuth, 2011). These findings leave us with some unanswered questions, and further cross-linguistic research is needed to fully understand what is at the root of these differences.

ACKNOWLEDGMENTS

Special thanks to Natacha Trudeau and Diane Poulin-Dubois for providing the QF-CDI data and to Yvan Rose for insightful comments. Additional thanks to Peter Milne for his assistance with programming.

This research was supported by a grant awarded to T. S. Zamuner from the University of Ottawa, Research Development Program and from SSHRC grant 410-2011-1961 awarded to T. S. Zamuner.

REFERENCES

Abercrombie, D. (1967). *Elements of general phonetics*. Edinburgh: Edinburgh University Press.

Bleses, D., Basbøll, H., Lum, J., & Vach, W. (2011). Phonology and lexicon in a cross-linguistic perspective: The importance of phonetics—A commentary on Stoel-Gammon's "Relationships between lexical and phonological development in young children". *Journal of Child Language, 38*, 61–68.

Charette, M. (2006). *Conditions on phonological government* (Vol. 58). Cambridge: Cambridge University Press.

Charles-Luce, J., & Luce, P. A. (1990). Similarity neighbourhoods of words in young children's lexicons. *Journal of Child Language, 17*(1), 205–215.

Coady, J. A., & Aslin, R. N. (2004). Young children's sensitivities to probabilistic phonotactics in the developing lexicon. *Journal of Experimental Child Psychology, 89*(3), 183–213.

Content, A., Mousty, P., & Radeau, M. (1990). Brulex. Une base de données lexicales informatisée pour le français écrit et parlé [BRULEX: A computerized lexical data base for the French language/BRULEX]. *Année Psychologique, 90*(4), 551–566.

De Cara, B., & Goswami, U. (2002). Similarity relations among spoken words: The special status of rimes in English. *Behavior Research Methods, Instruments, & Computers, 34*(3), 416–423.

De Cara, B., & Goswami, U. (2003). Phonological neighbourhood density: Effects in a rhyme awareness task in five-year-old children. *Journal of Child Language, 30*, 695–710.

Dell, F. (1984). L'accentuation des phrases en français. In F. Dell, D. Hirst & J.- R. Vergnaud (eds.), *Forme sonore du langage*, 65–122. Paris: Hermann.

Demuth, K. (2007). The role of frequency in language acquisition. In I. Gülzow & N. Gagarina (eds.), *Frequency effects in language acquisition*, 528–538. Berlin: Mouton de Gruyter.

Demuth, K. (2011). Interactions between lexical and phonological development: Cross-linguistic and contextual considerations—a commentary on Stoel-Gammon's 'Relationships between lexical and phonological development in young children'. *Journal of Child Language, 38*, 69–74.

Demuth, K., & Johnson, M. (2003). Truncation to subminimal words in early French. *Canadian Journal of Linguistics/La revue canadienne de linguistique, 48*(2), 211–241.

Fikkert, P. (2007). Acquiring phonology. In P. de Lacy (ed.), *Handbook of phonological theory*, 537–554. Cambridge, MA: Cambridge University Press.

Freedman, S., & Barlow, J. A. (2012). Using whole-word production measures to determine the influence of phonotactic probability and neighborhood density on bilingual speech production. *International Journal of Bilingualism, 16*(4), 369–387.

Garlock, V. M., Walley, A. C., & Metsala, J. L. (2001). Age-of-acquisition, word frequency, and neighborhood density effects on spoken word recognition by children and adults. *Journal of Memory and Language, 45*(3), 468–492.

Gladfelter, G., & Goffman, L. (2013). The influence of prosodic stress patterns and semantic depth on novel word learning in typically developing children. *Language Learning and Development, 9*(2), 151–174.

Hayes, B. (1995). *Metrical stress theory: Principles and case studies*. Chicago: University of Chicago Press.

Hirst, D., & Di Cristo, A. (1998). *Intonation systems: A survey of twenty languages*. Cambridge: Cambridge University Press.

Kirjavainen, M., Nikolaev, A., & Kidd, E. (2012). The effect of frequency and phonological neighbourhood density on the acquisition of past tense verbs by Finnish children. *Cognitive Linguistics, 23*(2), 273–315.

Lichtenberk, F. (1983). *A grammar of Manam*. Honolulu: University of Hawaii Press.

Luce, P. A., & Pisoni, D. B. (1998). Recognizing spoken words: The neighbourhood activation model. *Ear & Hearing, 19*, 1–36.

Maekawa, J., & Storkel, H. L. (2006). Individual differences in the influence of phonological characteristics on expressive vocabulary development by young children. *Journal of Child Language, 33*(3), 439–459.

Marinelli, C. V., Traficante, D., Zoccolotti, P., & Burani, C. (2013). Orthographic neighborhood-size effects on the reading aloud of Italian children with and without dyslexia. *Scientific Studies of Reading, 5*, 1–17.

Metsala, J. L., & Walley, A. C. (1998). Spoken vocabulary growth and the segmental restructuring of lexical representations: Precursors to phonemic awareness and early reading ability. In J. L. Metsala & L. C. Ehri (eds.), *Word recognition in beginning literacy*, 89–120. Mahwah, NJ: Erlbaum.

Peereman, R., & Content, A. (1999). LEXOP: A lexical database providing orthography–phonology statistics for French monosyllabic words. *Behavioral Research Methods Instruments & Computers, 31*, 376–379.

Rose, Y. (2000). *Headedness and prosodic licensing in L1 acquisition of phonology*. Ph.D. Dissertation. McGill University.

Rose, Y., & Inkelas, S. (2011). The interpretation of phonological patterns in first language acquisition. In M. van Oostendorp, C. Ewen, E. Hume &

K. Rice (eds.), *The Blackwell companion to phonology, 3*, 2414–2438. Malden, MA: Wiley-Blackwell.

Rose, Y., & MacWhinney, B. (to appear). The PhonBank Project: Data and software-assisted methods for the study of phonology and phonological development. In J. Durand, U. Gut & G. Kristoffersen (eds.), *The Oxford handbook of corpus phonology*, 380–400. Oxford: Oxford University Press.

Rose, Y., MacWhinney, B., Byrne, R., Hedlund, G., Maddocks, K., O'Brien, P., & Wareham, T. (2006). Introducing Phon: A software solution for the study of phonological acquisition. In D. Bamman, T. Magnitskaia & C. Zaller (eds.), *Proceedings of the 30th Annual Boston University Conference on Language Development*, 489–500. Somerville, MA: Cascadilla Press.

Rose, Y., & Wauquier-Gravelines, S. (2007). French speech acquisition. In S. McLeod (ed.), *The international guide to speech acquisition*, 364–385. Clifton Park, NY: Thomson Delmar Learning.

Sosa, A. V., & Bybee, J. (2008). A cognitive approach to clinical psychology. In M. Ball, M. Perkins, N. Muller & S. Howard (eds.), *Handbook of clinical linguistics*, 480–490. Oxford: Blackwell.

Sosa, A. V., & Stoel-Gammon, C. (2012). Lexical and phonological effects in early word production. *Journal of Speech, Language, and Hearing Research, 55*(2), 596–608.

Stoel-Gammon, C. (2011). Relationships between lexical and phonological development in young children. *Journal of Child Language, 38*(1), 1–34.

Stokes, S. F. (2010). Neighborhood density and word frequency predict vocabulary size in toddlers. *Journal of Speech, Language and Hearing Research, 53*(3), 670–683.

Stokes, S. F., Bleses, D., Basbøll, H., & Lambertsen, C. (2012). Statistical learning in emerging lexicons: The case of Danish. *Journal of Speech, Language, and Hearing Research, 55*(5), 1265–1273.

Stokes, S. F., Kern, S., & dos Santos, C. (2012). Extended Statistical Learning as an account for slow vocabulary growth. *Journal of Child Language, 39*, 105–129.

Storkel, H. L. (2004). Do children acquire dense neighborhoods? An investigation of similarity neighborhoods in lexical acquisition. *Applied Psycholinguistics, 25*, 201–221.

Storkel, H. L. (2009). Developmental differences in the effects of phonological, lexical, and semantic variables on word learning by infants. *Journal of Child Language, 36*, 291–321

Trudeau, N., Frank, I., & Poulin-Dubois, D. (1997). *Les Inventaires MacArthur-Bates du développement de la communication: Mots et gestes*. Montreal, Québec.

Trudeau, N., Frank, I., & Poulin-Dubois, D. (1999). Une adaptation en français québécois du MacArthur Communicative Development Inventory. *Revue d'orthophonie et d'audiologie, 23*(2), 61–73.

Vitevitch, M. S. (2002). The influence of phonological similarity neighborhoods on speech production. *Journal of Experimental Psychology: Learning, Memory, and Cognition, 28*(4), 735.

Vitevitch, M. S., Luce, P. A., Pisoni, D. B., & Auer, E. T. (1999). Phonotactics, neighbourhood activation, and lexical access for spoken words. *Brain and Language, 68*(1–2), 306–311.

Vitevitch, M. S., & Rodríguez, E. (2005). Neighborhood density effects in spoken word recognition in Spanish. *Journal of Multilingual Communication Disorders, 3*, 64–73.

Walker, D. 1984. *The pronunciation of Canadian French.* Ottawa: University of Ottawa Press.

Wang, N. M., Wu, Ch.-M., & Kirk, K. I. (2010). Lexical effects on spoken word recognition performance among Mandarin-speaking children with normal hearing and cochlear implants. *International Journal of Pediatric Otorhinolaryngology, 74*(8), 883–890.

Zaba, A., & Schmidt, T. (2011, May). Neighborhood density and word frequency in child German. In *LSA Annual Meeting Extended Abstracts* (No. 1).

Zamuner, T. S. (2003). *Input-based phonological acquisition.* New York: Routledge.

Zamuner, T. S. (2009). The structure and nature of phonological neighbourhoods in children's early lexicons. *Journal of Child Language, 36*, 3–21.

Zamuner, T. S., Gerken, L. A., & Hammond, M. (2005). The acquisition of phonology based on input: A closer look at the relation of cross-linguistic and child language data. *Lingua, 10*, 1403–1426.

Ziegler, J. C., & Goswami, U. (2005). Reading acquisition, developmental dyslexia, and skilled reading across languages: A psycholinguistic grain size theory. *Psychological Bulletin, 131*(1), 3–29.

3

DEVELOPMENT OF WORD-INITIAL CONSONANT CLUSTERS IN VALLEY ZAPOTEC
Universal vs. Language-Specific Effects of Sonority

Joseph Paul Stemberger and Mario E. Chávez-Peón

Limitations on complexity are a recurring theme in the phonological systems of all human languages, including the complexity of consonant sequences in syllable onsets. In adult languages (recently overviewed in Zec, 2007), syllable onsets may be limited to a single consonant; if two consonants are allowed, there are generally severe restrictions on which consonants may appear and in which order. Common restrictions are that clusters should begin with a consonant that is low in sonority and continue with a consonant higher in sonority (the Sonority Sequence Principle (e.g. Sievers, 1881), henceforth "the SSP"), and that the difference in sonority between the two consonants should be relatively large. A standard sonority hierarchy is based on manner of articulation, from low to high sonority: stops, fricatives, nasals, liquids, and glides. The most common clusters cross-linguistically begin with an obstruent (especially with a stop) and end with a sonorant (especially a liquid or glide), but a common exception cross-linguistically involves coronal fricatives, especially /s/, with clusters such as /sp/ violating the SSP (a higher-sonority fricative followed by a lower-sonority stop).

Sonority is not well-defined. It is related to the features of the segment but is not reducible to those features. Bernhardt and Stemberger (1998) take sonority as a measure of how vowel-like a segment is but raise the question of whether the "global" sonority of a segment contributes to behavior, or just the features themselves. In their view, each feature has a high-sonority value typical of vowels ([−consonantal,+sonorant,+continuant,+voice]) and a low-sonority

49

value typical of consonants ([+consonantal,−sonorant,−continuant, −voice]). Yavaş (2013) concludes for the acquisition of /sC/ clusters in several languages that global sonority is not important but rather the feature [continuant].

Children show sensitivity to complexity, eliminating onset consonant clusters early in development by deleting one consonant, by epenthesizing a vowel to separate them, by coalescing the two consonants into one consonant combining features from each segment, or by other low-frequency resolutions. The SSP is relevant in two ways (e.g. Smit, 1993; Fikkert, 1994; Bernhardt & Stemberger, 1998; Ohala, 1999; Goad & Rose, 2004; Yavaş, 2013): clusters that abide by the SSP may develop before clusters that do not, and they may be reduced in a different fashion. In many languages, children most often delete the second consonant (C2: liquids or glides) from clusters such as /pl/ and /kw/ and do not commonly coalesce them into one consonant, while in sonority-reversed clusters such as /sp/, children most often delete the first consonant (C1: /s/) but have a strong minority pattern involving coalescence (/sp/ [f]). Sonority-reversed clusters are in the minority (fewer cluster types and fewer words containing such clusters: type frequency) in European languages such as English (Germanic), Italian (Romance), and Slovenian (Slavic), and perhaps the predominance of rising-sonority clusters leads to these differences in acquisition. Even though Slavic languages such as Slovenian have a larger number of sonority-reversed clusters ([sp, ʃp, zb, ʋr, ʍs, . . .]), clusters with equal sonority (sonority plateaus: [pt, mn, tk, . . .]), and rising-sonority clusters with smaller sonority differences ([mr, ml, pʃ, kʃ, . . .]), rising-sonority clusters with large differences are predominant in the adult language (Unuk, 2003; and below), and Slovenian children typically show the same pattern of reduction of clusters such as /pl/ to C1 and /ʃk/ to C2 (Kogovšek et al., 2011).

Valley Zapotec is typologically quite different (Munro & Lopez, 1999; and references below). Native tautomorphemic onset clusters (i.e. where both consonants are in the same morpheme) fall into the following groups: (1) clusters ending in the glides /w, j/, which obey the SSP; (2) the stop-liquid clusters /bl/ and /bɾ/; (3) rising-sonority clusters with smaller differences (/bz, ʃn, . . ./); (4) sonority plateaus (/bd, mn, . . ./); and (5) sonority reversals[1] (/nd, st, wɾ, . . ./). Additional C-liquid clusters have been borrowed within Spanish words (/fɾ, pl, . . ./), but they remain low in type frequency after 400 years of language contact (as is often the case with borrowed phonological patterns). Zapotec clusters that do not contain a C2 glide typically violate the SSP. Table 3.1 presents information about word-initial clusters where C2 is [+consonantal]

Table 3.1 Differences in the statistics of three languages, focusing on clusters where C2 is [+consonantal]: the proportion of different clusters of each type and the proportion of word types for each type of cluster

	Cluster types			Word types		
	English	Slovene	Zapotec	English	Slovene	Zapotec
n	25	101	53	968	2755	190
C-liquid large rise	0.64	0.25	0.21	0.73	0.58	0.30
Small rise	0.16	0.33	0.11	0.06	0.16	0.12
Plateau	0.00	0.13	0.13	0.00	0.06	0.19
Reversal	0.20	0.30	0.54	0.20	0.20	0.38

and highlights the statistical differences between Valley Zapotec, English, and Slovenian. These are counts of tautomorphemic clusters found in word-initial position in monosyllables in Valley Zapotec (counted from Munro & Lopez, 1999) and English (from a private list of all monosyllables in English, excluding proper names); for Slovenian, using the *Slovar slovenskega knjižnega jezika* dictionary (Bajec, 1998), we have counted both monosyllables and disyllables where the rime of the second syllable contains only inflectional affixes (because excluding this group of disyllabic words would exclude almost all verbs and feminine and neuter nouns). The number of clusters of each type in the inventory gives a picture of the diversity of clusters in the language, and the number of words containing clusters of each type gives a picture of how commonly different types of clusters are used.

English is heavily weighted towards clusters where the C2 is /ɹ/ or /l/, with a modest proportion of clusters with sonority reversals; this is true for both cluster types and word types. Valley Zapotec, almost the inverse of English, has a larger number of cluster types, with a modest proportion of clusters where C2 is /ɾ/ or /l/ and a large proportion of clusters (for both cluster types and word types) with sonority plateaus and reversals. Slovenian is intermediate; it resembles Zapotec in terms of cluster types but resembles English in terms of word types. In English and Slovenian, C-liquid clusters are more strongly supported and more "basic", and children reduce these clusters to C1, while more commonly reducing other cluster types to C2. In Valley Zapotec, C-liquid clusters are less common and do not stand out as different.

Given the typologically unusual nature of complex onsets in Zapotec, it is an obvious place to look for language-specific developmental patterns. In this chapter, we make a preliminary exploration of the first-language acquisition of Zapotec onset clusters. Examples of words containing clusters of different types are provided in the appendix, along with one child pronunciation from our data.

Valley Zapotec adds an additional interesting characteristic in terms of clusters created by inflectional morphology. In most European languages, inflectional affixes are typically suffixes, and clusters that result from inflection are word-final or intervocalic. Studies of English report a tendency to resolve word-final clusters by omitting the suffix, so that e.g. the /ks/ in *rocks* is more likely to be reduced to [k] (homophonous to the singular *rock*) than to [s] (losing the /k/ of the base noun; Bernhardt & Stemberger, 1998; Song, Sundara, & Demuth, 2009). Valley Zapotec inflectional affixes are all prefixes, and every verb begins with an aspectual prefix in adult speech. Children generally use progressive forms at first: a syllabic prefix *ca-* which never creates consonant clusters. Perfective and irrealis forms eventually follow, involving single-consonant prefixes that often create word-initial consonant clusters. We investigate whether there is a tendency to omit the prefix in perfective and irrealis forms, or whether clusters tend to be reduced in the same way whether tautomorphemic (in the same morpheme) or heteromorphemic (in different morphemes). The development of consonant clusters derived through inflection may be affected by the development of inflectional morphology in addition to the development of clusters per se. This will be discussed below.

A BRIEF SKETCH OF VALLEY ZAPOTEC PHONOLOGY

The variant of Valley Zapotec spoken in San Lucas Quiaviní has a complex phonetic and phonological system (Munro & Lopez, 1999; Chávez-Peón, 2010; Munro, Lillehaugen, & Lopez, 2008; Lillehaugen, 2003, 2004, 2006; Lillehaugen et al., 2013). Like other Zapotec languages (e.g. Arellanes, 2009), Quiaviní Zapotec has a fortis-lenis contrast in its consonant inventory, rather than a strict voiced-voiceless opposition. Fortis obstruents /p t k ts tʃ s ʃ ʂ f x/ are always voiceless and relatively long, and stops are never fricated. Lenis obstruents /b d g z ʒ ʐ/ are variably voiced and relatively short. Lenis "stops" are variably fricated: /b/ [b b̥ β β̥ ɸ], /d/ [d d̥ ð ð̥ θ], /g/ [g g̥ ɣ ɣ̊ x̌]. For sonorants, the main difference between fortis and lenis consonants is duration, with fortis (/m: n: ŋ: l:/) being longer than lenis (/m n ŋ l w j/); Munro and Lopez (1999) are uncertain about the fortis/lenis status of /r ɾ/.

Valley Zapotec has six monophthongal vowels: /i ɨ u e o a/, which may bear tone and non-modal phonation. There are two level tones (high and low) and two contour tones (rising and falling). Distinctive non-modal voice includes breathy, laryngealized, and glottalized vowels. There are many diphthongs, in which the order of the subparts is contrastive: e.g. [au] vs. [ua]. There is a contrast between complexity in the onset with a glide (*zhye'et* /ʒjet/ 'cat') vs. complexity in the nucleus with a diphthong (*zhi'eb* /ʒieb/ 'goat').[2] Complexity within the vowel leads to transcriptions that may mislead readers into thinking that there are more syllables than there actually are; the diminutive for 'cat', /'ʒjetę'ę/, has only two syllables, where the second vowel /e/ is laryngeally very complex.

As for prominence, there is one stressed syllable for most words, which is the final syllable of the word, with two exceptions: (1) subject pronominal clitics have no stress and are part of the phonological word of the verb, creating Sw feet; and (2) nouns may end in an unstressed diminutive suffix (creating Sw feet). Most nouns and adjectives are (stressed) monosyllables, with an onset consisting of a single consonant, (less commonly) a two-consonant cluster, or (rarely) a three-consonant cluster; very few nouns or adjectives begin with a vowel. A glottal stop never appears at the beginning of a syllable, except in the marginal word-form *àà'* [ʔąʔ] 'yes'. Some nouns begin with an initial unstressed syllable, and relatively few of these start with a consonant cluster. Verb roots can begin with one or two consonants, and vowel-initial verb roots are also common; but verbs must begin with an aspectual prefix, which adds an onset or an initial unstressed syllable to vowel-initial roots, so no inflected verb forms begin with a vowel.

The exact make-up of clusters containing lenis "stops", relative to sonority, is variable, because /b d g/ can be realized variably as [b d g] or [β ð ɣ] in almost all environments (with a statistical skewing towards stops after pauses and [−continuant] phones and towards fricatives after [+continuant] phones; Stemberger & Chávez-Peón, in preparation). (Only in the nasal-stop clusters /nd/ and /ŋg/ are the lenis consonants nonvariably stops.) This variability only subtly affects the sonority relations in rising-sonority clusters before glides or liquids (e.g. /gj, bɾ/), in that the degree of difference in sonority varies. Other clusters, however, may vary between small-difference rising-sonority clusters, sonority plateaus, and sonority reversals. The cluster /bz/ can be stop-fricative [bz] (small-difference rising-sonority) or fricative-fricative [βz] (a sonority plateau). The cluster /bd/ can be stop-stop [bd] (a sonority plateau) or fricative-stop [βd] (a sonority reversal); we are unsure whether this cluster can be stop-fricative [bð] (small-difference rising-sonority) or fricative-fricative [βð] (a sonority plateau) but, if so, only infrequently. It is often not possible to know whether the child "intended" a stop or fricative variant, especially when the cluster is sim-plified via the deletion of the initial lenis stop (e.g. /bz/ [z]). We address below whether the similar behavior of small-difference rising-sonority, sonority-plateau, and sonority-reversal clusters could be related to this variability.

Methods

Subjects

We present results from six monolingual Valley Zapotec-learning chil-dren under the age of 3;0: Carlos-2 (1;8), Carlos-1 (1;11), Eleuterio (2;2), Vivian (2;8), Guadalupe (2;10), and Floriselda (2;11), from the town of San Lucas Quiaviní. All children in this community have some exposure to Spanish and a few to English, but they are functionally monolingual in Valley Zapotec until at least 4;0 (when some children begin bilingual preschool) and most often until 6;0 (when all children begin Spanish-only primary school). (The project as a whole involves 51 different children aged 1;3–6;0, with a few sessions with older chil-dren; partly cross-sectional, partly coarse-grained longitudinal, with ca. 130 hours of high-quality audio-video recordings).

Materials and Procedures

Recording sessions took place in the child's home and lasted up to 50 minutes. Background noise was generally low; the recordings are excellent for transcription and acoustic analysis. All sessions were videotaped using a Panasonic DVC30 mini-DV digital video camera, giving high-quality video with balanced stereo audio recording. Video provided contextual information (including pointing and eye gaze) to help identify the child's intended words, and facial information to aug-ment phonetic transcription. We used two Countryman wireless micro-phones on vests worn by the child and the interacting adult (making them relatively unobtrusive, so that the child did not play with them). Receivers were mounted on the camera, where the recording volume was continuously monitored. Stereo recording allows us to capture both the child and adult utterances at appropriate volume and leads to more accurate phonetic transcription.

We employed an assistant who is fluent in both English and this vari-ant of Valley Zapotec (and Spanish). We communicated with the assis-tant in English, who translated between us and the mothers (few of whom know English) and interacted with the child.

For the most part, data were collected in structured tasks designed to sample a wide variety of words with specific phonological charac-teristics. Nouns and adjectives were elicited with toys and pictures. In some instances where the child did not answer, an adult would prompt further or model the correct answer. In some instances, the child would spontaneously use the word without being asked or would use the word again in free speech. Verbs were elicited using video clips, with questions manipulating verbal aspect in the child's responses: progressive aspect (often corresponding to present time), perfective aspect (often corresponding to past time), and irrealis aspect (often corresponding to future time). Perfective and irrealis forms often begin with heteromorphemic consonant clusters, but young children often produce progressive aspect in situations where adults would use perfective or irrealis aspect, so heteromorphemic clusters cannot be reliably elicited in the age range examined in this chapter. More extended narratives (telling a story from wordless picture books) were collected but are not included in this chapter. There were occasional periods where the adult and child interacted in a natural fashion, but it is difficult to elicit such activity reliably with all children, especially for children less comfortable with the situation. All tasks involved production of real words.

Sessions were transcribed in Phon (Rose & MacWhinney, 2014) by research assistants, and then by the first author. Records containing target words with onset clusters in adult speech were exported to Praat (Boersma & Weenink, 2011), where transcriptions were compared to the acoustics. Differences between the transcribers were settled via acoustic analysis, and some transcriptions were altered on the basis of acoustic analysis.

The focus of this analysis is whether the child produced a cluster or reduced the cluster to C1, C2, or neither, and not on the accuracy of feature realization. For example, if a child produces /gj/ as [ðj] (fronting of velar [ɣ]) or /bɾ/ as [bj] (gliding of the liquid), and shows similar substitutions for singleton /g/ and /ɾ/, this is counted as producing the cluster. Similarly, given similar substitutions for singletons, /gj/ as [ð] would be counted as reduction to C1 (with fronting), and /bɾ/ as [j] would be counted as reduction to C2 (with gliding). In some instances, output that could be analyzed as coalescence (e.g. /bz/ as [d], with the manner of articulation of /b/ and the place of articulation of /z/) is counted as reduction to C2 (in this instance), if the child also produced singleton /z/ as [d] (stopping). Harmony with consonants later in the word was viewed as independent and did not affect analysis as e.g. reduction to C1.

We did not independently analyze whether the child had mastered both consonants in the cluster (when they appeared as singletons). In most instances of reduction, the child had independent mastery of both consonants. Where mastery of one of the consonants was an issue, a liquid or fricative was usually involved. It is unlikely that mastery of the constituent segments influences which consonant is deleted. For example, one child produced two tokens of *bra'u* 'lizard' as [jau], reducing the cluster to /ɾ/ (with gliding), despite the fact that the child had mastered both the stop and fricative variants of lenis /b/. This factor does not underlie the main effects reported below.

The number of different words and tokens of each word varied greatly from child to child. Pictures and toys are never fully successful in eliciting a unique target word (in any language), and some children produce more tokens of words than others. Verbal aspects other than progressive (/ka-/) are not consistently elicitable from children at this age, and so we have relatively few tokens of morphologically complex clusters in this chapter.

We analyze the results statistically using Fisher's exact test (for 2x2 contingency tables), contrasting e.g. the proportion of C-glide clusters vs. sonority-reversed clusters that are produced as clusters. Results are reported as significant ($p < .05$), marginally significant ($.05 < p < .12$), or nonsignificant ($p > .12$).

Results

Tautomorphemic Two-Consonant Clusters

Analysis of results as a group is shown for tautomorphemic two-consonant clusters in Table 3.2, with more detail for cluster types (Tables 3.3–3.5) or output type (Tables 3.6–3.7).

Table 3.2 Tautomorphemic CC-clusters in initial stressed syllables, by sonority type (summed across children)

Type	Realization								
	CC	C1	C2	C-coalescence	Ø	?	Vocalization/ V-coalescence	Epenthesis	Other
C-glide n = 189	54	71	17	0	7	8	5	27	0
Other rising n = 34	7	7	14	1	5	0	0	0	0
Plateau n = 69	5	9	51	2	0	1	0	0	1
Reversal n = 108	4	3	93	0	1	6	0	0	1
TOTAL = 400	70	90	175	3	13	15	5	27	2

Table 3.3 Break-down for other rising-sonority clusters in initial stressed syllables

Type	Realization						
	CC	**C1**	**C2**	**C-coalescence**	**Ø**	**?**	**Other**
C-liquid $n = 9$	0	3	4	0	2	0	0
Stop-fricative $n = 22$	6	4	9	0	3	0	0
Fricative-nasal $n = 3$	1	0	1	1	0	0	0
TOTAL = 34	7	7	14	1	5	0	0

Table 3.4 Break-down for sonority plateaus in initial stressed syllables

Type	Realization						
	CC	**C1**	**C2**	**C-coalescence**	**Ø**	**?**	**Other**
Stop-Stop $n = 14$	0	2	10	2	0	0	0
Stop-affricate $n = 1$	0	0	0	0	0	0	1
Nasal-nasal $n = 54$	5	7	41	0	0	1	0
TOTAL = 69	5	9	51	2	0	1	1

Table 3.5 Break-down for sonority reversals in initial stressed syllables

Type	Realization						
	CC	**C1**	**C2**	**C-coalescence**	**Ø**	**?**	**Other**
Fricative-stop $n = 8$	0	0	7	0	0	0	1
Nasal-obstruent $n = 94$	4	1	85	0	1	3	0
Glide-C $n = 6$	0	2	1	0	0	3	0
TOTAL = 108	4	3	93	0	1	6	1

As can be seen from Table 3.2, we have more tokens of target clusters ending in a glide ($n = 189$), followed by sonority-reversed clusters ($n = 108$), sonority plateaus ($n = 69$), and rising-sonority clusters ending in segments other than glides ($n = 34$). We have only nine tokens of target rising-sonority clusters ending in liquids.

Table 3.6 Proportion of tokens in initial stressed syllables where two consonants are realized as two separate segments or less

Type	Number		
	2	**1**	**Ø**
C-glide	0.475	0.446	0.079
Other rising	0.206	0.647	0.147
Plateau	0.085	0.901	0.014
Reversal	0.046	0.889	0.065
TOTAL = 397	0.262	0.668	0.071

Table 3.7 Distribution of tokens in initial stressed syllables where only one consonant is produced

Type	Which C		
	C1	**C2**	**C-coalescence**
C-glide	0.807	0.193	0.000
Other rising	0.318	0.636	0.045
Plateau	0.143	0.825	0.032
Reversal	0.031	0.969	0.000
TOTAL = 265	0.328	0.660	0.011

Sonority has a big impact on whether a cluster is actually produced (Table 3.2). The difference between the two rising-sonority groups is not significant (C-glide 54/189 vs. other rising 7/34), nor between the two unusual-sonority groups (plateaus 5/69 vs. reversals 4/108), but all other differences are significant or marginally significant (C-glide vs. plateaus, $p < .001$; C-glide vs. reversals, $p < .001$; other-rising vs. plateaus, $p = .058$; other rising vs. reversals, $p < .005$). C-glide clusters are different from all other clusters in having additional resolutions that realize both consonants without maintaining a cluster: vowel epenthesis (all involving the epenthetic vowel [i] between the C and a /j/) and shifting the glide into the following vowel nucleus (either creating legal diphthongs such as /ju/ [iu] or coalescing into a vowel with features of the glide and the target monophthong, e.g. /wa/ as [ʊ]). If these alternative ways of realizing both cluster consonants in separate segments are included with actual clusters (Table 3.6), C-glide is significantly different from other rising-sonority clusters ($p < .01$).

Both members of the cluster were deleted in 7.1% of tokens (with a 50–50 split between true vowel-initial syllables vs. beginning with a glottal stop).[3] Both realizations are interesting, because one (no onset) is of very low frequency in adult Valley Zapotec, and the other (glottal stop) occurs in word-initial position only in marginal words such as *àà̩a'* [ʔa̩ʔ] 'yes'. Realizations with a glottal stop mostly involve words in which the vowel targets contain a glottal stop ("checked" vowels), while onsetless realizations appear elsewhere. There is a nonsignificant tendency for more deletion of both consonants in rising-sonority clusters (20/223) than in plateaus and reversals (8/177).

When one consonant is produced, there are three possible outputs: the first consonant (C1), the second consonant (C2), or coalescence into a consonant that combines features from both target consonants. Different types of clusters reduce in different ways (Table 3.7). C-coalescence is too uncommon to evaluate interaction with cluster type. C-glide clusters reduce primarily to C1; reduction to the glide involved /gj/ in every token except one (which involved /nj/). All other cluster types reduce primarily to C2. The degree of reduction to C2 increases from C-glide to other rising ($p < .001$) and from other rising to plateaus[4] ($p < .05$), but there is no significant difference between plateaus and reversals. Tables 3.3–3.5 reveal no obvious difference in different cluster types within each sonority level. Even C-liquid clusters are not biased towards C1, though the small number of tokens does not allow us to demonstrate that statistically.

The minority instances of reduction to C1 appear to reflect a feature preference: reduction to a labial rather than to an anterior coronal. For non-glide rising-sonority clusters, plateaus, and reversals, only a third of tokens (.339) involved a target sequence of a labial followed by a coronal consonant (e.g. /bz/, /bd/, /mn/, /wɾ/), with most of the remaining clusters involving two consonants of the same place of articulation. Almost all reductions to C1 involved labial-coronal sequences (17/19); these reduce to C1 (17/60) significantly more often than non-labial sequences (2/117), $p < .001$. This was true even of C-liquid clusters, where two of the three reductions to C1 involved the labial-coronal cluster /pl/. More than just sonority is involved.

Effects of Stress: Initial Unstressed Syllables

There were only a few words with consonant clusters in an initial unstressed syllable, all with the stop-glide cluster /gj/ (e.g. *gyizhi'iilly* /ɡji'ʒiːlːj/ 'chair'). Of the 17 tokens in which the unstressed vowel was produced (excluding all instances of weak syllable deletion), deletion of the entire cluster ($n = 6$) and a glottal stop ($n = 8$) were the dominant realizations, with reduction to C1 ($n = 2$) or to C2 ($n = 1$) being less common.[5] The numbers are too small to statistically contrast realization as CC vs. C1 vs. C2, but full deletion and glottal-stop productions are more common in the unstressed syllables (14/17 tokens) than in the stressed syllables (15/220 tokens), $p < .001$. Reduction is more extreme in unstressed than in stressed syllables.

Effects of Intervocalic Position (after Aspectual Prefixes)

There were a few tokens ($n = 11$) of root-initial stop-glide clusters which were intervocalic because of a prefix (e.g. *nigyehsih* /ni'gjẹsi/ 'he is sleeping'). The proportion of tokens with clusters (.272) was comparable to word-initial position. But when reduced to a single consonant, most tokens (7/8) contained the C2 /j/ (e.g. *nigyehsih* /ni'gjẹsi/ [tʌ'jɛs:i]), significantly more reduction to the glide than in initial stressed syllables ($p < .001$).

Heteromorphemic Two-Consonant Clusters

There were 37 tokens of two-consonant clusters in which the first consonant was an aspectual prefix and the second was part of the verb root; e.g. *btyée'pyih* /btjẹpji/ 'he whistled'.

A minority appeared with a cluster, and most of these were C-glide clusters, consistent with tautomorphemic clusters. A higher percentage of tokens for C-glide targets were realized as clusters for these inflected forms (.556) than for similar clusters in monomorphemic forms (.245), but the numbers are too small to evaluate statistically. A marginally significant higher percentage of tokens were realized with no onset or with a glottal stop for inflected forms (.162) than for monomorphemic

Table 3.8 Heteromorphemic CC-cluster realization in initial stressed syllables, by sonority type (summed across children)

Type	Realization								
	CC	C1	C2	C-coalescence	Ø	ʔ	Vocalization/ V-coalescence	Epenthesis	Other
C-glide $n=9$	5	1	0	0	1	2	0	0	0
Other rising $n=8$	1	0	7	0	0	0	0	0	0
Plateau $n=8$	1	1	6	0	0	0	0	0	0
Reversal $n=12$	0	2	7	0	3	0	0	0	0
TOTAL = 37	7	4	20	0	4	2	0	0	0

forms (.071), p = .057. To evaluate reduction to C1 vs. C2, we eliminated C-glide clusters, since they reduced to a single C in only one token. For the other three types of clusters, both heteromorphemic and tautomorphemic clusters tended to reduce to C2 and were not significantly different. Note that one sixth of all tokens in which the cluster reduced to a single C were reduced to C1, containing the consonant of the aspectual prefix and losing the first consonant of the base.

Three-Consonant Clusters

There were only two instances of tautomorphemic clusters with three consonants, both reduced to single consonants: /str/ [t] and /wbw/ [β]. The /wbw/ cluster shows reduction to the /b/ (fricative variant [β]); deletion of the second /w/ follows the dominant reduction pattern for C-glide clusters, and deletion of the first /w/ follows the dominant reduction pattern for reversed-sonority clusters. The /str/ cluster showed deletion of /s/ (the dominant reduction pattern for /st/ clusters) and of /ɾ/ (a minority pattern for C-liquid clusters).

There were seven tokens of CCC heteromorphemic clusters, all beginning with two true consonants and ending in a glide. The first consonant (the prefix) deleted in six tokens (.857), comparable to the .870 deletion rate of C1 in similar heteromorphemic CC clusters; the remaining token involved vocalization of an initial glide (/jkw/ as [ɛkw]), leading to a vowel-initial form. In three tokens, the C3 glide (in a C-glide cluster at the beginning of the verb root) deleted, so that the cluster was reduced to the non-glide consonant, with four tokens successfully involving a cluster; this is reminiscent of C-glide clusters in Table 3.1 (the appropriate comparison, since both consonants are within the same morpheme).

Individual Differences

Our data come from only six children, with some children (especially the youngest) attempting few words containing clusters, and with some clusters appearing in the speech of few children. It is thus difficult to be sure about individual differences. All children showed the patterns described above for C-glide clusters (though only two children ever used epenthesis). All children produced few clusters and showed a bias to reduce sonority plateaus and sonority reversals to C2. For rising-sonority clusters where the C2 was not a glide, there was possibly variability. Some children had more stop-fricative clusters than others or reduced more to C1 than to C2. One child reduced C-liquid clusters to C1, while three others reduced them more to C2. But the number of tokens is too small to really address between-child variability, and different children produced different target words (so we cannot rule out differences between lexical items); we must await the analysis of data from a larger number of children.

Discussion and Conclusion

The phonology of onset consonant clusters in Valley Zapotec is quite different typologically from the majority of languages, in that there are many clusters with sonority plateaus and sonority reversals, as well as rising-sonority clusters with smaller-than-usual sonority differences (such as stop-fricative clusters). More typical languages such as English predominantly have rising-sonority clusters with large differences, with the primary exception being clusters starting with coronal fricatives. Zapotec-learning children acquire clusters in a way that is different from children learning English and other European languages. As shown in Table 3.1, the cluster statistics of English and Slovenian are weighted towards C-liquid clusters, while Valley Zapotec is weighted towards sonority plateaus and reversals. In English and Slovenian, C-liquid clusters are more strongly supported and more "basic", and children reduce the clusters to C1, while more commonly reducing other cluster types to C2. In Valley Zapotec, C-liquid clusters are less common and do not stand out as different, and children tend to reduce them to C2, as they do with other cluster types where C2 is [+consonantal]. The details as to how these statistical differences lead to differences in the way that children learn and reduce clusters remain to be worked out.

Rising-sonority clusters that end in a glide (/j, w/) are common in Valley Zapotec. Acquisition resembles that of European languages in two ways. (1) When reduced to a single consonant, they are far more likely to be reduced to C1 (whether stops, fricatives, or nasals). (2) Along with other rising-sonority clusters, they are more likely to be produced as clusters than clusters with sonority plateaus or reversals. The cluster /gj/ was an exception, with a minority pattern involving reduction to C2 ([j]). Munro and Lopez (1999) remark that the stop is sometimes difficult to perceive in /gj/. Phonetic variation in adult /gj/ may be relevant. In addition to common realizations such as [gj, g̊j, ɣj, ɣ̊j, xj], there are adult tokens with place assimilation of /g/ to a true palatal ([ɟj, ɟ̊j]). Child reductions of /gj/ to [j] might reflect these assimilated clusters; since palatal stops and fricatives never occur outside of clusters in adult pronunciations, they are not independently learned by the child as a singleton-consonant onset, so perhaps the independently available [j] is output instead. It is interesting that /gj/ is also more likely to reduce to [j] between vowels; Bernhardt and Stemberger (2002) report a tendency for English-learning children to favor medial consonants that are sonorant continuants. Recent studies (e.g. Kogovšek et al., 2011) have reported greater reduction of consonant clusters in initial unstressed syllables; our data suggest that this is also true of Valley Zapotec.

Children are more likely to vocalize the glide in C-glide clusters than in European languages: (a) creating a diphthong (so that /ju/ is realized as [iu]); (b) coalescing it with the vowel (/wa/ as [ʊ]), which has also been observed with target diphthongs such as /au/ and /ua/; and (c) epenthesizing [i] between the C and the /j/, which can also be viewed phonologically as changing the timing of the /j/ to include an unstressed (low-amplitude) steady state before the glide articulation, with no insertion of non-target vowel features. We observed one token of the heteromorphemic cluster /jkw/ where the first glide vocalized to the unstressed vowel [ɛ]. Glides are acting more vowel-like than in English. There is a contrast in Zapotec between onset /j/ and nucleus /i/ in diphthongs, e.g. *zhye'et* /ʒjet/ 'cat' vs. *zhi'eb* /ʒieβ/ 'goat'. Perhaps having such a contrast facilitates cross-over from onsets to nuclei during phonological development.

Other rising-sonority clusters, including C-liquid clusters, differ from C-glide clusters. They are similar only in the rate of production as clusters (mostly contributed by stop-fricative clusters such as /bz/). Vocalization and epenthesis are not attested in our data. When reduced to a single consonant, they are more likely to be reduced to C2; almost all exceptions involve labial-coronal sequences being reduced to the labial C1. C-liquid clusters do not differ from stop-fricative clusters, though the numbers are too small for this to be a secure result. We suggest that the low type and token frequency of C-liquid clusters leads to them behaving more like stop-fricative clusters than like C-glide clusters, an interesting difference from their behavior in European languages.

Clusters with more unusual sonority (plateaus and reversals) show significantly lower rates of production as clusters than do rising-sonority clusters, and a significantly greater tendency to be reduced to C2. Again, almost all reduction to C1 involved labial-coronal sequences. This is reminiscent of the tendency for English /s/-stop clusters (and German /ʃ/-stop clusters and Slovenian /sC, zC, ʃC, ʒC/ clusters) to be reduced to C2. A common theoretical assumption is that there is a difference in syllable structure between rising-sonority and sonority-reversed clusters: in /pl/ both consonants are in the onset, while in /sp/ only the /p/ is in the onset and the /s/ is external to the syllable and attaches directly to the foot. Goad and Rose (2004) suggest that consonants that are external to the onset are more likely to be deleted, but when two consonants are in the onset, C1 is more likely to be retained. If we were to extend this explanation to our data, we could say that both consonants in C-glide clusters are in the onset (and C1 tends to be retained) but that C1 in all other cluster types (including C-liquid clusters such as /bɾ/) is not part of the onset and hence tends to delete. The novel conclusion here would be that clusters such as /br/ can be complex onsets in some languages but are treated like /sp/ clusters in other languages.

Not everyone assumes a difference in representation between clusters such as /pl/ and /sp/. Stemberger and Treiman (1986), examining speech errors involving clusters in a laboratory task and from natural speech, show that English-speaking adults process both types of clusters in a somewhat parallel fashion. The statistically predominant errors are similar for both types of clusters (/pl/ to /p/ more than to /l/, and /sp/ to /s/ more than to /p/; /p/ to /pl/ more than /l/ to /pl/, and /s/ to /sp/ more than /p/ to /sp/), though there was slightly more tendency for interactions between /p/ and /sp/ than between /l/ and /pl/. They conclude that syllable structure is parallel in the two types of clusters, with both consonants in the onset. Bernhardt and Stemberger (1998) point out that the difference between /pl/ and /sp/ in acquisition can be explained just as easily by assuming that there is a preference to reduce the cluster to the consonant lower in sonority, and also discuss the possibility that there could be preferences to reduce any cluster to C1 (preserving the consonant at the beginning of the word) or to C2 (preserving the contiguity between C2 and the vowel). For Zapotec, a tendency to preserve the consonant that is lower in sonority leads to a prediction that /gj/ will be reduced to [g] and /nd/ to [d], as observed. No prediction is made for sonority plateaus (since in /bd/ the consonants are equal in sonority), and the statistical reduction to C2 suggests an effect of contiguity (retention of the consonant that immediately precedes the vowel). Where both tendencies pull in the same direction (sonority reversals), the reduction to C2 is strongest. When they are pitted against each other (in C-glide clusters), it is the sonority constraint that predominates. When only contiguity is relevant (in sonority plateaus) or when sonority differences are smaller (as in stop-fricative and C-liquid clusters), contiguity is predominant, but preferences for labial consonants lead to C1 winning on occasion. It is not necessary to presuppose differences in syllable structure between the different sorts of clusters.

We concur with Yavaş (2013) that differences in reduction are not being driven by differences in syllable structure. The Zapotec data do not show reduction to [−continuant] as the main effect, as Yavaş suggested for other languages. Both fricative-stop and stop-fricative clusters tend to reduce to C2, reducing to a stop vs. a fricative respectively. Contiguity with the following vowel affects reduction. This is a minority option for children learning European languages (where rising-sonority clusters predominate in the adult languages) but the dominant pattern for children learning Valley Zapotec.

Zapotec-learning children also seem to reduce initial clusters to nothing or to a glottal stop more than children learning European languages. All six children had a number of tokens of this. No verbs or adjectives ever begin with a vowel in adult Zapotec, and only a few borrowed nouns (such as *uba* 'grape') are vowel-initial. Words in adult Zapotec do not begin with a glottal stop (other than the marginal word *ááa'* 'yes'); glottal stops appear only as part of checked and rearticulated vowels (e.g. Chávez-Peón, 2010: 216). Nonetheless, children reduce clusters (and some singleton-consonant onsets) to no consonant; the glottal-stop tokens primarily seem to be the shift of a glottal stop from internal to the vowel into onset position, in order to supply an onset, itself a rather interesting phenomenon that cannot be observed in languages without the complex voice quality distinctions of Zapotec. Why Zapotec children have a tendency to delete both members of onset clusters is unclear.

Studies of the production of clusters containing suffixes in English suggest a tendency to omit the suffix and produce the final consonant of the base (Bernhardt & Stemberger, 1998; Song et al., 2009). Our data show a similar tendency for the prefixal consonant to be omitted from onset clusters in Zapotec. However, there is a large minority of tokens in which it is the prefixal consonant that is retained; this possibly reflects the same minority tendency to output labial consonants that is evident in tautomorphemic clusters, showing the role of phonology in the acquisition of morphology. In addition, C-glide clusters are more often successfully produced as clusters when they are heteromorphemic, suggesting joint contribution of phonology and the need to mark verbal aspect. The strong bias to reduce all clusters except C-glide clusters to C2 (as also for tautomorphemic clusters), combined with the high rate of successful cluster production for C-glide clusters, prevents us from demonstrating that there is an extra tendency towards C2 by omitting prefixal consonants. There is a greater tendency to delete both members of the cluster in inflected forms than in monomorphemic forms, suggesting that inflection also comes with a cost that increases the likelihood of deviation from the adult target. Morphology in some ways enhances the ability to output clusters and in others makes it more difficult to output any consonant at all, an over-emphasis of both extremes.

Our results resemble those previously reported for European languages, showing shared (possibly universal) tendencies. But we also observe differences that result from absolute and statistical phonological differences, including the possibility that C-liquid clusters behave more like reversed-sonority clusters in Zapotec than they do in European languages. Further exploration of typically diverse languages is clearly of value.

ACKNOWLEDGMENTS

This research has been supported by grants from the Social Sciences and Humanities Research Council of Canada and from the University of British Columbia (Hampton), as well as a Doctoral Scholarship granted to the second author by CONACYT (Consejo Nacional de Ciencia y Tecnología). We would like to thank the families in San Lucas Quiaviní who have participated in this study, and our Zapotec assistants: Felipe Lopez, Francisco Lopez, Manuel Núñez, Brígida Núñez, and Misael Martínez. We would like to thank the additional researchers and research assistants who have been involved with this project: Felicia Lee, Diana Gibrael, John Lyon, Masaki Noguchi, Lauren Quinn, and Andrea Ordaz-Nemeth.

NOTES

1 Adult pronunciation allows an optional epenthetic vowel [a] before some clusters; no tokens of this appeared in the child data analyzed here.

2 For San Pablo Güiá Zapotec, Arellanes (2009: 309–314) considers both types of glides to be part of the nucleus, with two distinct types of diphthongs: asymmetric /je/ and symmetric /ie/. For this study, we treat C-glide sequences as complex onsets.

3 Deletion is also observed for target word-initial singleton consonants. We have yet to investigate what factors influence such deletion.

4 A caveat regarding the data on sonority plateaus: the nasal-nasal clusters mostly involved the word *mnìi'iny* 'child', which has a less-common adult pronunciation with only /n/. Child productions with [n] could be either reduction of /mn/ to C2 (parallel to /bd/) or the less-common adult variant pronunciation. A quarter of the child tokens (with [mn] or [m]) clearly involve target /mn/. If some portion of the realizations with [n] reflect an adult /n/ pronunciation, then the percentage of tokens with CC and C1 realizations is greater than reflected in these tables, but our main conclusions are unaffected.

5 The deletion of word-initial unstressed syllables also occurs when the syllable has a singleton-consonant onset. It is beyond the scope of this paper whether weak syllables that begin with clusters are more prone to deletion.

REFERENCES

Arellanes, F. (2009). *El sistema fonológico y las propiedades fonéticas del zapoteco de San Pablo Güilá. Descripción y análisis formal.* Ph.D. dissertation. El Colegio de México.

Bajec, A. (1998). *Slovar slovenskega knjižnega jezika* (Electronic edition). Ljubljana, Slovenia: SAZU.

Bernhardt, B. H., & Stemberger, J. P. (1998). *Handbook of phonological development: From the perspective of constraint-based nonlinear phonology.* San Diego, CA: Academic Press (now Bingley, UK: Emerald).

Bernhardt, B. M., & Stemberger, J. P. (2002). Intervocalic consonants in the speech of children with phonological disorders. *Clinical Linguistics & Phonetics, 16*, 199–214.

Boersma, P., & Weenink, D. (2011). *Praat: Doing phonetics by computer* [Computer program]. Version 5.2.16, retrieved 20 February 2011 from http://www.praat.org/.

Chávez-Peón, M. E. (2010). *The interaction of metrical structure, tone and phonation types in Quiaviní Zapotec.* Ph.D. dissertation. University of British Columbia.

Fikkert, P. (1994). *On the acquisition of prosodic structure.* The Hague, the Netherlands: Holland Academic Graphics.

Goad, H., & Rose, Y. (2004). Input elaboration, head faithfulness, and evidence for representation in the acquisition of leftedge clusters in West Germanic. In R. Kager, J. Pater, & W. Zonneveld (Eds.), *Constraints in phonological acquisition* (pp. 109–157). Cambridge, UK: Cambridge University Press.

Greenberg, J. H. (1965). Some generalizations concerning initial and final consonant sequences. *Linguistics, 18*, 5–34.

Kogovšek, D., Ozbič, M., Stemberger, J. P., Bernhardt, B. M., Košir, S., & Zimic, M. (2011). Crosslinguistic study of protracted phonological development: Preliminary Slovenian data. Paper presented at the International Child Phonology Conference, York, June 15–18, 2011.

Lee, F. (2006). *Remnant raising and VSO clausal architecture: A case study of San Lucas Quiavini Zapotec* (Vol. 66). Dordrecht, the Netherlands: Springer.

Lillehaugen, B. D. (2003). *The categorical status of body part prepositions in Valley Zapotec languages.* M.A. thesis. University of California, Los Angeles.

Lillehaugen, B. D. (2004). The syntactic and semantic development of body part prepositions in Valley Zapotec languages. In J. Castillo (Ed.), *Proceedings from the sixth Workshop on American Indigenous Languages,* Santa Barbara Papers in Linguistics 14: 69–92.

Lillehaugen, B. D. (2006). *Expressing location in Tlacolula Valley Zapotec.* Ph.D. dissertation. University of California, Los Angeles.

Lillehaugen, B. D., Munro, P., Lopez, F. H., Ruiz, R. A., & Ruiz, J. A., with C. Batten, H. Felker, A. Mannix, K. Donovan McCormick, & R. E. Weissler. (2013). *Tlacolula Valley Zapotec talking dictionary*, pilot version. Salem, OR: Living Tongues Institute for Endangered Languages. http://www.talkingdictionary.org/zapotec [August 2013].

Munro, P., Lillehaugen, B. D., & Lopez, F. H. (2008). *Cali Chiu? A course in Valley Zapotec.* Los Angeles: Department of Linguistics, University of California, Los Angeles.

Munro, P., & Lopez, F. H., with O. V. Méndez Martínez, R. García & M. R. Galant. (1999). *Di'csyonaary x:tèe'n dìi'zh sah Sann Lu'uc (San Lucas Quiaviní Zapotec dictionary/Diccionario Zapoteco de San Lucas Quiaviní).* Los Angeles, CA: UCLA Chicano Studies Research Center Publications.

Ohala, D. K. (1999). The influence of sonority on children's cluster reductions. *Journal of Communication Disorders, 32*, 397–422.

Phon. Version 1.6.1, retrieved from http://childes.psy.cmu.edu/phon/.

Rose, Y., & MacWhinney, B. (2014). The PhonBank project: Data and software-assisted methods for the study of phonology and phonological development. In J. Durand, U. Gut, & G. Kristoffersen (Eds.), *Handbook of corpus phonology* (pp. 380–401). Oxford, UK: Oxford University Press.

Sievers, E. (1881). *Grundzüge der Phonetik.* Leipzig, Germany: Breitkopf and Hartel.

Smit, A. B. (1993). Phonologic error distributions in the Iowa–Nebraska articulation norms project: Word-initial consonant clusters. *Journal of Speech, Language, and Hearing Research, 36*, 931–947.

Song, J. Y., Sundara, M., & Demuth, K. (2009). Phonological constraints on children's production of English third person singular –s. *Journal of Speech, Language, and Hearing Research, 52*, 623–642.

Stemberger, J. P., & Treiman, R. (1986). The internal structure of word-initial consonant clusters. *Journal of Memory and Language, 25*, 163–180.

Stemberger, J. P., & Chávez-Peón, M. E. (in preparation). Development of variability of lenis stops in Valley Zapotec. Unpublished manuscript, University of British Columbia and Centro de Investigaciones y Estudios Superiores en Antropología Social.

Unuk, D. (2003). *Zlog v slovenskem jeziku.* Ljubljana, Slovenia: Rokus.

Yavaş, M. (2013). What explains the reductions in /s/-clusters: Sonority or [continuant]? *Clinical Linguistics & Phonetics, 27*:6, 394–403.

Zec, D. (2007). The syllable. In P. de Lacy (Ed.), *The Cambridge handbook of phonology* (pp. 161–194). Cambridge, UK: Cambridge University Press.

APPENDIX

Examples of Valley Zapotec onset clusters

Cluster type	Adult	Gloss	Child example
(1) C-glide			
stop + glide	/giax/	'tree'	[ja:x]
fricative + glide	/ˈʒjetȩʔȩ/	'cat (diminutive)'	[ˈdʒɛte]
nasal + glide	/njis/	'water'	[njɛs:]
(2) Other rising sonority			
stop + liquid	/ˈpladȩʔȩ/	'plate (diminutive)'	[ˈba̧:bɛʔ]
fricative + liquid	/fɾes/	'strawberry'	[ɛɕ]
nasal + liquid	/nɾaʒ/	'orange'	[ɹa:ɕ]
stop + fricative	/bzinj/	'mouse'	[ʒ̧ɪn]
fricative + nasal	/ ʃnia/	'red'	[na]
(3) Sonority + plateaus			
stop + stop	/bdi̧/	'ant'	[ḑi̧]
nasal + nasal	/ˈmninji̧ʔi̧/	'child (diminutive)'	[ˈminjʔi̧]
(4) Reversed sonority			
fricative + stop	/stebj/	'again'	[ˈtibi]
nasal + stop	/ŋga̧ʔa̧/	'green'	[ga̧ʔa̧]
nasal + fricative	/nsual/	'blue'	[suʌl]
glide + liquid	/wɾilj/	'yard'	[ˈβa:ḑla]
glide + stop + glide	/wbwiʒ/	'sun'	[βiɕ]
fricative + stop + liquid	/ˈstreli̧ˈi̧/	'star (diminutive)'	[ˈdeiʔɹ̧]

The table below summarizes the possible onset consonant sequences in Quiaviní Valley Zapotec. The only sequences not attested in adult speech are stop + nasal and glide + glide, but others were absent from our child data.

C1	C2				
	Stop	Fricative	Nasal	Liquid	Glide
Stop	√	√	*	√	√
Fricative	√	√	√	√	√
Nasal	√	√	√	√	√
Liquid	√	√	√	√	√
Glide	√	√	√	√	*

4

MARKEDNESS IN FIRST LANGUAGE ACQUISITION

Paula M. Reimers

MARKEDNESS

In first language acquisition cross-linguistic studies show remarkable similarities between the patterns produced by young children, although the phonologies of their target languages can vary greatly. Earliest word forms are more or less similar across languages, but they differ in ways which are often regarded as systematic and predictable. Reduplication is one such example, as can be seen in Table 4.1, and occurs most frequently during the earliest stage and coincides with the transition from babbling to first words.

Reduplication is not restricted to child language and occurs frequently in adult languages around the world. There is a fundamental difference, however, between reduplication in adults and children: While it has a clear grammatical function in adult languages, infants do not reduplicate to change the meaning of a word. The fact that all phonological processes observed in first language acquisition are strategies that are also found in adult languages (Johnson & Reimers, 2010, pp. 1–19) has led linguists to assume that child phonology is no different from any adult phonology. Furthermore, universally observed patterns in first language acquisition where any normally developing child is capable of mastering any language equally well, within a relatively short period of time, without explicit instruction, have prompted the view that simplification strategies are governed by general principles provided by Universal Grammar (UG) where markedness plays a crucial role.

Since the term *markedness* was first introduced formally by Trubetzkoy in 1939 in the study of adult language typology, it has been

Table 4.1 Reduplication in Child Languages

Language	Child Form	Target Form		Source
ENGLISH	[dada]	[dædɪ]	'daddy'	Ingram, 1974
	[baba]	[blænkət]	'blanket'	
FRENCH	[pɔpɔ]	[po]	'pot'	Ingram, 1974
	[nene]	[ne]	'nose'	
GERMAN	[nana]	[naːze]	'nose'	Dressler et al., 2005
	[bebe]	[bɛr]	'bear'	
Jordanian	[bobo]	[boːt]	'shoes'	Daana, 2009
ARABIC	[baba]	[baab]	'door'	
Mandarin	[tʰaŋ tʰaŋ]	[tʰaŋ kʷoʊ]	'sweet/candy'	S. Chen, personal
CHINESE	[maʊ maʊ]	[maʊ tsɪ]	'hat'	communication, 2008
JAPANESE	[dʒudʒu]	[dʒuːsu]	'juice'	Reimers (unpublished data)
	[meːmeː]	[osembeː]	'rice cracker'	Ota, 2001
MALTESE	[baba], [nana]	[banana]	'banana'	H. Grech, personal
	[gaga]	[gazaza]	'dummy/ pacifier'	communication, 2004
RUSSIAN	[gɔm-gɔm]	[bʲiˈgɔm]	'running'	Dressler et al., 2005
	[kap-kap]	[ˈkapətʲ]	'to drip'	
SWEDISH	[gaːgaː], [dada]	[tak]	'thank you'	Vihman, 1996
	[dædːæ]	[tɪtʊt]	'peek-a-boo'	
ZUNI	[titi]	[ʃiwe]	'meat'	Kroeber, 1916
	[wewe]	[watʃita]	'dog'	

extended to other fields and areas. It is generally used in explanations of universals and naturalness and appears in numerous domains but mainly in phonetics, descriptions of specific languages, typological studies, first language acquisition, and language change, where the term *unmarkedness* is commonly used to indicate simplicity or commonness as opposed to complexity or rarity (see Reimers, 2006, for detailed discussion of markedness criteria). In view of the fact that markedness continues to occupy a substantial position in phonological theory (e.g. Rice, 2007) and is heavily relied upon in child phonology models based on UG, one way to validate the claim that humans are biologically programmed to acquire language would be through an identification of UG markedness and its manifestation. However, there are difficulties in linguistically based markedness accounts in coming to terms with observations from acquisition.

While the Jakobsonean markedness theory (Jakobson, 1941/1968) has difficulties with variability in child language (any evidence for UG should be found as uniformity across children) and the Stampean markedness theory (Stampe, 1972/1979) faces problems in accounting for child language phenomena which have no phonetic basis, optimality theory (Prince & Smolensky, 2004) appears to offer more than just a remedy to the difficulties that the previous theories faced through the flexibility provided by its architecture: Since evaluation of the structure (markedness) is separated from repair (constraint ranking), which varies according to the child, variability in child language is explained as markedness constraints being satisfied in different ways across children (and languages) at different stages of development. However, the assumption of the initial state ranking, in which markedness constraints disfavouring complex structures (e.g. prompting 'cat' to surface as [ta]) are ranked above faithfulness constraints favouring the surface or output form to be the same as the input (e.g. 'cat' surfacing as [kæt]), cannot be valid for the stage in which first words appear in children, since perception precedes production and phonology has already taken a turn towards language specificity at the onset of production.

There is adequate empirical evidence in both perceptual and production studies that the onset of speech, which occurs during the second year of life, cannot be equated with the initial state of the grammar: The perception of 9-month-old infants seems to prefer the more common sound patterns of their native language (Jusczyk, Luce, & Charles-Luce, 1994); the capacity to perceive a rich set of phonetic contrasts becomes restricted to those that are phonemic in the ambient language at 10 months (Werker & Tees, 1984); certain marked segments of high frequency in a language appear earlier in children acquiring that language (e.g. the palato-alveolar affricate is acquired earlier by Spanish-acquiring children than English-acquiring children), and certain low frequency segments can appear later in children in spite of them being unmarked (e.g. Finnish children acquire /d/ later than children acquiring other languages due to its low frequency) (Macken, 1995); the different occurrence frequencies of initial consonants in Quiché versus English are reflected in the child productions of these languages (Pye, Ingram, & List, 1987); while English-acquiring children tend to depalatalise [ʃ, ʧ, ʤ] to surface as [s, ʦ, ʣ] (e.g. Stampe, 1972/1979), Japanese-acquiring children (e.g. Kobayashi, 1981) tend to do the opposite; while the first onset consonant cluster to be acquired in most Dutch children is an obstruent-sonorant cluster and an /s/-obstruent cluster for some, most Portuguese children seem to start with /s/-obstruent clusters (Fikkert & Freitas, 1997); codas appear earlier in children acquiring English than in children acquiring Spanish, which has fewer coda occurrences than English (e.g. Roark & Demuth, 2000); the early production of coda consonants by English-acquiring children shows their sensitivity to input frequency over the markedness properties of the coda (Zamuner, 2003); Dutch children first acquire the most frequent syllable structure in Dutch (Levelt & van de Vijver, 2004). Consequently, it is now widely acknowledged that linguistic input plays an important role in phonological acquisition. Furthermore, when the influence of the ambient language is taken into account and the initial state of the grammar is modified to an earlier stage than the onset of production, another problem crops up: The child's earliest underlying representations may not contain the full set of phonological features to which markedness refers.

The difficulties of UG markedness not being able to provide an adequate explanation for child language could be due to at least two possibilities. One possibility is to suppose that recurrent properties of adult and child languages are not the result of a cognitive concept of markedness embodied in UG. However, while cross-linguistic similarities in the early stages of acquisition predicted by non-UG-based accounts are limited to explanations of statistical learning (ambient language influence) and immaturity that lie outside phonology, children do exhibit patterns which cannot be attributed to the effect of the linguistic input or articulatory immaturity. For example, not all of the most frequent phonemes in a language appear in the child's phonemic inventory (e.g. Moskowitz, 1970; Pye et al., 1987), which does not always develop according to the degree of articulatory difficulty (e.g. Menn, 1976).

The other possibility is to circumvent the rejection of UG and consider whether the existence of counter-examples to the predictions made by a markedness theory is due to child data containing other factors interfering with such predictions. With abundant perception and production studies showing how infants are sensitive to what goes on in their linguistic environment, it is reasonable to consider that production data are contaminated primarily by the influence of the ambient language, which increases with the amount of exposure. Thus, if we are to investigate markedness in terms of what the child brings to the task of language learning, ideally we should be looking at a stage where there is no ambient language influence at all. However, since such a stage could be before the development of the auditory capacity is complete in the foetus, making such a task infeasible, we can only take the initial state of the grammar as far back as possible. Hence, we now turn to perceptual studies where we might find some clues regarding the child's underlying representation and the role played by markedness in phonological acquisition.

THE INITIAL STATE

Compared to speech production, the study of infant speech perception is relatively new. Since the finding in 1971 by Eimas, Siqueland, Jusczyk, & Vigorito that 1- and 4-month-old American infants could discriminate the English voicing contrast between [ba] and [pa], the amount of research undertaken on the infant perceptual capacity is now vast. Subsequent research showed that infants, ranging from newborn to six months, are also capable of perceiving phonetic contrasts other than voicing, including those not found in their native language (e.g. Streeter, 1976), differences in place of articulation (Eimas, 1974), [r]-[l] distinction (Eimas, 1975), speech versus non-speech distinction (Morse, 1972), and speaker differences (e.g. Kuhl, 1979), which all seemed to corroborate the innate ability of infants to discriminate contrasts in any potential human language.

However, since Werker and Tees (1984) reported that the remarkable ability of the "universal" learner in perception undergoes a gradual decline with increased exposure to the native language, other studies followed substantiating this development of infants tuning in to their target language before the appearance of first words and confirming that they have surpassed the initial state by this time. Consequently, the position of UG-based acquisition models equating the onset of speech with the initial state of the grammar was weakened and led to questioning of the innateness of the universal learner. Nevertheless, considering one of the postulations of the innateness hypothesis that language is unique to humans, if it is the case that UG is behind the universal speech perception ability exhibited by the youngest infants, we should expect it to be specific to humans.

After Kuhl and Miller (1975) observed that chinchillas, like human infants, are capable of discriminating "phonemes", subsequent studies of human speech processing in animals found that several other kinds of non-human species are just as capable as human infants in the categorical processing of human speech. Moreover, a study of the perceptual and neurobiological mechanisms of human newborns and cotton-top tamarin monkeys by Ramus, Hauser, Miller, Morris, and Mehler (2000) found that sound boundaries perceived by monkeys occur in the same place as in humans. With perceptual studies showing similarity between humans and non-humans in segmental perception, if we are to maintain the position that only the human infant is pre-programmed to acquire language, their performances must be interpreted as *the ability to perceive phonetic differences*.

Defining phonetics as the categorisation of raw acoustics, phonetics is not specific to humans and not part of UG. Thus, we have phonetics on one side and language-specific phonology on the other. When speech sounds reach the listener's ear, each sound is given a phonetic representation in the phonetic component, which is where animals "perceive" human speech, parrots "speak", and humans imitate speech sounds with no semantic content. For comprehension, the phonetic representation is then transformed into phonological representation, which is under the control of language-specific grammar that is linked with the semantic component. During the earliest stages of acquisition, the infant can only perceive phonetic representations without converting the phonetic values into phonemes. The role played by UG is then to provide the learner with a mechanism to internalise or phonologise the phonetic representations, which occurs at a later stage. Thus, our search for how markedness guides the infant in the pre-production stage must be steered away from segments. This is not refuting the innateness of universal phonological features but suggesting that there seems to be no evidence for segmental markedness in the initial state and that our search should be taken to the prosodic aspect of phonology.

A useful starting point is a study by Ramus et al. (2000) which investigated for the first time whether or not the mechanisms enabling the perception of prosody are unique to humans. Languages can be classified into three rhythm types (Ladefoged, 1975; Pike, 1945): *stress-timed* (e.g. English and most Germanic languages), *syllable-timed* (e.g. Turkish and most Romance languages), and *mora-timed* (e.g. Japanese). Studies have shown that newborns can discriminate languages with different rhythms, e.g. English versus Japanese, but not languages belonging to the same linguistic rhythm group, e.g. Spanish versus Italian (e.g. Nazzi, Bertoncini, & Mehler, 1998). Ramus et al. tested the ability to discriminate Dutch versus Japanese using the same habituation-dishabituation task for French newborn infants and tamarin monkeys. Similarities and differences between the monkey and the human auditory systems were studied through head-orientation responses to natural speech production by four speakers as well as synthesised (i.e. computerised) speech, played forward and backward, in which all speech cues other than rhythm were removed. The conclusion was that since both newborns and tamarins were able to discriminate Dutch and Japanese in forward natural and synthesised speech, but failed to do so in backward natural and synthesised speech, newborns and tamarins process speech in the same way.

However, there was a subtle difference in the result figures of forward speech responses between newborns and tamarins. Newborns responded better to synthesised speech and were confused by speaker variability in natural speech, while tamarins responded better to natural speech and hesitated more with synthesised speech. The assumption that the initial state does not contain any internalised or phonologised phonetic representations, but only internalised rhythm, provides an explanation for why only newborns, but not tamarin monkeys, could discriminate between Dutch and Japanese in synthesised speech samples containing only rhythm: Since the only aspect of speech that is internalised in newborns is rhythm, the discrimination task was made easier for newborns when other "noises", such as speaker variability and phonetics, were removed from the stimuli; also, since the discrimination in tamarins with no internalisation relies on the combination of cues from all aspects of acoustics, rhythm alone was not adequate to perform the task successfully. In addition to the fact that only humans can move their bodies to rhythm (Pinker & Jackendoff, 2005), further support for this assumption is found in the ability of people with hearing impairment to sing, dance, and use rhythm linguistically in the form of poetry.

Thus, without explicit evidence that the ability of infants to discriminate segmental contrasts is specific to humans, but with adequate evidence that rhythm is specific to humans, the only way to uncover markedness is by assuming that UG equips infants with an internalised rhythm.

THE INTERNALISED RHYTHM

Since infants can discriminate all three rhythm types (stress-timed, syllable-timed, and mora-timed) at birth and this three-way distinction is not possible without a certain amount of linguistic exposure if the internalised rhythm consisted of evenly distributed beats, it is reasonable to assume that UG provides a default setting, which could be either the trochaic or the iambic rhythm.

Let us first consider the possibility that the default setting is trochaic and refers to the Iambic/Trochaic Law in Hayes, 1995, which is a reformulation of the results of earlier perceptual studies on well-formed rhythmic structure. The Iambic/Trochaic Law, which is based on non-linguistic perceptual abilities, states that elements contrasting in intensity naturally form groupings with initial prominence and elements contrasting in duration naturally form groupings with final prominence (Hayes, 1995, p. 80). The Iambic/Trochaic Law does not claim any trochaic bias but only postulates a perceptual mechanism, which imposes a trochaic structure on the input when we hear alternating patterns of intensity and an iambic structure when we hear alternating patterns of duration. Since the durational cue in speech is perceivable only through the durational contrast between syllables or vowels, which is optimised at the average speaking rate (Nazzi et al., 1998), and speaker variability interferes with speech perception in newborns (Ramus et al., 2000), we could assume that durational contrast is irrelevant and that intensity, which does not require a comparison of the syllable-internal structure, is coupled with the internalised rhythm, taking the form of initial prominence, namely the trochaic rhythm.

In fact, the trochaic rhythm has been suggested as being the unmarked rhythm in acquisition studies. However, leaving aside the numerous production studies supporting the trochaic bias in "speaking children", since their linguistic exposure has probably exerted sufficient influence on the grammar to have changed the initial setting, perceptual studies do not provide adequate support for postulating the trochaic rhythm as the default as they tend to be in trochaic languages. Furthermore, while Jus-czyk, Cutler, and Redanz (1993) did not find English-acquiring infants to show a preference for the trochaic stress pattern until the second half of their first year, a study by Vihman (2002) investigating English-acquiring infants showed that there is no preference for trochaic over iambic disyllables at either 6, 9, or 12 months of age. Hence, it is difficult to assume a UG default rhythm.

A default rhythm requires the internalisation to have three levels: the rhythm-bearing unit, the grouping of these units into pairs, and the prominent member of the pair defining the trochaic or iambic default setting. When the default setting is taken out of the equation, we are left with pairs of rhythm-bearing units, which may seem unnecessary since there is no need to define the prominent beat. Nevertheless, there is ample evidence to suggest that the infant is equipped with something that resembles a foot structure without any further specification than binarity. In production, constructing disyllabic words by adding dummy syllables to the target monosyllabic words is not an uncommon phenomenon in children. Also, studies of prosodic development have claimed that children operate at the foot level when their output does not exceed the size of a foot (Demuth & Fee, 1995; Fikkert, 1994). Thus, the internalised rhythm in the initial state can be assumed to be:

(XX) (XX) (XX) . . .

However, the pairing of rhythm-bearing units is still inadequate to explain the ability of newborns to discriminate all three rhythms. Although the traditional classification into stress-, syllable-, and mora-timed languages is not problem-free due to the existence of a few languages which do not seem to belong to any of the classes (see Reimers, 2006, pp. 190–193, for details), what is apparent in the literature of typological studies is that the rhythm-bearing unit seems to play an extremely significant role. While the discussion of classification revolves around how the components which constitute rhythm are organised by each language, and there are no clear phonetic or acoustic correlates of intensity due to its manifestation in different forms, e.g. duration, stress, tone, pitch, etc., it is impossible to have rhythm without reference to a structural unit which bears it.

The question is then what constitutes the rhythm-bearing unit. Since morae are syllable weight units, which may or may not need to be distinguished by a language (CVC-syllables count as heavy in some languages and light in others), and there are no reports on whether newborn infants are sensitive to duration and quantity, it is difficult to assume the existence of the mora in the initial state of the grammar. Furthermore, it has been suggested that while adult Japanese phonology operates with the mora as the timing unit, Japanese-acquiring children, who have not yet been influenced by the mora-based orthography, seem to use a different timing unit before the mora develops in their phonology (Kubozono, 1993). Thus, it seems feasible to assume that the rhythm-bearing unit is the syllable and that the three rhythm classes can be categorised in terms of syllables: Stress-timed languages can be identified through the dominant CVC-syllables allowing complex onsets and codas, mora-timed languages as having almost only CV-syllables, and syllable-timed languages as being in between, with more CV-syllables and more restrictions on the onset and coda than stress-timed languages. Since distinguishing the three rhythmic types requires the infant to evaluate the proportion of CV- versus CVC-syllables, the only way to modify the internalised, unbiased, binary-footed rhythm in order to accommodate the innate ability of newborns to distinguish linguistic rhythm is by assuming that one of these two syllable shapes is given by UG as the default or basic syllable.

THE BASIC SYLLABLE

Whether it is in the form of a rule (e.g. the CV-rule in Ito, 1986), a template (e.g. the coda condition in Ito, 1986), a principle (e.g. the Minimal Onset Satisfaction Principle in Roca & Johnson, 1999), or optimality theory constraints (ONSET and NOCODA in Prince & Smolensky, 2004), the CV-syllable is enshrined as the basic syllable. However, it is logically not possible for the infant to distinguish all three linguistic rhythm classes from birth if CV were the basic unit in the initial prosodic hierarchy consisting of only syllables and unbounded feet. There would be two steps between the basic CV-syllable and distinguishing the three rhythm classes: The infant needs to acquire the distinction between the mora-timed and the stress-timed rhythms before the syllable-timed (or between the mora-timed and the syllable-timed before the stress-timed) rhythm can be discriminated, since the newborn equipped with the basic CV-syllable would easily distinguish the CV-dominant mora-timed rhythm, while the other two rhythms would be more difficult to distinguish. Thus, it is worth exploring the possibility that the basic syllable given by UG contains a coda constituent.

The unchallenged status of the basic CV-syllable is based purely on typological studies and transcriptions of infant productions. Jakobson's typological observation that there are no languages that disallow syllables with initial consonants or final vowels lies at the heart of the basic CV-syllable, favouring onsets and disfavouring codas. While the basic CV-syllable would predict more restrictions on the coda than the onset, no languages that disallow onsets or open syllables, and even the existence of languages that allow only CV-syllables, there is evidence against these: Some Australian languages seem to have more constraints on the onset than the coda (Blevins, 1995), and the set of possible coda consonants in Kashaya (formerly known as Southwestern Pomo), spoken in northern California, is larger than that of onset consonants (Blevins, 2006); Kunjen, another Australian language, disallows onsets (Blevins, 1995); the native vocabularies of Olgol and Oykangand, two different Australian language families, as well as several subgroups of Austro-Asiatic languages, disallow open syllables (Blevins, 2006); although Hua (Haiman, 1998) is often cited as a CV-only language, it is not a pure CV-language since vowel-only syllables are not exactly rare (Haiman, personal communication, 2004). Thus, syllable typology does not provide a robust base for the CV-syllable.

As for the applicability of child production as evidence for the basic CV-syllable, it is important to note how syllable tokens produced by infants are transcribed by adults. The major problem with transcription data is that they are products of indirect representation of the articulatory gestures. Since the acoustic signal contains complex cues from which the transcriber must extract articulatory information, it is difficult to tease apart phonological errors from phonetic distortions. Consequently, transcription data could contain phonological contrasts produced by the child but not perceived by the listener. In fact, since the idea that children's speech contains contrasts that are neutralised by the listeners' perceptual capacity was introduced by Macken and Barton (1980), instrumental analyses have revealed various cases of covert contrasts in the speech of children with both normative and disordered phonological development (e.g. Scobbie, Gibbon, Hardcastle, & Fletcher, 2000).

It is then conceivable, and perhaps inevitable, that the smallest tokens of any syllable-final consonant, e.g. a glide or a glottal stop, are likely to be lost in child data transcriptions due to their perceptual insalience. This is indeed witnessed by cases of disagreement between multiple transcribers regarding the presence of glottal segments in word margins (e.g. between four transcribers in Vihman, Macken, Miller, Simmons, & Miller, 1985, p. 401). An acoustic measurement of the infant output could be a solution to this predicament. However, since the syllable-final segment can be anything from a full consonant to an articulatory closure associated with a stop consonant that cannot manifest itself with any sonority values, it may not appear at all on such measurements. Thus, based on the difficulty in detecting syllable-final consonants in terms of perception and measurement, it is plausible to suppose that early child production may not be adequately dominated by CV-syllables so as to support the claims of universality for the CV-syllable.

The objective here is not to criticise the vast amount of cross-linguistic data, whose contribution to the research into child language is invaluable, but to provide arguments for the plausibility of assuming that the default syllable may not be CV. Thus, having stipulated the reasons for the existence of the basic syllable and why it is thought that the CV-sequence does not necessarily have to be the basic syllable, we now turn to the assumption that the syllable given by UG contains a coda constituent. Since the coda constituent of the basic syllable can be filled with anything that is less sonorous than a vowel, up to a full consonant, it would be most appropriate to label this basic syllable as CVX.

THE CVX-SYLLABLE

First, the assumption of the basic CVX-syllable finds support in infant perception. The fact that infants do not seem to be able to define syllable boundaries precisely in the very early stages (Jusczyk, 1997) suggests that syllable boundaries are perceptually fuzzy in infants. Since infants have been exposed to human speech sounds in the womb (mainly through the voice of their mothers) and they know that speech consists of falling sonority after each peak, which goes up again to the next peak, CVX as the basic syllable would provide a better continuum than CV by being closer to the sonority profile of running speech, as shown below.

```
      V           V           V           V
          X           X           X           X
  C           C           C           C
```

If it were the case that infants are equipped with CV as the basic syllable, then syllable boundaries should be clearly definable, since every vowel would mark the end of the syllable:

Thus, from the point of view of infants, who cannot define clear syllable boundaries but are capable of perceiving the sonority profile as a continuous flow, CVX seems to be the more plausible basic syllable.

In terms of learnability, the assumption that the child equipped with the basic CV-syllable must acquire the coda if the target language is a CVC language (e.g. English) may seem logically just as plausible as the assumption that the child equipped with the basic CVX-syllable must learn to delete the coda if the target language is a CV language (e.g. Japanese). However, the implications of these two assumptions are not the same. With CV as the basic syllable, the learner must acquire the coda constituent before s/he can perceive or produce codas. But since the coda constituent is already there with the basic CVX-syllable, "acquiring the coda" is reduced to learning the language-specific phonotactics, i.e. learning to have an empty coda or what is allowed in the coda. In these terms, the assumption of CVX as the basic syllable seems to possess a greater generality.

Although it has been argued that the grammar has surpassed the initial state by the time first words appear in children, earliest production data can still be thought to provide a window into UG since their deviation from their target forms is systematic. Therefore, it is not surprising to find uniformity in Vihman's (1992) cross-linguistic data of the first syllables in babbling. If children are governed by the basic CV-syllable, an obvious implication is that earliest utterances should be dominated by CV-syllables in all children. Subsequently, occurrences of earliest words containing VC, geminates, or, indeed, CVC, should be rare, especially if these are not found in the ambient language.

Already in 1966, Weir observed that Chinese infants tend to organise their early utterances into monosyllabic CVC shapes marked prosodically by tone. More recently, a cross-linguistic study by Vihman and Velleman (2000) of the development of geminates using acoustic analysis found that American, Finnish, and French infants were all producing geminates at the earliest stage. The development went in the direction of the medial consonants becoming shorter if the native language did not contain them (English and French) and the medial consonant becoming longer if there was gemination in the target language (Finnish). Moreover, in a study of the acquisition of geminate stops in Finnish, Japanese, and Welsh infants by Kunnari, Nakai, and Vihman (2001), the mean length of medial stops in infants acquiring Welsh, which has no geminates as opposed to Finnish and Japanese, was greater than that of the other infants at the onset of word production, including babbling. The basic CV-syllable, but not the basic CVX-syllable, cannot explain why the CVC-syllable should be preferred by Chinese infants or why geminates are produced by children whose target languages do not contain them.

The most crucial support, however, for the basic CVX-syllable comes from Vihman's unpublished data of Japanese children collected in 1987 in the Stanford Child Phonology Project.[1] If the basic syllable given by UG is CV and the target language consists largely of CV-syllables, we would expect the data of Japanese infants to contain only CVs. Some of the Japanese data from the Stanford Child Phonology Project, which can be found in the appendix of Vihman (1996), are reproduced in Table 4.2.

Table 4.2 Vihman's Japanese data (Stanford Child Phonology Project)

Emi (14 months)

atta/haitta	[(ha)ta]	'here it is!/put it in/on'
ba	[pa]	'peek-a-boo'
bu:	[bu::]	'vroom'
hai	[haʔ]	'here (yes)'
mama	[mam:a:]	'mama'
nenne	[nen:e]	'sleep'
wanwan	[wawa]	'doggie'

Haruo (15 months)

bubu	[bubu]	'car'
ija	[ɪjæʔ]	'no'
kore	[gɔɛ]	'this'
oiʃo	[(oɪ) ʃɔʔ]	'oof!'

Kazuko (14 months)

ba	[baʔ]	'peek-a-boo'
bubu	[βaʔpa]	'car'
dʒu:su	[ʒuʃu]	'juice'
jaru	[ja(ɣ)u]	'do it!'

Kenji (12 months)

dore	[dɔ:li]	'which(?)'
kore	[koje], [kole], [koɾe]	'this'
nainai	[nja:naja], [na(i)na(i)]	'no-no, all gone'
njannjan	[njəʔnjəʔ]	'kitty, meow'

Vihman's data above clearly show that there are CVC-syllables in the production of the Japanese infants. When the faithfulness to the adult form is considered and when such tokens are disregarded, CVC-syllables are minimal: There is only Emi's [haʔ], Haruo's [(oɪ) ʃɔʔ], [ɹjæʔ], and Kazuko's [baʔ], [βaʔpa]. Crucially, however, some Japanese infants are substituting CVs with CVCs. The most interesting ones are Kazuko's forms. While an explanation can somehow be forced for words containing more than pure CV-syllables, there is no reason to convert a pure CV target into CVC in 'peek-a-boo' and a pure CVCV into CVCCV in 'car' if the basic syllable is CV. Kazuko's case is not unique to Vihman, 1996. Kobayashi's (1981) data includes a 135-word-long list from one girl, who produced 38 words at 18 months of age. Four of them were:

/basʊ/ → [bʊʃ]   /nani/ → [naːn]   /kɒrɛ/ → [kɒʔ]   /ɹja/ → [jaʔ]

Moreover, when the narrow (unpublished) transcriptions of Vihman's Japanese infants are taken into consideration, not only did they all have CVC-syllables in the form of a full consonant or a diacritic consonant taking the shape of a glottal stop, glides, or [h], but also more than half of the input CV-syllables were produced as CVC-syllables (see Reimers, 2006, for detailed analysis and discussion).

The linguistic behaviour of Japanese infants above can be taken as supporting the basic CVX-syllable. However, a proper evaluation of the basic CVX-syllable requires an investigation of infants acquiring a language with more CVC inputs than Japanese, since the basic CVX-syllable should facilitate the production of input CVC-syllables. Hence, the unpublished American data (narrow transcription) of the Stanford Child Phonology Project were studied and compared with their Japanese peers. In order to focus on the coda element, diphthongs and vowel lengthening were ignored and counted as single Vs; the coda nasals in Japanese and coda liquids in American English were excluded in this count due to their lack of saliency as true consonants; the rare cases of extremely long Japanese target words were also excluded. The results are summarised in Table 4.3.

Taking the input first, it is not the case that closed syllables are extremely limited in the Japanese target words or that the American input words are clearly dominated by closed syllables. However, the input figures in the table presented above are consistent with syllable type analyses based on the Switchboard corpora of spoken American English by Greenberg (1997) and of Japanese by Arai and Greenberg (1997).

Table 4.3 Comparison of American and Japanese infants' output syllable shapes

Narrow transcription data		INPUT syllable		OUTPUT syllable	
		CV	CVC	CV	CVC
American infants	4-word point	50%	50%	64%	36%
	25-word point	42%	58%	67%	33%
Japanese infants	4-word point	69%	31%	52%	48%
	25-word point	81%	19%	74%	26%

In terms of the output, the Japanese infants were clearly producing more CVCs than their American peers at the 4-word point. With CV as the basic syllable, we should not expect to find a significant difference in the CV-CVC ratio between the input and output data for the Japanese infants at this stage. The Japanese 4-word point dataset was analysed with the basic CV-syllable as the null hypothesis and tested against an alternative hypothesis with CVX as the basic syllable (*t*-tests were conducted under the assumption that the variance is different in the two data sets, input and output). The analysis revealed that there is statistical support for the basic CVX-syllable, since the null hypothesis could be rejected at a 5% significant level ($p = 0.0387$). Furthermore, the Japanese 4-word point was compared to the 25-word point and examined as to whether the influence of the ambient language (input) increases with time. If there is an ambient language effect, there should be a significant difference in the ratios between the 4- and 25-word points. Since the tests, conducted under the assumption that the variance is different in the 4-word point and the 25-word point data set, showed that the *p* value was 0.0087 with the null hypothesis that there is no ambient language effect, the null hypothesis could be rejected at a 1% significance level, thus statistically supporting ambient language influence.

As for the output data of the American infants, they were producing considerably more CVs than CVCs at both word points and more CVs than their Japanese peers at the 4-word point. Again, two hypotheses were tested to see whether the American data support the basic CV- or CVX-syllable. However, neither one of them could be rejected. Moreover, the ambient language influence test did not reveal any significant results. These tests suggest that the American data may not be as reliable as the Japanese data due to a ceiling effect causing the ambiguous statistical figures for the American data. For example, the considerable difference in the number of monosyllabic and polysyllabic input words between American and Japanese children at both word points could be thought of as contributing to the ceiling effect: There were approximately twice as many monosyllabic as disyllabic input words at both word points in the American data and at the Japanese 4-word point; the number of disyllabic input words was almost four times the number of monosyllabic input words, increasing to almost eight times at the 25-word point, at which time there were eight times more polysyllabic input words in the Japanese data than those of the American infants.

While some very interesting speculations can be made regarding the ceiling effect of the American data, the focus should be on the conclusion we can draw from the Japanese data that the assumption of the basic CV-syllable is statistically not supported, and not on the inconclusiveness of the American data. Since the ambient language influence was shown to be effective at the 25-word point compared to the 4-word point in the Japanese infants, it follows that the role played by UG markedness in terms of the basic syllable is greater at the 4-word point. Also, the assumption that the basic syllable given by UG is CVX is consistent with the data. Furthermore, one could assume that the substitution pattern of CV with CVC in Japanese infants is a result of them attempting to manifest the mora-based rhythm of Japanese through word-final coda constituents. However, this can only be if UG gives them the basic CVX structure, of which the coda constituent can further be exploited to discover the language-specific timing unit, the mora, required by the prosodic phonology of Japanese.

CONCLUSION

This chapter investigated markedness in first language acquisition. In addition to the fact that any normally developing child is capable of mastering any language equally well, within a relatively short period of time, without explicit instruction, observations of universal patterns in first language acquisition have supported the view that simplification strategies by children are governed by general principles provided by UG where markedness plays a crucial role. While markedness continues to occupy a substantial position in phonological theory and is heavily relied upon in child phonology models, there are problems for linguistically based markedness accounts to come to terms with observations from acquisition, thus contributing to the on-going "nature or nurture" debate. The main problem is that the initial state of the grammar, where we would expect to be able to identify UG markedness, cannot be equated with the onset of speech production since child production data exhibit ambient language influence. Consequently, the initial state had to be taken as far back as possible, which steered our investigation towards infant perceptual studies.

Assuming that markedness guides the infant in language development from birth, perceptual studies led us to postulate that the initial state does not contain any segments but only the sense of rhythm. Since newborn infants are capable of distinguishing between stress-timed, syllable-timed, and mora-timed languages, but there is no evidence for a UG default setting of the internalised rhythm, the role played by the basic syllable was claimed to be extremely significant by virtue of it being the rhythm-bearing unit. Although the CV-syllable is enshrined as the basic syllable, it is logically not possible for all three rhythm classes to be distinguished at birth with CV as the basic unit, since the distinction between mora-timed rhythm with predominantly CV-syllables and stress-timed (or syllable-timed) rhythm must be made first. Hence, it was suggested that the basic syllable given by UG contains a coda constituent and the plausibility of the basic CVX-syllable was explored. Support for the basic CVX-syllable was found in the explanations of fuzzy syllable boundaries in infants, the facilitation of coda acquisition, earliest words containing both open and closed syllables as well as geminates, and Japanese infants' first words taking the form of CVC for CV target words. Thus, the conclusion of this chapter is that although UG markedness is thought to guide phonological acquisition, when ambient language influence is taken into account and the initial state of the grammar is modified to an earlier stage than the onset of production, the child's earliest underlying representations may not contain the full set of phonological features to which a markedness theory refers but only rhythm in which the basic syllable given by UG consists of an onset, a nucleus, and a coda constituent.

NOTE

1 Marilyn Vihman kindly invited me to see her unpublished data (videos and transcriptions) for the first time in 1999, after which I was privileged to become involved in the task of re-evaluating the original transcriptions of the Japanese data together with Satsuki Nakai, her assistant at the time.

REFERENCES

Arai, T., & Greenberg, S. (1997). The temporal properties of spoken Japanese are similar to those of English. In Kokkinakis, G., Fakotakis, N., & Dermatas, E. (Eds.). *Fifth European Conference on Speech Communication and Technology, Eurospeech 1997*, 1011–1014. Rhodes, Greece: ISCA.

Blevins, J. (1995). The syllable in phonological theory. In Goldsmith, J. (Ed.). *The handbook of phonological theory*, 206–244. Oxford: Blackwell.

Blevins, J. (2006). Syllable typology. In Brown, K. (Ed.). *Encyclopaedia of language and linguistics* (2nd ed.), 333–337. Oxford: Elsevier.

Daana, H. A. (2009). *The development of consonant clusters, stress and plural nouns in Jordanian Arabic child language.* Doctoral dissertation, University of Essex, UK.

Demuth, K., & Fee, J. (1995). Minimal words in early phonological development. Ms., Brown University and Dalhousie University.

Dressler, W. U., Dzuibalska-Kolaczyk, K., Gagarina, N., & Kilani-Schoch, M. (2005). Reduplication in child language. In Hurch, B. (Ed.). *Studies on reduplication*, 455–574. Berlin: Mouton de Gruyter.

Eimas, P. (1974). Linguistic processing of speech by young infants. In Schiefelbusch, R., & Lloyd, L. (Eds.). *Language perspectives: Acquisition, retardation, and intervention*, 55–73. Baltimore, MD: University Park Press.

Eimas, P. (1975). Auditory and phonetic coding of the cues for speech: Discrimination of the [r-l] distinction by young infants. *Perception and Psychophysics 18*, 341–347.

Eimas, P., Siqueland, P., Jusczyk, P., & Vigorito, J. (1971). Speech perception in infants. *Science 171*, 303–306.

Fikkert, P. (1994). *On the acquisition of prosodic structure.* Dordrecht: Holland Institute of Generative Linguistics.

Fikkert, P., & Freitas, M. J. (1997). Acquisition of syllable structure constraints: Evidence from Dutch and Portuguese. In Sorace, A., Heycock, C., & Shillcock, R. (Eds.). *Language acquisition: Knowledge representation and processing. Proceedings of GALA 97*, 217–222. Edinburgh: Edinburgh University Press.

Greenberg, S. (1997). On the origins of speech intelligibility in the real world. *Proceedings of the ESCA Workshop on Robust Speech Recognition for Unknown Communication Channels (Pont-a-Mousson, France)*, 23–32.

Haiman, J. (1998). Hua (Papuan). In Spencer, A. J., & Zwicky, A. M. (Eds.). *The handbook of morphology*, 539–562. Oxford: Blackwell.

Hayes, B. (1995). *Metrical stress theory: Principles and case studies.* Chicago: University of Chicago Press.

Ingram, D. (1974). Phonological rules in young children. *Journal of Child Language 1*, 49–64.

Ito, J. (1986). *Syllable theory in prosodic phonology.* Doctoral dissertation, University of Massachusetts, Amherst. Published 1988. New York: Garland.

Jakobson, R. (1941/1968). *Child language, aphasia and phonological universals.* Keiler, A., Trans. The Hague: Mouton.

Johnson, W., & Reimers, P. (2010). *Patterns in child phonology.* Edinburgh: Edinburgh University Press.

Jusczyk, P. W. (1997). *The discovery of spoken language*. Cambridge, MA: MIT Press.

Jusczyk, P. W., Cutler, A., & Redanz, N. J. (1993). Infants' preference for the predominant stress patterns of English words. *Child Development 64*, 675–687.

Jusczyk, P. W., Luce, P. A., & Charles-Luce, J. (1994). Infant's sensitivity to phonotactic patterns in the native language. *Journal of Memory and Language 33*, 630–645.

Kobayashi, C. (1981). Dialectal variation in child language. In Dale, P. S., & Ingram, D. (Eds.). *Child language: An international perspective*. Baltimore, MD: University Park Press.

Kroeber, A. L. (1916). The speech of a Zuni child. *American Anthropologist 18, 4*, 529–534.

Kubozono, H. (1993). Kodomo no shiritori to mor no kakutoku [Children's shiritori and the acquisition of mora]. *Nihongo no mora to onsetsu koozoo ni kanusru soogooteki kenkyuu [General studies on structures of Japanese mora and syllable] 2*, 130–137.

Kuhl, P. K. (1979). Speech perception in early infancy: Perceptual constancy for spectrally dissimilar vowel categories. *Journal of the Acoustical Society of America 66*, 1668–1679.

Kuhl, P. K., & Miller, J. D. (1975). Speech perception by the chinchilla: Voiced-voiceless distinction in alveolar plosive consonants. *Science 190*, 69–72.

Kunnari, S., Nakai, S., & Vihman, M. M. (2001). Cross-linguistic evidence for the acquisition of geminates. *Psychology of Language and Communication 5*, 13–24.

Ladefoged, P. (1975). *A course in phonetics*. New York: Harcourt Brace Jovanovich.

Levelt, C., & van de Vijver, R. (2004). Syllable types in cross-linguistic and developmental grammars. In Kager, R., Pater, J., & Zonneveld, W. (Eds.). *Constraints in phonological acquisition*, 204–218. Cambridge: Cambridge University Press.

Macken, M. (1995). Phonological acquisition. In Goldsmith, J. (Ed.). *The handbook of phonological theory*, 671–696. Oxford: Blackwell.

Macken, M., & Barton, D. (1980). The acquisition of the voicing contrast in Spanish: A phonetic and phonological study of word-initial stop consonants. *Journal of Child Language 7*, 433–458.

Menn, L. (1976). Evidence for an interactionist discovery theory of child phonology. *Papers and Reports on Language Development 12*, 169–177.

Morse, P. (1972). The discrimination of speech and nonspeech stimuli in early infancy. *Journal of Experimental Child Psychology 14*, 477–492.

Moskowitz, A. (1970). The two-year-old stage in the acquisition of phonology. *Language 46*, 426–441.

Nazzi, T., Bertoncini, J., & Mehler, J. (1998). Language discrimination by newborns: Towards an understanding of the role of rhythm. *Journal of Experimental Psychology: Human Perception and Performance 24, 3,* 756–766.

Ota, M. (2001). Phonological theory and the acquisition of prosodic structure: Evidence from child Japanese. *Annual Review of Language Acquisition 1,* 65–118.

Pike, K. L. (1945). *The intonation of American English.* Ann Arbor: University of Michigan Press.

Pinker, S., & Jackendoff, R. (2005). What's special about the human language faculty? *Cognition 95, 2,* 201–236.

Prince, A., & Smolensky, P. (2004). *Optimality theory constraint interaction in generative grammar.* Oxford: Blackwell.

Pye, C., Ingram, D., & List, H. (1987). A comparison of initial consonant acquisition in English and Quiche. In Nelson, K. E., & van Kleek, A. (Eds.). *Children's language 6,* 175–190. Hillsdale, NJ: Lawrence Erlbaum.

Ramus, F., Hauser, M. D., Miller, C., Morris, D., & Mehler, J. (2000). Language discrimination by human newborns and by cotton-top tamarin monkeys. *Science 288,* 349–351.

Reimers, P. M. (2006). *The role of markedness in the acquisition of phonology.* Doctoral dissertation, University of Essex, UK.

Rice, K. (2007). Markedness in phonology. In de Lacy, P. (Ed.). *Cambridge handbook of phonology,* 79–97. Cambridge: Cambridge University Press.

Roark, B., & Demuth, K. (2000). Prosodic constraints and the learner's environment: A corpus study. In Howell, S. C., Fish, S. A., & Keith-Lucas, T. (Eds.). *Proceedings of the 24th Boston University Conference on Language Development, Vol. 2,* 597–608. Somerville, MA: Cascadilla Press.

Roca, I., & Johnson, W. (1999). *A course in phonology.* Oxford: Blackwell.

Scobbie, J. M., Gibbon, F., Hardcastle W. J., & Fletcher, P. (2000). Covert contrast as a stage in the acquisition of phonetics and phonology. In Broe, M., & Pierrehumbert, J. (Eds.). *Papers in laboratory phonology V: Language acquisition and the lexicon,* 194–207. Cambridge: Cambridge University Press.

Stampe, D. (1972/1979). *How I spent my summer vacation: A dissertation on natural phonology.* Doctoral dissertation, University of Chicago. Republished with annotations in 1979 as *A dissertation on natural phonology.* New York: Garland.

Streeter, L. A. (1976). Language perception of two-month-old infants shows effects of both innate mechanisms and experience. *Nature 259,* 39–41.

Trubetzkoy, N. (1939/1969). *Grundzüge der Phonologie/Principles of phonology.* Baltaxe, C. A., Trans. Berkeley: University of California Press.

Vihman, M. M. (1992). Early syllables and the construction of phonology. In Ferguson, C. A., Menn, L., & Stoel-Gammon, C. (Eds.). *Phonological development: Models, research, implications.* Timonium, MD: York Press.

Vihman, M. M. (1996). *Phonological development: The origins of language in the child.* Cambridge, MA: Blackwell.

Vihman, M. M. (2002). The relationship between production and perception in the transition into language. End of award report, Economic and Social Research Council, UK. www.esrc.ac.uk/my-esrc/grants/R000238236/read

Vihman, M. M., Macken, M. A., Miller, R., Simmons, H., & Miller, J. (1985). From babbling to speech: A re-assessment of the continuity issue. *Language 61*, 397–445.

Vihman, M. M., & Velleman, S. L. (2000). Phonetics and the origins of phonology. In Burton-Roberts, N., Carr, P., & Docherty, G. (Eds.). *Phonological knowledge: Its nature and status*, 305–339. Oxford: Oxford University Press.

Weir, R. (1966). Some questions on the child's learning of phonology. In Smith, F., & Miller, G. A. (Eds.). *The genesis of language*, 153–172. Cambridge, MA: MIT Press.

Werker, J. F., & Tees, R. C. (1984). Cross-language speech perception: Evidence for perceptual reorganization during the first year of life. *Infant Behavior and Development 7*, 49–63.

Zamuner, T. S. (2003). *Input-based phonological acquisition.* New York: Routledge.

5

A COMPARISON OF FRICATIVE ACQUISITION IN GERMAN- AND CANADIAN ENGLISH-SPEAKING CHILDREN WITH PROTRACTED PHONOLOGICAL DEVELOPMENT

**B. May Bernhardt, Roswitha Romonath and
Joseph Paul Stemberger**

The primary question addressed in this book is to what degree patterns of phonological acquisition reflect crosslinguistic ('universal') tendencies versus language-specific trends. Acquisition patterns have many influences, among them perception, articulatory complexity, phoneme and/or feature frequency, word types and individual differences (age, gender, cognitive level, other developmental or environmental factors). This chapter examines the question for singleton German and English fricative data from two cohorts of preschool children with protracted phonological development (PPD; alternatively, speech sound disorders). The following introduction outlines challenges for fricative acquisition and reviews previous research.

Fricatives are one of the more challenging sound classes for speech acquisition.[1] In terms of auditory perception, lower-energy fricatives can be difficult to distinguish from similar-sounding segments, e.g., [f]/[θ], [v]/[b], [ð]/[d] (Miller & Nicely, 1955). In terms of speech production, active articulators need to be positioned so that air will be forced through apertures of varying degrees of narrowness, creating turbulences with different characteristics of pitch and loudness. In terms of articulatory ease, control of lip apertures (labial fricatives) may be less challenging than control of tongue apertures (lingual fricatives). Regarding lingual fricatives, speakers may find it easier to configure the tongue with relatively flat central apertures (i.e., ungrooved, distributed), such as for [θ, ð, ɬ, ʐ, ɕ, z, ç, j, x, ʁ], directing airflow over a broad area. The often more challenging higher-energy sibilants [s, z, ʃ, ʒ] require a centrally grooved tongue configuration (tighter aperture for [s, z] than for [ʃ, ʒ]), with stabilization of the tongue against both sides of the palate along the teeth (Bernhardt & Stemberger, 1998). Such gradations of phonetic control can take years to learn, with some adults still showing relatively ungrooved, lower-energy /s/ and /z/ (Fox & Dodd, 1999; Van Borsel, Van Rentergem & Verhaeghe, 2007). Voiced fricatives present an additional challenge because of their competing demands on air pressure: sub-glottal pressure must be high enough to allow voicing but low enough to allow intraoral turbulence, i.e., frication (Bernhardt & Stemberger, 1998).

The perceptual and articulatory challenges for fricative acquisition could lead to a similar timeline for development of the same fricatives across languages (universal tendencies). However, if a particular segment (phoneme) or feature is relatively more frequent in a language, it may be mastered earlier. For example, Ingram (1988) observed earlier acquisition of the relatively frequent /v/ in Swedish, Estonian and Bulgarian compared with English, where it is relatively infrequent. The frequency and 'functional load' of a particular segment or feature (its appearance in phonological oppositions) in a particular language may override articulatory ease/complexity as a determinant of the order of acquisition (Pye, Ingram & List, 1987). The effect of frequency is itself a 'universal' tendency but plays out as a language-specific factor. Whether type or token frequency may be more relevant is debated, however (see Richtmeister, Gerken & Ohala, 2011). Frequency effects may also affect mismatch patterns in acquisition. Leonard (1992) suggested that substitutions tend to come from children's phonetic inventories and the input language inventory/ies, suggesting that different inventories might result in different mismatch patterns.

Most data concerning speech sound acquisition derive from cross-sectional studies addressing all phonemes of the language, and differences across studies make generalization difficult. Participant groups vary in size, age group, population (typical/atypical) and dialect. Data vary in terms of linguistic description and transcription precision, number of exemplars per target, word position coverage and word length/complexity/frequency. Criteria for acquisition may cite emergence, customary use or mastery levels, with levels ranging from 75% to 90% or 100% accuracy by segment, word position, child or group.

Table 5.1 summarizes the general age of acquisition findings for German and English fricatives and their features. (See the section 'Method' for segment-feature correspondences.)

Table 5.1 Age range (in years) for acquisition of fricatives and their feature set in German and English

Fricative	German[a]	English[b]	Features
f	2;0–3;7 (2;6 >, 90% criterion[c])	WI: 2;4–3;11 WF: 5;6[d]	Manner: [+continuant] & [–sonorant] Laryngeal: [–voiced], [+spread glottis] Place: [Labial] ([+labiodental])
v	2;0–3;7	3;0–9;0	Manner: [+continuant] & [–sonorant] Laryngeal: [+voiced] Place: [Labial] ([+labiodental])
θ		4;0–8;0	Manner: [+continuant] & [–sonorant] Laryngeal: [–voiced], [+spread glottis] Place: [Coronal] ([+anterior], [–grooved])
ð		4;0–7;0+	Manner: [+continuant] & [–sonorant] Laryngeal: [+voiced] Place: [Coronal] ([+anterior], [–grooved])
s	2;0–6;0[e]	3;0–9;0[e]	Manner: [+continuant] & [–sonorant] Laryngeal: [–voiced], [+spread glottis] Place: [Coronal] ([+anterior], [+grooved])
z	2;0–6;0[e]	4;0–9;0[e]	Manner: [+continuant] & [–sonorant] Laryngeal: [+voiced] Place: [Coronal] ([+anterior], [+grooved])
ʃ	3;0–4;1	3;6–7;0	Manner: [+continuant] & [–sonorant] Laryngeal: [–voiced], [+spread glottis] Place: [Coronal] ([-anterior], [+grooved])
ʒ	3;0–7;0		Manner: [+continuant] & [–sonorant] Laryngeal: [+voiced] Place: [Coronal] ([–anterior], [+grooved])
[ç/x] Allophones	2;0–4;1 ([x] 2;6> at 90% criterion[c])		Manner: [+continuant] & [–sonorant] Laryngeal: [–voiced], [+spread glottis] Place, [ç]: [Coronal] ([–anterior], [–grooved]) & [Dorsal] ([–back]) Place, [x]: [Dorsal] ([+back])

Note: WI = word-initial; WF = word-final. Features are based on Bernhardt & Stemberger (1998) and Ullrich (2011).

[a]German age range based on Grohnfeldt (1980); Fongaro-Levorin (1992); Fox & Dodd (1999), at a 75%–90% criterion.

[b]English age range based on Smit (2007: General American English); Dodd et al. (2003: British English, 90% criterion).

[c]Fox & Dodd (1999).

[d]Smit et al. (1990): 90% criterion, word-initial and word-final positions.

[e]A proportion of children in English produce /s/ and /z/ as slightly ungrooved $[s^\theta]$/$[z^\theta]$ up to age 9 (Smit et al. [1990], 90% mastery criterion). For German, Fox and Dodd (1999) observed up to 40% of the children with [θ]/[ð] replacements for /s/ and /z/ and classified these as phonetic differences rather than phonological mismatches.

The age of acquisition summary for English is based on Smit (2007) and Dodd et al. (2003). Smit (2007) cites, among others, Templin (1957), Prather, Hedrick and Kern (1975), Arlt and Goodban (1976) and Smit et al. (1990). For German, the age of acquisition summary is based primarily on Grohnfeldt (1980), Fongaro-Levorin (1992) and Fox and Dodd (1999), with either a 75% or 90% criterion level for acquisition (90% considered mastery). (Other German studies examined include Hacker & Weiß, 1986; Fox & Dodd, 2001; and Kehoe & Lleó, 2002.) Table 5.1 shows a wide age range for fricative acquisition, with earlier acquisition of fricatives in German. The degree to which these facts reflect differences in study design is unclear, however, and they must be interpreted cautiously. Overall, labiodental /f/ appears to be mastered earliest, at least word-initially in English, with the labiodental /v/ also relatively early in German (congruent with Ingram, 1988). For coronal fricatives, tongue grooving and the [anterior] (alveolar-palatoalveolar) contrast appear to be particularly challenging. For German, the ungrooved palatal/dorsal allophones ([ç]-[x])[2] appear in the mid-range of acquisition. Kehoe and Lleó (2002) observed no word position differences for acquisition of /ʃ/ by typically developing (TD) German-speaking children, but see Hacker and Weiß (1986) further on.

In terms of mismatch patterns, some early features may be affected during development. Early on, stop substitutions are common (Fongaro-Levorin, 1992; Fox & Dodd, 1999; Smit et al., 1990). Concerning place of articulation, both major place substitutions, e.g., [Labial] /f/ > [Coronal] [s], and subsidiary place changes may occur, e.g., palatoalveolar [−anterior] /ʃ/ > alveolar [+anterior] [s]; [+grooved] /s/ > [−grooved] [θ] or alveopalatal [ɕ]). Changes in laryngeal features may also occur in either direction (Bernhardt & Stemberger, 1998). Often (and most simply), when a manner mismatch occurs, laryngeal and major place feature(s) (Labial, Coronal, Dorsal) continue to match the target, e.g., /f/ > [Labial] [pʰ] or /v/ > [Labial] [w], /z/ or /ʒ/ > [Coronal] [d]. However, major place and laryngeal features may also change along with the manner, e.g., [Labial] /f/ > [Coronal] [s], [t], [d]; [Coronal] /s/ > [Labial] [p], [b] or [Dorsal] [k]; [Labial] /v/ > [Coronal] [d], [z], [s] (Bernhardt & Stemberger, 1998).

By age, different types of mismatch patterns have been observed. For English TD children, Smit et al. (1990) noted fewer fricative deletions after 3;0, and Haelsig and Madison (1986), a general decline in mismatches after 3;6. Ingram (1978) examined patterns for 15 TD children (aged 7 months to 3;4) and 15 with PPD (aged 3;0 to 6;6). For the TD group, mismatch patterns by developmental phase first included deletion and stop substitutions, then [+continuant] consonants (one or two fricatives; glide or liquid substitutions) and, finally, changes only in subsidiary place ([anterior], [grooved]). Smit et al. (1990) noted that more than 10% of TD children showed 'dentalized' /s/ at age 9;0.

For German, Fox and Dodd (1999) observed deletion of word-initial /v/ up to age 2;0 (TD). Place changes (fronting, backing) and manner changes (stop substitutions) appeared until age 3;0, and fronting of sibilants until 3;11.

For children with PPD, Ingram (1978) observed developmental patterns similar to those of the TD group but more persistent and pervasive mismatches (e.g., continued deletion, use of stops), more multiple feature mismatches (e.g., /f/ > [t], /s/ > [l]) and a greater proportion of less common substitutions, e.g., lateralized fricatives, ingressive airflow fricatives and voiceless nasals. For 15 German-speaking children with PPD (ages 4;6–6;8), Hacker and Weiß (1986) noted that /ʃ/ was least accurate, with increasing proportions of mismatches in order for [x/ç], /f, v, s, z, ʃ/. Most mismatches involved only one feature change (79%). Mismatches increased from word-initial to -medial to -final position, although [x] showed fewer mismatches word-finally than word-medially. Over 50% of mismatches concerned place (e.g., [−anterior] /ʃ/ > [+anterior] [s]), and 37% manner (stops); other mismatches were infrequent.

Detailed crosslinguistic data are lacking, especially for children with PPD. The current study thus set out to compare fricative acquisition in German versus English for children with PPD. A number of predictions were made regarding universal, language-specific and other tendencies:

UNIVERSAL

1. Stops would be the most common manner substitutions, but other manner substitutions would occur (nasals and liquids least frequently).
2. Major place features would show higher match proportions than subsidiary place features overall.
3. Age and developmental level: developmental level and age would be relevant in match proportions and mismatch types.

BOTH UNIVERSAL AND LANGUAGE-SPECIFIC

1. Labiodental /f/ would show the highest accuracy in both languages (articulatorily least challenging), but labiodental /v/ would be advanced in German, reflecting the higher frequency of labiodentals in German compared with English.
2. Positional differences in mismatch types would occur both within and across languages, but the literature was unclear on what to expect.

3. English-speaking children would show more mismatches for laryngeal features because of the necessary contrast in voicing word-finally in English (German having only voiceless obstruents word-finally).

LANGUAGE-SPECIFIC

1. Substitutions would partially reflect differences in the two languages' phonetic inventories, i.e., more palatal/dorsal substitutions in German and more interdental substitutions in English.

METHOD

Participants

Participants included 30 English-speaking Canadian children (British Columbia) and 30 German-speaking children (Cologne) identified by local speech-language pathologists as having PPD. (See Table 5.2.)

Samples were balanced for gender across languages (7 females; 23 males). The mean age for the German and English samples respectively was 49.73 months and 48.27 months, with the German girls being

Table 5.2 Participant characteristics for the German and English cohorts with protracted phonological development

	Mean age (months)	# female (Mean age, SD)	# male (Mean age, SD)	# with mild language delay	Mean Whole Word Match[c] (SD)
German	49.73 (SD 8.25)	7 (46.7, SD 7.1)	23 (50.7, SD 8.5)	20[a]	18.97% (11.8)
English	48.27 (SD 7.23)	7 (53, SD 10.03)	23 (48.9, SD 5.7)	13[b]	12.70% (10.9)

Note: No significant differences on *t*-tests comparing age (overall; male sample: $p = .4669$; $p = .0753$) or on Mann-Whitney U ($p = .31$) for the female samples.

[a]Based on a standardized speech-language assessment (SETK 3-5—*Sprachentwicklungstest für drei- bis fünfjährige Kinder*; Grimm, 2001). The children scored within or above average on the Kaufman and Kaufman Assessment Battery for Children (cognitive development) (Kaufman & Kaufman, 1994).

[b]Based on the *Clinical Evaluation of Language Fundamentals—Preschool* (CELF-P; Wiig, Secord & Semel, 1992), *Peabody Picture Vocabulary Test* (PPVT; Dunn & Dunn, 1997) and a short language sample. Four English speakers showed a mild delay on the CELF-P or PPVT, and 13 in morphosyntactic production.

[c]Whole Word Match = proportion of words that match the adult target exactly (small deviations in sibilant placement and slight devoicing considered acceptable). This was a significant difference by *t*-test ($p = .034$).

younger than the English girls and the German boys slightly older than the English boys (although not significantly). Some children had other mild delays in language acquisition (typically involving production of sentences/morphology) but no other developmental concerns.

Speech Samples

For English, the Photo Articulation Test (Lippke et al., 1997) provided a single word elicitation sample of all phonemes across word positions in 80 words with a variety of CV shapes and stress patterns. For German, the assessment tool Nichtlineare phonologische Diagnostik was used (NILPOD [Nonlinear phonological assessment]: Ullrich, 2011). NILPOD samples all phonemes across word positions in 105 words with a variety of CV shapes and stress patterns. English samples were collected using a Marantz PMD430 tape recorder and PMZ table-top microphone, and German samples with a CANON 3CCD Camcorder XM2 PAL and Sennheiser microphone MKH 416 P48 U. A Whole Word Match for the entire set of single word speech samples from each language showed a mean of 18.9% (SD 11.8) for the German children and 12.7% (SD 10.9) for the English-speaking children, a significant difference in severity of PPD: $t(58) = 2.14$, $p = .037$.[3]

Fricative Singleton Samples

Singleton fricatives common to the two languages by word position were examined in monosyllables and trochaic disyllables. The sets of fricatives were (a) word-initial /f/, /v/, /z/, /ʃ/; (b) word-medial (intervocalic[4]) /s/, /z/, /ʃ/; and (c) word-final /f/, /s/, /ʃ/. English words consisted of *fish* (/ˈfɪʃ/), *fork* (/ˈfɔɹk/), *knife* (/ˈnaɪf/), *feather(s)* (/ˈfɛðɚ(z)/), *vacuum* (/ˈvæːkjum/), *whistle* (/ˈwɪsl̩/), *house* (/ˈhaʊs/), *zipper* (/ˈzɪpɚ/), *shoe* (/ˈʃuː/), *station* (/ˈsteɪʃn̩/), *brush* (/ˈbɹʌʃ/) (and, for some children, *this* /ˈðɪs/, *yes* /ˈjɛs/). The German words included *Fenster* ('window' /ˈfɛnstɐ/), *Fisch* ('fish' /ˈfɪʃ/), *Vögel* ('birds' /ˈføːgəl/), *Schiff* ('ship' /ˈʃɪf/), *Schaf* ('sheep' /ˈʃaːf/), *Wasser* ('water' /ˈvasɐ/), *Wippe* ('seesaw' /ˈvɪpə/), *Schlüssel* ('key' /ˈʃlʏsəl/), *Glas* ('glass' /glaːs/), *Bus* ('bus' /bʊs/), *Saft* ('juice' / ˈzaft/), *Sonne* ('sun' /ˈzɔnə/), *Nase* ('nose' /ˈnaːzə/), *Pfirsich* ('pear' /ˈ(p)fɪɐzɪç/), *Schuh* ('shoe' /ˈʃuː/), *Schatz* ('treasure' /ˈʃats/), *Flasche* ('bottle' /ˈflaʃə/), *Dusche* ('shower' /ˈduːʃə/), and *Frosch* ('frog' /ˈfʁɔʃ/).

Narrow phonetic transcriptions were completed in Germany by two master's students in phonetics and in Canada by two master's students in speech-language pathology. Transcription conventions were determined with the project leaders at the outset with consultation throughout the process. Transcription reliability for the German data was 89.3% for all segments, and in English, just over 90%. Although the transcriptions were reliable within language, an examination of the transcripts showed differences arising because of within-language conventions for acceptability of productions, particularly in terms of degree of tongue grooving expected for sibilants, and which symbols to use for ungrooved coronal fricatives, e.g., a slightly ungrooved [s$^\theta$][5] (acceptable) variant versus a fully ungrooved [θ] (less acceptable), an ungrooved alveopalatal [ɕ] or an ungrooved palatal [ç]). The English and German samples were entered into the Computerized Articulation and Phonology Evaluation System (CAPES; Masterson & Bernhardt, 2001) for basic computation of inventory and mismatch patterns, and then into spreadsheets for further quantitative and statistical analysis (Microsoft Excel 2010; SPSS 12.0 2003). Spreadsheet data entries were confirmed by a second research assistant.

For analysis, nonlinear feature frameworks were adopted from Bernhardt and Stemberger (1998) and Ullrich (2011). (See Table 5.1.) Each feature category is described below in turn, and the rubric for feature mismatch coding outlined.

Features are organized into three categories: Manner, Place and Laryngeal. Manner features are considered the 'highest' level features in the 'geometry' (at the 'Root node', mediating between the relevant features and prosodic position of a phoneme). Only relevant features for a specific fricative are designated: e.g., the feature [Labial] is not designated for /s/ because the primary articulator for /s/ is the tongue tip.

By manner, fricatives are [+continuant] (like glides and vowels) and [−sonorant] (like stops). English and German do not have lateral or nasal fricatives, and thus [−lateral] and [−nasal] are not specified for fricatives. A change in either [+continuant] ([−continuant] stop) or [−sonorant] ([+sonorant] glide, nasal or lateral) was tallied as a mismatch for fricative manner. An affricate substitution was tallied as a change in [+continuant] (addition of [−continuant]). Lateral or nasal substitutions result in a change from unspecified to specified values, e.g., [−lateral] > [+lateral], but these were not tallied as additional mismatches; i.e., only the change to [+sonorant] was tallied.

Place is described using privative (non-binary) features for *major place* and binary features for *subsidiary place*. The major place features for English and German fricatives include [Labial] for /f/, /v/; [Coronal] (tongue tip or blade) for /θ/ and /ð/ (English), /s/, /z/, /ʃ/ (both), /ʒ/ (English), [ç] (German); and [Dorsal] (tongue approximating velar or uvular areas), in German for [ç]-[x], /ʁ/. Most fricatives have only one major place, with the exception of palatals (both [Coronal] and [Dorsal]: German [ç]). Examples of major place substitutions were [f] or [k] for /s/; [ç] for other coronals, i.e., adding [Dorsal].

The subsidiary feature for [Labial] fricatives in German and English is designated as [+labiodental] (for /f/ and /v/) (with [−round] assumed as a default). Because labiodental stops are rare in adult languages, substitution of [p] or [b] for the labiodentals was not counted as a mismatch for subsidiary place, even though the subsidiary feature was absent. Substitution of [w] for /v/ or /f/, however, results in the default value of [round] changing to the specified [+round], and was therefore tallied as a subsidiary feature mismatch. The [Coronal] fricatives in English and German contrast in anteriority. For fricatives common to the two languages, /s/ and /z/ are [+anterior] and /ʃ/ [−anterior]. English also has [−anterior] /ʒ/ and German [−anterior] [ç]. A change in value for Coronal [anterior] was considered a subsidiary place mismatch. However, a slight backing or fronting of a sibilant (intermediate between /s/ and /ʃ/) was considered a change in phonetic precision and not a feature mismatch. Both languages have grooved ('strident') and ungrooved fricatives: in English, [+grooved] /s/, /ʃ/, /z/, /ʒ/ and [−grooved] /θ/ and /ð/, and in German [+grooved] /s/, /ʃ/, /z/ and [−grooved] [ç]. Changes in values for [grooved] were considered subsidiary place mismatches. [θ]/ [ð], [ɕ]/[ʑ] or [ɬ]/[ɮ] were considered mismatches for [+grooved] sibilants. Slightly ungrooved [sθ] or [zð] were also not tallied as mismatches for [+grooved]. Subsidiary features automatically change when major place features change (because they are dependents of major place features) and were therefore not counted as additional mismatches: e.g., /s/ > [f] also implies the loss of [+anterior] and [+grooved], but these were ignored because they are irrelevant to [f].

Laryngeal features comprise both [voiced] and [spread glottis]. Voiceless fricatives are designated as [−voiced] and [+spread glottis], whereas voiced fricatives have the opposite values. A mismatch involving voicing does not necessarily imply a change in [spread glottis]. For example, an unaspirated stop is [−spread glottis] and thus matches [spread glottis] for voiced fricatives (even though there is a mismatch for [voiced]). A [+spread glottis] aspirated stop was considered a match for the [+spread glottis] voiceless fricative, whereas an unaspirated stop was considered a mismatch. Partial devoicing for voiced fricatives was not counted as a mismatch. German has no word-final voiced fricatives and thus fewer opportunities for Laryngeal mismatches overall.

While features are considered independent entities (since Goldsmith, 1979/1976), segments are composed of features from all categories. Thus, mismatches may affect one of the categories or any combination of the categories. A [tʰ] for /s/ is thus a mismatch only for Manner, but a [d] for /f/ is a mismatch for Manner, Place and Laryngeal features. Analyses considered all changes involving each category, and various combinations thereof (i.e., Place and Manner, Laryngeal and Manner, all three, etc.). (For further detail on features, see Bernhardt and Stemberger, 1998; Ullrich, 2011.)

RESULTS

Fricative production is compared across words and children for the two languages, first in terms of overall matches, then within word position. Because there were unequal numbers of tokens for most targets between the languages, the proportions of match were compared between languages. (Raw numbers appear in the substitution charts.)

Overall Match Proportions

The mean match proportion overall was 34.8% for the German sample and 31.3% for the English sample (a non-significant difference overall and by individual word positions) (See Figure 5.1.) Among individual consonants, /f/ had the highest match across positions for both languages (approximately 75% for German and 46% for English) with a significantly higher proportional match for both /f/ and /v/ in German (multivariate analysis of variance: $F[1,57] = 13.006$, $p = .001$). The coronal fricatives showed matches in the 15%–30% range with slight non-significant differences between the languages (/s/ slightly higher in German and /z/ and /ʃ/ slightly higher in English).

Considering mismatch types, place mismatches were more frequent in German and laryngeal mismatches more frequent in English,

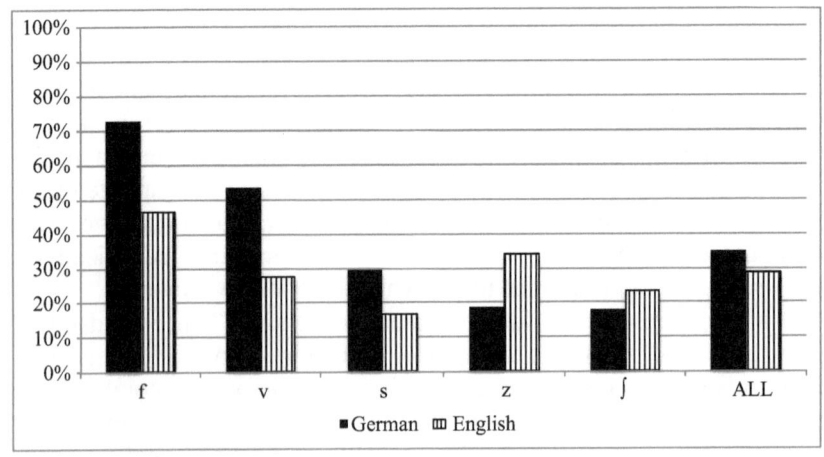

Figure 5.1 Overall fricative match proportions for German- and Canadian English-speaking children with protracted phonological development.

significant differences on repeated measures between-subject ANO-VAs: Place ($F[1,57] = 28.171$, $p < .001$); Laryngeal ($F[1,57] = 4.294$, $p = .043$). Manner mismatch proportions, although more common for the English sample, just missed significance between languages: Manner ($F[1,58] = 8.63$, $p = .054$). The English-speaking children had a significantly higher proportion of multiple feature mismatches per consonant (Manner & Place & Laryngeal): ANOVA ($F[1,58] = 11.328$, $p = .001$) and a near-significant difference between two feature mismatch types per segment (Manner & Laryngeal, Manner & Place, or Place & Laryngeal) ($F[1,58] = 3.325$, $p = .073$).

Word-Initial Fricatives

Figure 5.2 shows the match proportions of word-initial /f/, /v/, /z/ and /ʃ/.

The labiodentals had the highest match in German (67% for /f/, about 10% higher than /v/), and a higher match than in English, which showed a 48% match for /f/ versus a 23% match for /v/. In English, /z/ had the next-highest match proportion (10% lower than /f/), about 15% higher than for German. The /ʃ/ was equivalent across languages (17%–18%). A repeated measures ANOVA confirmed significant differences in match proportions between consonant types ($F[1,16] = 36.809$, $p < .001$) and in the interaction of group and consonant type ($F[1,16] = 2.61$, $p = .032$). Age and gender were not significantly related to match outcomes.

Tables 5.3 and 5.4 show segmental mismatch patterns. The German sample showed no deletions. Glottal stop substitutions appeared only

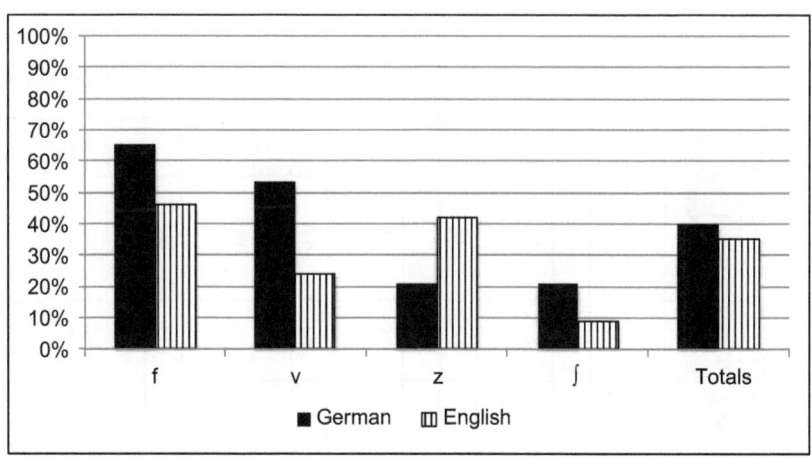

Figure 5.2 World-initial fricative match proportions for German- and Canadian English-speaking children with protracted phonological development.

Table 5.3 Word-initial subtitutions by manner in German (G) and English (E) (raw numbers)

Fric.	Lang.	Total targets	Total mismatch	p	pʰ	b	b̥	t	tʰ	d	d̥	c	k	kʰ	g	ʔ	ts	tθ	tɕ	tʃ	dʒ	tç	tɬ	ps	pɛ	pç	ʃm	l	m	n	w	j	ɹ	ʋ	ɥ	h
f	G	93	30			2	1		4					1			3								1	1								2	1	3
	E	89	47	1		**10**		1	1	8			1			**14**													2		4					
v	G	64	28			5			1	2							1												1				1		3		7
	E	29	21			15				1						1														2			1			
z	G	61	47						3	10	1						3											1		2		2				3
	E	31	17							4					1	4					1	1									2	1				
ʃ	G	121	93		1			**12**		3		1			1		7	3	6	4		1	2	1			1	1							1	4
	E	33	27						1	1	3						3				4	1	1				1									3

Note: Glottal stop was considered deletion. Total = Total for Tables 5.3 and 5.4. **Bold** indicates higher proportions.

Table 5.4 Word-initial substitutions by other fricatives in German (G) and English (E) (raw numbers)

Fric.	Lang.	Total targets	Total mismatch	ɸ	f	θf	v	vw	s	θ	ð	ð̥	sθ	ɬ	lʒ	ʃ	s>	ʃɣ	ɕ	ç	j	x	ʁ	sç	çj
f	G	93	30			1	1							6				1	1					1	
	E	89	47																						
v	G	64	28		1		2							2									2		
	E	29	21					1					1			2									
z	G	61	47		2		1		3	2	9	1		1	2						2				1
	E	31	17					1					2							1					
ʃ	G	121	93	2					8	10	1			13					8	2	1	1		1	
	E	33	27						1		1		5				1			1					

Note: Shaded columns contain acceptable variants (slightly degrooved [sθ] or backed [s>]).

for English and were coded conservatively as deletions (10% of total mismatches); glottal onsets are a default onset in vowel-initial single words in English and therefore ambiguous as to their status as substitutions or deletions.

Manner feature mismatches did not differ significantly between the languages, although the English speakers had proportionally more. Stops were frequent substitutions across languages; affricates were relatively frequent substitutions for German coronal fricatives. Laryngeal mismatches had similar proportions overall for the two languages (30%–40% of targets), with the only significant difference between languages occurring for /v/, for which the German children had proportionally more laryngeal mismatches (multivariate ANOVA: $F[1,53] = 10.303, p = .002$).

For place, the German children had proportionally higher matches across consonants (one-way ANOVA, $F[1,57] = 12.667, p = .001$) and for /v/ and /z/ (multivariate): /v/ ($F[1,53] = 5.363, p = .024$, and /z/ ($F[1,53] = 4.479, p = .039$). The labiodentals had more *major* place changes (i.e., Labial > Coronal) than the coronals in both languages; this differed significantly between languages for /v/ (one-way ANOVA, $F[1,57] = 10.190, p = .002$). The German children overall had a higher proportion of [Dorsal] substitutions and ungrooved interdentals and lateral fricatives; the proportion of subsidiary place differences thus was significantly higher for German: one-way ANOVA for /z/ ($F[1,56]$, $p < .001$) and for /ʃ/ ($F[1,56] = 13.542, p = .001$). Age and gender were not significant.

Word-Medial Position

Overall, the English-speaking children had a non-significantly higher word-medial match proportion (Figure 5.3). This reflected slightly higher matches for /z/ and /ʃ/, a significant difference favoring English: one-way ANOVA $F(1,55) = 4.661, p = .043$.

Regarding specific mismatches (Tables 5.5, 5.6), English speakers frequently used stop substitutions (commonly [d]). Stops were also common substitutions for German children, who also showed affricates and sonorant substitutions. An [h] substitution appeared infrequently for the English-speaking children. For place, the German speakers showed degrooving of sibilants (including both ungrooved interdentals and lateral fricative substitutions) and [Dorsal] substitutions (palatals, velars, uvulars).

Overall, the English speakers had a greater proportion of manner and laryngeal mismatches and the German children a higher proportion of

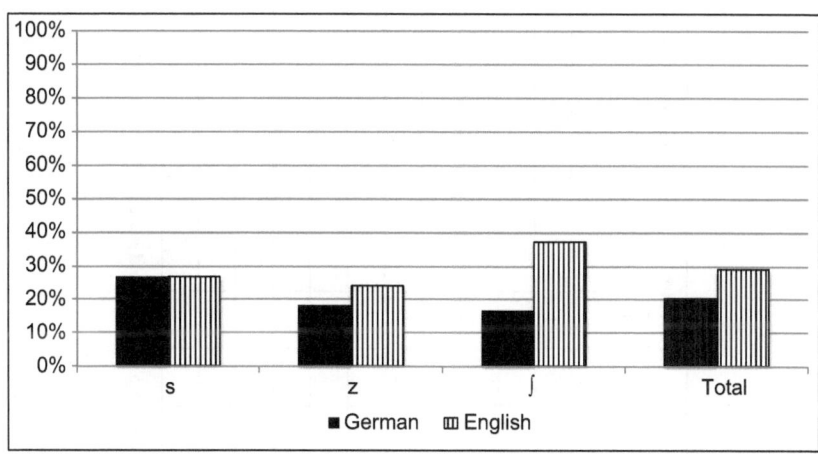

Figure 5.3 Word-medical fricative match proportions for German- and Canadian English-speaking children with protracted phonological development.

place mismatches. A multivariate analysis confirmed a significant difference for each mismatch type across consonants between languages (not for age or gender): Manner: $F(1,53) = 10.291$, $p = .002$; Place: $F(1,53) = 5.539$, $p = .012$; Laryngeal: $F(1,53) = 6.809$, $p = .022$. The English group also had a significantly greater proportion of segments with two mismatch types (Manner & Laryngeal, Place & Laryngeal, etc.) (one-way ANOVA $F[1,57] = 16.867$, $p < .001$).

Word-Final Position

Figure 5.4 shows word-final match proportions for /f/, /s/ and /ʃ/.

Again, labiodental /f/ was developmentally advanced, with German speakers having a significantly higher degree of accuracy (one-way ANOVA, $F[1,57] = 9.063$, $p = .004$). Sibilant accuracy levels were roughly equivalent between languages.

Table 5.7 displays mismatch types. Deletion was significantly more common in English (one-way ANOVA, $F[1,58] = 20.825$, $p < .001$), with younger children showing more deletion. Manner substitutions did not differ significantly between languages and followed the same pattern as for other positions: primarily stops but a few affricates and sonorants. The proportion of place changes was significantly higher for the German children ($F[1,58] = 8.998$, $p = .004$). The most common substitutions were other fricatives; tongue grooving was the

Table 5.5 Word-medial substitutions by manner of articulation for German (G) and English (E) (raw numbers)

Fric.	Lang.	Total target	Total mismatch	Stops									Affricates				Sonorants		
				t	tʰ	d	c	kʰ	ʔ	ʔʔ	ʔd	ʔz	ts	tʃ	tɬ	tɕ	j	ɲ	h
s	G	59	44	1		**1**	1	1					**5**	1		2			
	E	31	27	1		**8**			**4**	1	1								2
z	G	60	49		1	7		1					2					1	
	E	31	24			**8**			**5**	1		1		2			3		1
ʃ	G	59	49	1	**3**			2					**4**	1	2				
	E	29	18	1		**4**			**6**		1								

Note: For English, there was one deletion per fricative. Glottal stops were considered onsets. Total = Total for Tables 5.5 and 5.6. **Bold** indicates higher proportions.

Table 5.6 Word-medial substitutions by other fricatives for German (G) and English (E) (raw numbers)

Fric.	Lang.	Total targets	Total mismatch	f	β	θ	ð	s	st	z	sᶿ	θˢ	s>	zᶿ	ɫ	lʒ	ʃ	ʒ	ɕ	z	ç	χ
s	G	59	44	1		**15**						1			7		1		4		2	1
	E	31	27						1	1	1	1	3	1								
z	G	60	49	2	1	4	**17**	**3**							5	1			1	2		
	E	31	24				1											1				
ʃ	G	59	49	1		**13**		**8**				1			4				**8**			
	E	29	18							2		1									1	

Note: Shaded areas indicate acceptable variants ([s] slightly backed [>] or degrooved [sᶿ]; [zᶿ]; [θ] slightly grooved [θˢ]). **Bold** indicates higher proportions.

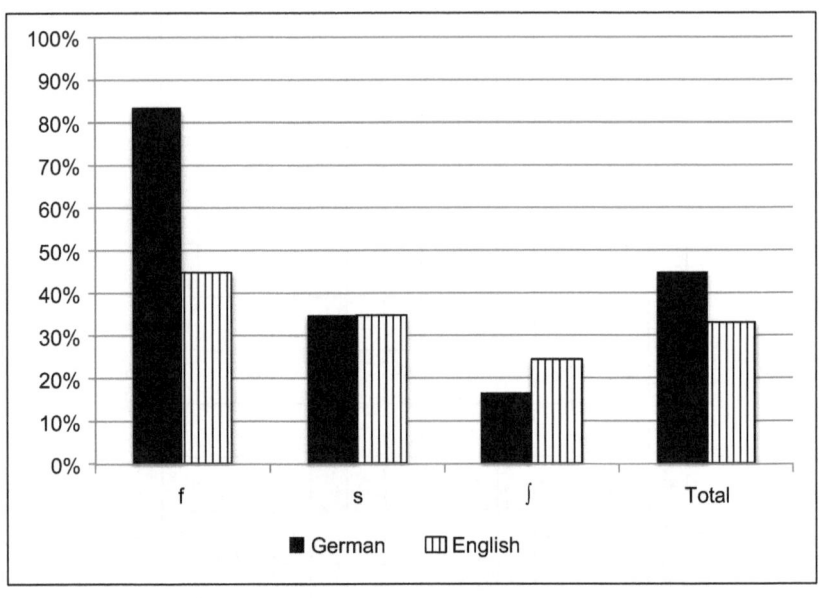

Figure 5.4 Word-final fricative match proportions for German- and Canadian English-speaking children with protracted phonological development.

primary feature challenge, especially for the German speakers, who showed more [+lateral] and [Dorsal] substitutions and, similarly to the English speakers, many ungrooved substitutions for the coronal fricatives.

DISCUSSION

This chapter addresses the issue of universal versus language-specific tendencies in the acquisition of fricatives by German-speaking and English-speaking children with PPD. Caution is advised in interpretation, because the words evaluated were necessarily different between languages (except for *Fisch/fish*), and it cannot be taken for granted that all words are equivalent (Clark, 1973) when comparing phonemes by position. Furthermore, the samples were relatively small, increasing the impact of individual differences, especially in samples of children with PPD, where heterogeneity may be higher than in TD samples (Bernhardt & Stemberger, 1998).

Table 5.7 Word-final mismatches for German (G) and English (E) fricatives (raw numbers)

Fric.	Lang.	Total targets	Total mismatch	Del.	Stops							Affric.		Sonorant		Other fricatives																	
					pʰ	p	t	tʰ	c	kʰ	ʔ	ts	tʃ	l	ʋ	f	s	θ	ʃ	s>	ʃ>	ɬ	tɬ	ls	ç	ɕ	z	sᶿ	θˢ	ɛs	st	x	χ
f	G	59	10	2	1	1	0			1					1							2			2								
	E	30	17	9	2	1	1	1								3									1								
s	G	56	39	1		1	1	2	1			3				2		13	1			6	1	2	4				1	1	1		
	E	70	62	28	1	1					2					2		6	4	2					1	1	1	13					
ʃ	G	60	50	1				2		1		3		1		3	11	11				3	1		2	8		1					
	E	80	63	26		2	2	2		1	2	1	6			6		2	2	2	1				2	2		10			1	1	1

Note: Shaded areas contain acceptable variants (slight backing [>], slight degrooving [sᶿ] or slight grooving [θˢ]). **Bold** indicates higher proportions.

Confounds were reduced in the study by (a) matching the groups for age, gender and typicality, (b) hiring phonetically trained students to do narrow transcriptions under supervision and according to a transcription protocol, (c) examining only those fricatives common to the two languages by word position in monosyllables and trochaic disyllables and (d) using a match-proportion analysis to reduce the impact of unequal numbers of tokens per target. However, the two samples of children differed in overall severity of PPD: the German children appeared significantly more advanced, with a 10% higher Whole Word Match.

Universal Tendencies (Articulatory Complexity)

As predicted, /f/ (a visible, labial voiceless fricative) was the most advanced fricative for both languages (despite being less frequent than /v/ in German and /s/ in English). For sibilants overall, the match proportions were lower than 40%, and thus the data are ambiguous as to the relative advancement of the three fricatives: /s/, /z/, /ʃ/. Both groups of children showed a slightly higher match for /z/ compared with /ʃ/ word-initially (Figure 5.2), and for /s/ compared with /ʃ/ word-finally. This met expectations that the default [+anterior] (alveolar) would be more advanced than the nondefault [−anterior] (palatoalveolar). The English-speaking children, however, had a slightly higher match for /ʃ/ word-medially than for /s/ and /z/ (despite /ʃ/ being less frequent). (See below.)

Other universal tendencies were observed for mismatch types. For the English-speaking children, who were overall developmentally less advanced, the highest proportion of deletion occurred word-finally as expected (onsets less likely to delete than codas). The least deletion occurred word-medially (although the glottal replacement in word-initial position may or may not have indicated deletion). Word-medially, [+continuant] fricatives are supported by the surrounding [+continuant] vowels, possibly enhancing the opportunity for fricative realization. The glottal stop (although [−continuant]) can function as a minimally specified syllable-boundary marker.

Regarding features, there was a predicted developmental trend, with manner mismatches and complex mismatches (combinations of Manner and/or Place and/or Laryngeal) more common in the developmentally less advanced children (English) and place mismatches more common in the more advanced children (German). Stops were the most common of the manner substitutions in both languages, and sonorants the least common (as expected). Subsidiary place substitutions were more common than major place substitutions (as expected), and many of the major place changes reflected place assimilation (harmony). Laryngeal mismatches were overall higher in onsets than codas for English (there were no voiced targets word-finally in the sample) and were slightly higher word-initially in German than word-medially (although there were more opportunities, i.e., both /v/ and /z/ word-initially but only /z/ word-medially). Because glottal stops were frequent word-medially in English and were counted as substitutions, not deletions, these probably affected the outcomes for laryngeal mismatches word-medially (not matching in [spread glottis] for voiceless fricatives).

Possible Language-Specific Frequency Effects

The German-speaking children showed more advanced production of /v/ as predicted by word-initial phoneme frequency (Institut für Informatik Universität Leipzig, 2013). Furthermore, /f/ was also more advanced than in English, despite a similar phoneme frequency level. Because sibilant development was overall equivalent between the languages, it seems unlikely that the higher match for /f/ in German reflects overall advanced development. The German /f/ may have benefited from the overall higher frequency of [+labiodental] in German, i.e., a feature frequency effect rather than a phoneme frequency effect. An unexpected difference between languages was the significantly higher proportion of devoicing of /v/ in substitutions in German, possibly influenced by the relative advancement of the voiceless counterpart, /f/, and the greater complexity of voiced fricatives articulatorily.

The palatoalveolar sibilant /ʃ/ and the voiced sibilant /z/ were slightly more advanced in English than their German counterparts. This was somewhat unexpected, because word-initial /z/ is far more frequent in German than English, and /s/ is far more frequent in English than /z/. An examination of word-initial /s/ in English (external to the current analysis) showed a match proportion of 7%, i.e., lower than for /z/. Thus, feature frequency for [+anterior] fricatives in English did not appear to enhance the accuracy of word-initial /z/, at least in terms of accuracy for /s/.

For mismatch patterns, there were significant differences between the languages, as noted above in the discussion of universal tendencies. The relatively high proportion of ungrooved substitutions for sibilants (both dental and lateral) in German is consistent with Fox and Dodd (1999) and may reflect more advanced development of the German group (subsidiary place features being the last to develop). In terms of manner mismatches, the German children showed more affricate substitutions than the English, possibly reflecting the higher proportion of affricates in German. Furthermore, the German speakers replaced fricatives with a higher proportion of [Dorsal] stops, affricates and fricatives than the English speakers, possibly reflecting the German phonetic inventory, which includes [ç]-[x] and /ʁ/. Overall, the English speakers showed more laryngeal mismatches, which was predictable from the higher type frequency of [+voiced] fricatives in English.

Other Factors

Other factors may also have promoted between-language differences. Word frequency and familiarity may or may not have influenced outcomes. The English test word for word-initial /z/ was *zipper*, a frequent word for children, which may have promoted higher matches for /z/ in English; however, the German test words *Sonne* ('sun') and *Saft* ('juice') are also frequent words for children, and *Sonne* has only coronal consonants. (*Saft* is arguably more complex, with its cluster and coronal-labial-coronal sequence.) The English word for word-medial /ʃ/ was *station*, a word with an initial cluster (which did not usually match the target), yet the /ʃ/ was overall more accurate than the /ʃ/ of *Dusche* and *Flasche* in German, both relatively frequent words, only one of which has an initial cluster. The word-medial /ʃ/ of *station* was also more accurate than the word-medial /z/ of *scissors* and the word-medial /s/ of *whistle* in English. Whereas adults say *whistle* less often to children than *scissors* or *station*, *scissors* is spoken to children more frequently than *station* according to MacWhinney and Snow (1990, CHILDES) (although gas and train stations may be interesting to children). The effects of word frequency across or even within languages are unclear relative to phoneme accuracy in acquisition but need to be considered as a possible confounding factor.

Finally, in participant sample sizes of 30, individual differences may affect the outcome, especially considering the wide age range (3 to 5 years). The English sample accounted for 9/10 of the lowest Whole Word Match scores (0%–5%) and only 4/10 of the highest Whole Word Match scores (28%–51%). Between-language differences for the various analyses reflect at least in part the significant difference between the groups' overall phonological development levels even though overall fricative match proportions were similar.

Conclusion

The data appear to show both universal and language-specific tendencies in the development of fricatives for children with PPD in German and English. The observed trends in the literature—the role of articulatory complexity and the roles of phoneme and feature frequency in overriding complexity—are supported by the current study. Future research is needed with larger sample sizes across a variety of languages and with similar types of words for elicitation.

ACKNOWLEDGMENTS

We would like to thank the Social Sciences and Humanities Research Council of Canada, the British Columbia Health Research Foundation and the University of Cologne, Germany, for project funding. We also acknowledge and thank the analysis assistants for the project, Amanda Pack and Clara Liu (English) and Angela Ullrich, Silvia Mack, Lisa Leonhardt and Janine Lebeter (German).

NOTES

1 The [−consonantal], [+sonorant] /h/ is not included in the study; fricatives are designated here as [+consonantal] and [−sonorant].
2 The palatal [ç] and dorsal [x] may be considered allophones, the latter occurring in the context of back vowels and the former in the context of front vowels (Wiese, 1996).
3 In Schmitt, Howard and Schmitt (1983) Whole Word Match means for English were 70% at age 3;0, 80% at age 4;0 and 90% at age 5;0.
4 Intervocalic consonants in the two languages might be alternately viewed as onsets (syllable-initial-within-word) or ambisyllabic (Bernhardt & Stemberger, 1998).
5 The symbol [s$^\theta$] indicates an alveolar or dental place of articulation with slightly less *grooving* than a typical [s]. The dental diacritic [s̪] is not used because children at this age generally produce /s/ in a dental location in any case (even though grooved) and the /s/ in many adult languages is a [+grooved] dental sibilant.

REFERENCES

Arlt, P.B. & Goodban, M.T. (1976). A comparative study of articulation acquisition as based on a study of 240 normals aged three to six. *Language, Speech, and Hearing Services in Schools, 7,* 173–180.

Bernhardt, B.H. & Stemberger, J.P. (1998). *Handbook of phonological development: From the perspective of constraint-based nonlinear phonology.* San Diego, CA: Academic Press (now published in Bingley, UK: Emerald).

Clark, H.H. (1973). The language-as-fixed-effect fallacy: A critique of language statistics in psychological research. *Journal of Verbal Learning and Verbal Behavior, 12*, 335–359.

Dodd, B., Holm, A., Hua, Z. & Crosbie, S. (2003). Phonological development: A normative study of British-speaking children. *Clinical Linguistics and Phonetics, 17(8)*, 617–643.

Dunn, L.M. & Dunn, L.M. (1997). *Peabody Picture Vocabulary Test.* Circle Pines, MN: American Guidance Service.

Fongaro-Levorin, S. (1992). *Der Erwerb des Lautsystems und die phonologischen Prozesse sich normal entwickelnder Kinder: Ein interlinguistischer Vergleich Deutsch/Portugiesisch.* Unpublished doctoral dissertation, Ludwig-Maximilians-Universität, Munich, Germany.

Fox, A.V. & Dodd, B.J. (1999). Der Erwerb des phonologischen Systems in der deutschen Sprache. *Sprache, Stimme und Gehör, 23*, 183–191.

Fox, A.V. & Dodd, B. (2001). Phonologically disordered German-speaking children. *American Journal of Speech-Language Pathology, 10*, 291–307.

Goldsmith, J. (1979/1976). *Autosegmental phonology.* Milton Park, UK: Garland. (Published version of MIT dissertation, 1976).

Grimm, H. (2001). *Sprachentwicklungstest für drei- bis fünfjährige Kinder.* Göttingen, Germany: Hogrefe.

Grohnfeldt, M. (1980). Erhebung zum altersspezifischen Lautbestand bei drei- bis sechsjährigen Kindern. *Die Sprachheilarbeit, 25*, 169–177.

Hacker, D. & Weiß, K.-H. (1986). *Zur phonemischen Struktur funktioneller Dyslalien.* Oldenburg, Germany: Verlag Arbeiterwohlfahrt.

Haelsig, P.C. & Madison, C.L. (1986). A study of phonological processes exhibited by 3-, 4-, and 5-year-old children. *Language, Speech and Hearing Services in Schools, 7*, 107–114.

Ingram, D. (1978). The acquisition of fricatives and affricates in normal and linguistically deviant children. In A. Caramazza & E. Zurif (eds.), *The acquisition and breakdown of language* (pp. 63–85). Baltimore, MD: Johns Hopkins University Press.

Ingram, D. (1988). The acquisition of word initial [v]. *Language and Speech, 31*, 77–85.

Institut für Informatik Universität Leipzig. (2013). Wortschatz Universität Leipzig. http//:corpora-informatik.uni-leipzig.de/?dict=de.

Kaufman, A. & Kaufman, N. (1994). *Kaufman-Assessment Battery for Children (K-ABC).* Amsterdam: Swets & Zeitlinger.

Kehoe, M.M. & Lleó, C. (2002). Intervocalic consonants in the acquisition of German: Onsets, codas or something else? *Clinical Linguistics & Phonetics, 16*, 169–182.

Leonard, L. (1992). Models of phonological development and children with phonological disorders. In C. Ferguson, L. Menn & C. Stoel-Gammon (eds.), *Phonological development: Models, research, implications* (pp. 495–507). Parkston, MD: York Press.

Lippke, B.A., Dickey, S.E., Selmar, J.W. & Soder, A.L. (1997). *Photo articulation test*—Third Edition. Austin, TX: Pro-Ed.

Masterson, J.J. & Bernhardt, B.H. (2001). *Computerized Articulation and Phonology Evaluation System* (CAPES). San Antonio, TX: Harcourt Assessment (copyright reverted to authors, 2013).

MacWhinney, B. & Snow, C. (1990). The Child Language Data Exchange System (CHILDES): An update. *Journal of Child Language, 17,* 457–472.

Microsoft. (2010). Microsoft Excel [computer software]. Redmond, WA: Microsoft.

Miller, G.A. & Nicely, P.E. (1955). An analysis of perceptual confusions among some English consonants. *Journal of the Acoustical Society of America, 27,* 338–352.

Prather, E.M., Hedrick, D.L. & Kern, C.A. (1975). Articulation development in children 2–4 years. *Journal of Speech and Hearing Disorders, 40,* 179–191.

Pye, C., Ingram, D. & List, H. (1987). A comparison of initial consonant acquisition in English and Quiche. In K.E. Nelson & A. van Kleeck (eds.), *Children's language,* Vol. 6 (pp. 175–190). Hillsdale, NJ: Lawrence Erlbaum.

Richtmeister, P., Gerken, L. & Ohala, D. (2011). Contributions of phonetic token variability and word-type frequency to phonological representations. *Journal of Child Language, 38,* 951–978.

Schmitt, L.S., Howard, B.H. & Schmitt, J.F. (1983). Conversational speech sampling in the assessment of articulation proficiency. *Language, Speech, and Hearing Services in Schools, 14,* 210–214.

Smit, A.B. (2007). General American English speech acquisition. In S. McLeod (ed.), *The international guide to speech acquisition* (pp. 128–147). Clifton Park, NY: Thomson Delmar Learning.

Smit, A.B., Hand, L., Freilinger, J.J., Bernthal, J.E. & Bird, A. (1990). The Iowa Articulation Norms Project and its Nebraska replication. *Journal of Speech and Hearing Disorders, 55,* 779–798.

SPSS Inc. (2003). *SPSS for Windows Version 12.0.* Chicago, IL: SPSS Inc.

Templin, M.C. (1957). *Certain language skills in children* (Monograph Series No. 26). Minneapolis: University of Minnesota, the Institute of Child Welfare.

Ullrich, A. (2011). *Evidenzbasierte Diagnostik phonologischer Störungen. Entwicklung eines Sprachanalyseverfahrens auf der Basis nichtlinearer phonologischer Theorien*. Unpublished doctoral dissertation, University of Cologne, Germany.

Van Borsel, J., Van Rentergem, S. & Verhaeghe, L. (2007). The prevalence of lisping in young adults. *Journal of Communication Disorders, 40,* 493–502.

Wiese, R. (1996). *The phonology of German.* Oxford: Clarendon.

Wiig, E., Secord, W. & Semel, E. (1992). *Clinical Evaluation of Language Fundamentals—Preschool.* San Antonio, TX: Pearson Assessment (formerly Harcourt).

6

PRE- AND POST-TREATMENT PRODUCTION OF SYLLABLE INITIAL /ʁ/-CLUSTERS BY CHILDREN SPEAKING QUÉBEC FRENCH

Susan Rvachew and Françoise Brosseau-Lapré

One motivation for the study of phonological acquisition across groups of children with different experiences, such as in cross-linguistic or clinical studies, is to allow the identification of universal constraints on well-formedness that explain patterns of acquisition within and between children. Given the hypothesis that linguistic constraints may be grounded in acoustic or articulatory phonetics, another motivation is the possibility of identifying variables that explain the emergence of these constraints, by taking into account both common patterns and individual differences in the child data (for discussion, see Fikkert & de Hoop, 2009).

In this chapter we describe children's productions of 15 words containing two-element /ʁ/-clusters, which in French are legal in word initial and word internal onsets (Dell, 1995). The children are preschool aged francophones who were receiving intervention for the remediation of their speech delay in Montréal, Québec, as part of a moderately large randomized controlled trial examining the impact of speech therapy on phonological awareness and emergent literacy outcomes. The 21 children described in this report are a subset of the total sample, selected because they received treatment specifically targeting /ʁ/-clusters, and thus we had access to pre- and post-treatment probes, obtained 6 weeks apart. The analyses applied to these data are necessarily post hoc given that the probes were administered for the purpose of measuring the efficacy of the treatment and not for the purpose of testing any linguistic hypotheses. Nonetheless, our meditation on the factors that may have influenced the children's patterns of errors and patterns of change in the production of these words (other than the specifics of the treatment program itself) may illuminate general principles of phonological development.

PHONOLOGICAL ACQUISITION IN FRENCH

MacLeod, Sutton, Trudeau, and Thordardottir (2011) describe consonant acquisition for 156 children aged 20 to 53 months speaking Québec French. These researchers employed a picture naming task to target all 20 consonants in the language, specifically, the nasals /m, n, ɲ/; the voiceless unaspirated stops /p, t, k/; the pre-voiced stops /b, d, g/; the voiceless and voiced fricatives /f, s, ʃ, v, z, ʒ/; the liquid /l/; the uvular fricative rhotic /ʁ/; and the glides /w, j, ɥ/. Mastery age was reported for each phoneme as the age at which a given consonant was produced accurately by 90% or more of the children in initial, medial, and final position of words. All consonants were mastered by 53 months of age except /s, ʃ, ʒ, j/, although customary production (i.e., produced correctly by 50% of the children) was achieved for these late developing phonemes before 53 months of age. With regard to clusters, /bl/, /fl/, and /kʁ/ were mastered in the word initial position during the preschool period. The children were still having some difficulties with /fʁ/ and /tʁ/ at the age of 53 months. Using a different word set (the Test de Dépistage Francophone de Phonologie), we examined consonant acquisition in children attending *maternelle* and *première année* classrooms in Québec (Rvachew et al., 2013). The /tʁ/ cluster was produced correctly by more than 90% of these children aged at least 67 months (unfortunately, the screening test does not sample /fʁ/). These data suggest that most phonemes are mastered earlier in French than in English (for comparison to English norms, see Smit, 1993) but that some ʁ-clusters are relatively late developing in (Québec) French.

POTENTIAL INFLUENCES ON /ʁ/-CLUSTER ACQUISITION IN FRENCH

We will consider factors that may influence the children's acquisition of /ʁ/-clusters across three levels of representation: acoustic-phonetic, articulatory-phonetic, and phonological. With respect to acoustic-phonetic representations, it has been established that perceptual salience plays an important role in early phonological development in English (Echols, 1993; Snow, 1998); specifically, patterns of syllable deletion and segment weakening by young children can be predicted by the prosodic structure of the target utterances, with unstressed syllables being particularly vulnerable to incomplete representation by the child. Although concerned with adult patterns of cluster simplification, Coté (2004) similarly suggests that predictable error patterns by speakers of Québec French are "perceptually motivated" (p. 151). In order to consider the potential impact of perceptual salience on error patterns observed in our data, we assessed the children's ability to produce syllable initial /ʁ/-clusters in five single-syllable words (hereafter denoted /^{cc}σ/), five 2-syllable words with the cluster in the first unstressed syllable (hereafter denoted /^{cc}σσ/), and five 2-syllable words with the cluster in the second stressed syllable (hereafter denoted /σ^{cc}σ/). Foot structure in French is right-headed, with the second syllable in 2-syllable words being perceptually more salient (Rose, 2000) due to the usual acoustic correlates of stress, with longer duration being a particularly reliable characteristic of these word final syllables (Fant, Kruckenberg, & Nord, 1991; Jun & Fougeron, 2002; Ménard & Thibeault, 2009). Although explanations for this phenomenon vary somewhat, it has been documented that deletions and misarticulations of consonants by toddlers increase in unstressed contexts (Rose, 2000; Vihman, 2006; Wauquier & Yamaguchi, 2014). Therefore, it is expected that even in this sample of older children, cluster accuracy will vary with prosodic pattern: specifically, accuracy should decline with prominence of the syllable in order from /^{cc}σ/ words to the /σ^{cc}σ/ words to the /^{cc}σσ/ words. Changes in accuracy over time might also proceed in this order with improvements being least for the /^{cc}σσ/ words compared with the other two word patterns.

With respect to articulatory-phonetic factors, the /ʁ/ is described as a uvular fricative phonetically although its phonetic and phonological status is highly unstable: in Québec French multiple phonetic variants are possible (specifically [ʁ, ʀ, r, ɹ]) within and between talkers, and the feature specification is ambiguous with respect to place, manner, and voicing (Coté, 2004; Martin, 1996; Rose & dos Santos, 2010). At least two studies have found that /l/-clusters are acquired earlier than /ʁ/-clusters in French, a finding that was attributed to the articulatory difficulty of this phoneme (Kehoe, Hilaire-Debove, Demuth, & Lleó, 2008; MacLeod et al., 2011). Rose (2000) further suggested that the "placelessness" of this phoneme plays a role in its late emergence: regardless of its phonological specification, the variable articulatory manner features in Québec French may create enough ambiguity in the input to complicate acquisition of productive accuracy, especially since all the variants might be considered to be composed of difficult articulatory gestures (Coté, 2004; Friesner, 2010; Rose & Wauquier-Gravelines, 2007; Sankoff & Blondeau, 2007). Therefore, we expect that the ability to produce this phone will be correlated with overall cluster accuracy and growth in cluster accuracy from time 1 to time 2. It is further expected that the coarticulatory challenge of producing two abutting consonants must be overcome by the child before these clusters can be correctly produced; examination of the forms that appear in the children's output may reveal a preference for productions involving Dorsal + [ʁ] (no change in articulatory place), followed by Labial + [ʁ] (coordination of separate articulators) and finally Coronal + [ʁ] (coordination of articulatory place within a single articulator) among those children who are capable of producing the [ʁ] (following from a review of studies of the development of inter- and intra-articulator coordination in Rvachew and Brosseau-Lapré, 2012).

Finally, we consider phonological factors in relation to the proposal put forward by Jongstra (2003), on the basis of an examination of cluster development in Dutch-speaking children, to explain within and between child variability in the acquisition of clusters. Jongstra suggested that some variability reflects different developmental stages: at an earlier stage, the child selects the onset head from the input on the basis of relative sonority so that the word *bras* 'arm' would be represented with /b/ in the onset (head) whereas the /ʁ/ would not be prosodified; this representation would lead to the production [ba]. At a later stage, both elements would be prosodified in the onset of the syllable resulting in an appropriate output, [bʁa]. This same child might, however, be confused about the prosodification of items with a flat sonority profile so that *front* 'forehead' might be represented with the /f/ as an appendix and the /ʁ/ as the head, resulting in [ʁɔ̃] until such time as the segments are reprosodified appropriately as a branching onset. This developmental proposal may explain not only differences between children but also apparent "regressions and reversals" that have been noted for cluster acquisition (McLeod, Van Doorn, & Reed, 2001a). For example, a child might progress along an uneven path with forms such as [fɔ̃] → [ʁɔ̃] → [fʁɔ̃] appearing along the way to mastery. We will examine our data in relation to Jongstra's proposal by considering patterns of reduction and coalescence errors at time 1 and time 2. In these analyses we will not try to settle the issue of the proper feature specification for the Québec French /ʁ/ but will generally assume that the sonority distance for stop + /ʁ/ clusters is greater than that for the fricative + /ʁ/ clusters, being open to the possibility that the latter represent a flat sonority profile.

METHOD

Participants

The participants were 21 preschool aged francophone children who were recruited from the greater Montréal area. These children were part of a larger sample that received treatment for speech delay and emergent literacy skills in the context of a randomized controlled trial. The children described in this report were selected because they misarticulated /ʁ/-clusters during the intake assessment and received treatment for this target during the course of the trial. Therefore, we had access to pre- and post-treatment /ʁ/-cluster probe data for analysis in this descriptive study. The children are described further in Table 6.1.

Procedures

All assessment sessions took place either in a quiet room at McGill University or in a testing room at the Montréal Children's Hospital. At intake the children were assessed by the second author, a certified speech-language pathologist, or by graduate speech-language pathology students under the supervision of the second author. During the intake assessment the nonverbal subtest of the Kaufman Brief Intelligence Test (Kaufman & Kaufman, 2004) was administered to ensure eligibility for participation in the study. The Échelle de Vocabulaire en Image de Pea-body (Dunn, Theriault-Whalen, & Dunn, 1993) was administered as a normed Canadian-French measure of receptive vocabulary. The Test Francophone de Phonologie (Paul & Rvachew, 2008), as described in Paul (2009), was used to assess accuracy of consonant production while naming pictures, with the global outcome expressed as the percentage

Table 6.1 Summary of Intake Test Scores for the 21 Participants

Test	Minimum	Maximum	Mean	SD
Age (months)	46.00	63.00	54.86	4.36
Percentage of French exposure at home	60.00	100.00	90.95	15.01
Percentage of French exposure at daycare	100.00	100.00	100.00	100.00
Kaufman Brief Intelligence Test (Nonverbal)	82.00	124.00	102.38	12.07
Échelles de Vocabulaire en Images de Peabody	69.00	133.00	92.71	16.35
PCC in conversation	56.27	94.39	76.88	9.08
Test Francophone de Phonologie—PCC	37.89	85.70	68.27	13.35

Note: PCC is percentage of consonants correct. More details about the intake assessment procedures are available in Brosseau-Lapré and Rvachew (2014).

of consonants correct (PCC). At this time the parent completed a number of questionnaires regarding the child's development including a detailed inventory of language exposure from birth in home and child care environments. Other measures of phonological processing abilities not reported here were also administered.

Approximately 4 to 6 weeks later, a pre-treatment assessment was conducted by a graduate student research assistant. A conversational speech sample was recorded while the child and examiner discussed the wordless book *You're a Good Dog, Carl* by Alexandra Day. This speech sample was used to calculate the PCC in conversation. Single-word probes were administered to assess articulation of phonemes or prosodic structures that would be targeted in speech therapy. The child was asked to name pictures of items to elicit productions of these therapy targets. Each child received treatment for three targets, and therefore three probes that each elicited 15 single-word productions were administered (the three targets per child are listed in Appendix A). Then the child received six treatment sessions, one per week, each targeting /ʁ/-clusters for one-third of the 45-minute treatment session. This treatment block was followed by a post-treatment probe (identical to the pre-treatment probe), administered in the 7th week. The probes were administered by a student who had no involvement in the child's treatment program and was unaware of the procedures that were used to help the child achieve improved speech accuracy or phonological processing skills. The procedure for administering the probes involved a delayed imitation task: the child was shown the probe items, five at a time, on a computer screen; the research assistant named all five items and then asked the child to do the same. The procedure was repeated for the remaining slides. The probe administration procedure was the same during the pre- and post-treatment assessments (hereafter referred to as time 1 and time 2 respectively). In this report we describe the data only for the /ʁ/-probe, which elicited (in order as shown) the following 15 words during time 1 and time 2: *bras* 'arm' /ˈbʁa/, *front* 'forehead' /ˈfʁɔ̃/, *crêpes* 'pancakes' /ˈkʁɛp/, *frites* 'fries' /ˈfʁit/, *griffes* 'claws' /ˈgʁif/, *cravate* 'tie' /kʁaˈvat/, *fromage* 'cheese' /fʁɔˈmaʒ/, *dragon* 'dragon' /dʁaˈgɔ̃/, *brochette* 'kebab' /bʁɔ̃ˈʃɛt/, *trophée* 'trophy' /tʁoˈfe/, *écran* 'computer screen' /eˈkʁɑ̃/, *citron* 'lemon' /siˈtʁɔ̃/, *micro* 'microphone' /miˈkʁo/, *batterie* 'drums' /baˈtʁi/, and *chevreuil* 'male deer' /ʃəˈvʁœj/.

Each assessment was videorecorded with a Sony Handycam HDR-XR520 or a JVC Everio GZ-MG360 videocamera (using the internal microphone and Dolby digital 5.1 sound recording system). Audio files were extracted from the video recordings and saved as .wav files. Narrow phonetic transcriptions of the participants' responses to the probe were completed by a research assistant, who reviewed each file at least three times. If a child produced the same target more than once, the clearer recording was transcribed; if productions of the same target were equally clear, the first one was transcribed. The second author completed narrow phonetic transcriptions of 20% of the probes independently. Transcription agreement with the second author for narrow transcription of the target consonants on the probes was 96% (range = 88% to 100%). The raw data are reproduced in Appendix B by child, word, and assessment time.

Results and Discussion

Acoustic-Phonetic Factors

The first analyses determined accuracy of cluster production as a function of syllable number and syllable stress. Three measures of cluster accuracy were calculated. The first is the most straightforward, being a simple count of the number of clusters produced completely correctly. The second measure is a count of the number of the segments included without regard to their accuracy; in other words, /bʁa/ → [bʁa] or [bwa] would both receive a score of 2, and /bʁa/ → [ʁa] or [ga] would both receive a score of 1. A final measure reflects the proportion of features that were matched across the two target segments, using feature specifications described in Bérubé, Bernhardt, and Stemberger (2013). For example, the target /dʁ/ was credited with a total number of 6 specified features: [+consonantal] and [+voice] for the first segment and [+consonantal], [+sonorant], [+continuant], and Dorsal for the second segment. If the child produced [d] in place of this cluster, a score of 2/6 would be assigned, crediting matches for [+consonantal] and [+voice] for the first segment but no matches for the features of the second segment. If, on the other hand, the child produced [gʁ], a score of 6/6 would be assigned, crediting a match for all features of both segments despite the incorrect segment in the C1 position.

Figure 6.1 presents the three measures of cluster production by word, aggregated across participants, and arranged by stress pattern. Focusing first on the time 1 data, it is apparent that all three measures of production accuracy show an advantage for stressed syllables, especially in single-syllable words, over the unstressed syllables. The numbers of correctly produced clusters on average were 9.6 (/^{cc}σ/ items), 7.4 (/σ^{cc}σ/ items), and 4.6 (/^{cc}σσ/ items), with the maximum score being 21. The average scores for number of segments included were 36.6 (/^{cc}σ/ items), 34.8 (/σ^{cc}σ/ items), and 31.4 (/^{cc}σσ/ items), with the maximum score being 42 when aggregating across children. Finally, feature

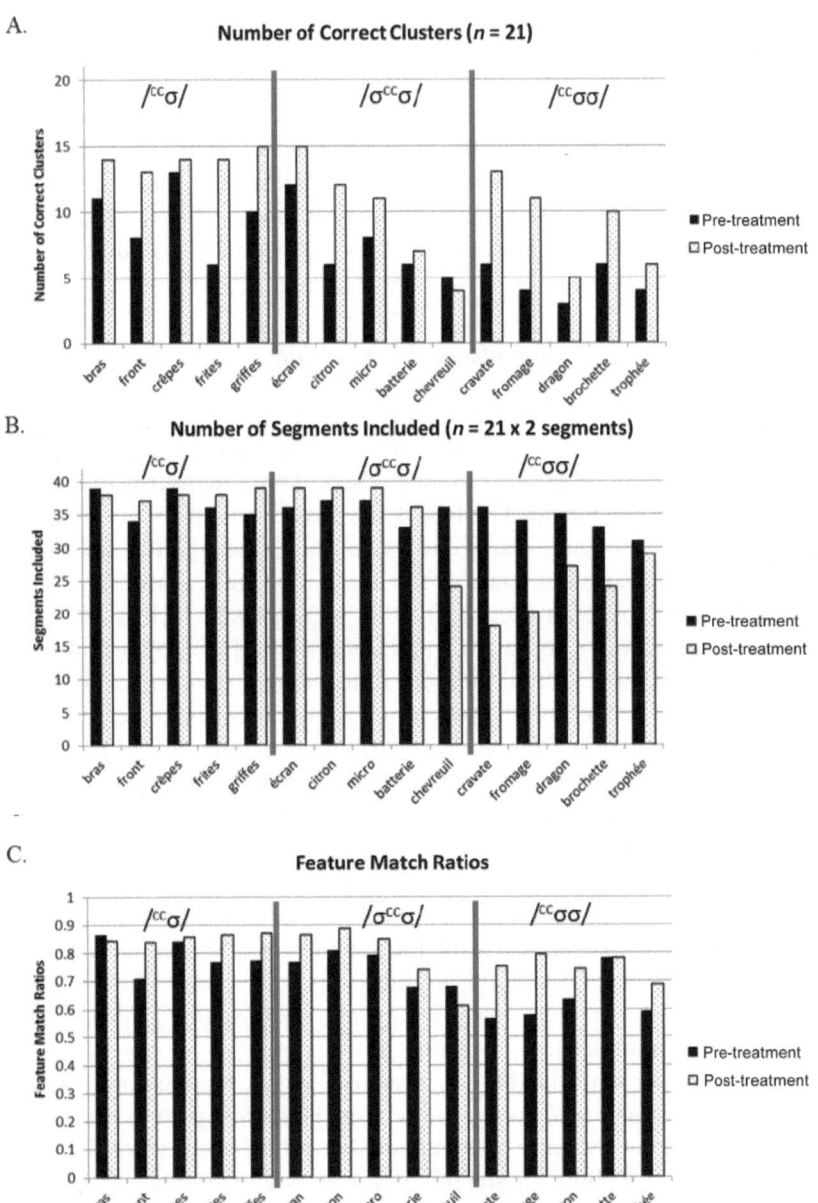

Figure 6.1 Three measures of cluster production accuracy by word aggregated across participants.

match ratios indicate a similar pattern, with the scores being 0.79 (/^{cc}σ/ items), 0.75 (/σ^{cc}σ/ items), and 0.63 (/^{cc}σσ/ items). Production accuracy is somewhat improved at time 2 by all three measures, but the same pattern is retained: the scores for the /^{cc}σ/, /σ^{cc}σ/, and /^{cc}σσ/ contexts were as follows: 14.0, 9.8, and 9.0 for the number of correctly produced clusters; 38.0, 36.4, and 34.8 for the number of segments included; and 0.85, 0.79, and 0.75 for feature match ratios.

These data clearly indicate that the children achieved greater accuracy in the production of these clusters in stressed syllables. When the target cluster occurred in the onset of a syllable that had less perceptual salience, however, less accuracy was observed on average. At the same time, considerable variability was observed within similar syllable types. For example, accuracy was higher for *brochette* than *dragon* and for *écran* than *batterie*.

Articulatory-Phonetic Factors

The first issue to be considered was the impact of having access to articulatory knowledge of the [ʁ] phone on cluster accuracy at time 1 and on improvements in cluster accuracy between time 1 and time 2. Although it seems rather banal to conclude that one cannot produce a correct /ʁ/-cluster without access to the /ʁ/ phone, the rule seems to be observed with surprising consistency given that the children received speech therapy to remediate their cluster errors. Two children produced no correct tokens of this phoneme and one child produced only one during the time 1 probe. These three children made no progress toward acquisition of these clusters when measured as the number of correct clusters at time 2. Participant 1101 reduced all clusters at times 1 and 2. Participant 2108 produced 12 simplified clusters (i.e., glides substituted for /ʁ/) and 2 reduced clusters at time 1, with the only improvement being an increase to 13 simplifications at time 2 (this child was reported to have 100% French exposure at home and daycare, and thus the glide substitution may reflect the influence of English in Québec society generally but not in this child's input specifically). Participant 5110 reduced all the target clusters on both probes except for one simplified token at time 1. The most impressive gains were made by children who produced only three correct tokens of /ʁ/ at time 1. Children who produced many correct tokens of /ʁ/ at time 1 showed only small improvements, largely because they tended to have very good accuracy at the single-word level prior to treatment.

Turning to the impact of coarticulatory factors, Table 6.2 presents the frequency with which specific types of production patterns were observed in the children's output. The correct realizations of the target

Table 6.2 Counts of Time 1 and Time 2 Types of Cluster Realizations by Target Type Aggregated across Children

Time 1 Target

	Time 1 Cluster Realizations (Count)																
	ʁ	LS	LF	LSg	LFg	LSʁ	LFʁ	CS	CF	CSg	CSʁ	DS	DSg	DSʁ	O	Total	Correct (%)
LSʁ	1	8		12		*17	1			1				2		42	40
LFʁ	4	1	23	1	18	1	*23		3					2	4	84	27
CSʁ	4							25		7	*19	6	4	17	2	84	23
DSʁ	3						1	6		3		25	16	*50	1	105	48
Total	12	9	23	13	18	18	25	32	3	10	20	32	22	71	7	315	35

Time 2 Target

	Time 2 Cluster Realizations (Count)																
	ʁ	LS	LF	LSg	LFg	LSʁ	LFʁ	CS	CF	CSg	CSʁ	DS	DSg	DSʁ	O	Total	Correct (%)
LSʁ	1	8		3		*25	1							2	2	42	60
LFʁ	3	9	13		10	1	*42							1	3	84	50
CSʁ	3	2						11		2	*30	7	3	21	4	84	36
DSʁ	1						1	1			4	15	10	*68	6	105	65
Total	8	19	13	3	10	26	44	12	0	2	34	24	13	92	15	315	52

Note: Target and actual cluster realizations are denoted with the first segment in capital letters and the second segment in lower case letters as follows: L = labial, C = coronal, D = dorsal, S = stop, F = fricative, g = glide (i.e., [w] or [j]), ʁ = uvular approximant/fricative, and O = other types that involved nasal, liquid /l/, or affricate substitutions as well as resyllabifications including epenthesis and metathesis. The asterisk (*) marks the correct match for place and manner in each row.

with respect to place and manner are marked with an asterisk in the table. It can be seen that correct productions increased from 35% to 52% from time 1 to time 2 overall. The pattern of correct responding corresponded to our expectations before and following treatment with correct tokens observed most frequently for Dorsal targets, followed by Labial targets and then least frequently for Coronal targets. Labial targets were probed with a frequency of 40%, but Labial types were observed in 33% of the output forms at time 1, increasing to 37% at time 2. Dorsal targets were probed with a frequency of 33%, but Dorsal types were observed in 40% of the children's productions at both time 1 and time 2. Coronal targets were probed with a frequency of only 27% but were observed even less often in the children's output, with Coronal types occurring in 10% and 15% of the children's productions at times 1 and 2 respectively. The under-representation of Labial and Coronal types in the children's output is almost entirely explained by the over-appearance of Dorsal types in these contexts. The preponderance of Dorsal types is not restricted to tokens with [ʁ] in the C2 position but also occurs for tokens that involve simplification to a glide; in these cases, the glides were [w] or [j] with the occurrences being 15:7 at time 1 and 7:6 at time 2 for these two options respectively. Furthermore, this pattern of Dorsal types appearing frequently in place of Coronal targets and occasionally in place of Labial targets occurred for reduced realizations of the cluster as well as those realizations that included two segments. These last two observations suggest that ease of coarticulation between a Dorsal stop and the [ʁ] is not the only probable explanation for the preponderance of Dorsal + [ʁ] types in the children's productions, and therefore we turn our attention to phonological factors.

Phonological Factors

Jongstra (2003) proposed a "sonority stage" as an early period of cluster development in which children select the least sonorant segment as the head of the onset; during this stage, the second segment in the input would not be prosodified and would be omitted from the output. As mentioned previously, Participants 1102 and 5110 reduced every cluster at times 1 and 2 (with the anomaly of a single /bʁ/ → [bw] production by Participant 5110 at time 1). The remaining 59 productions examined for these two children involved production of the C1 consonant (e.g., /fʁ/ → [f]) or a close match to the C1 consonant (e.g., /dʁ/ → [g]). Given the assumption that the true fricatives /f, v/ are less sonorant than /ʁ/, these cases are consistent with Jongstra's prediction with respect to their reduction patterns. It is not clear that these two children can be characterized as being at a uniformly "early" stage of phonological development: Participant 1102 obtained a PCC of 37.89 on the Test Francophone de Phonologie, suggesting profoundly delayed phonological development; on the other hand, Participant 5110 obtained a PCC of 80.70 on this test, indicating a more advanced level of phonological development overall although this child had significant difficulties with prosodic structure (involving, for example, syllable marking and inclusion of word final and word internal codas despite good knowledge of consonantal segments). Nonetheless, consistent cluster reduction shows that these two children presented with significant phonological delay, and it is also clear that they made very slow progress in speech therapy.

Jongstra (2003) further proposes that children progress to the "head" stage, during which time both segments are prosodified with the relationship between head and dependent determined according to the sonority distance between the segments. Initially there may be confusion about the prosodification of items that involve two segments that are very close in sonority. In particular, onsets with a relatively flat sonority profile may be prosodified with the C1 segment represented as an appendix and the C2 segment as the head. Following from data on reduction of /s/-clusters in English (e.g., Yavaş & McLeod, 2010), it is reasonable to assume that C1 will be particularly vulnerable to deletion in these contexts, leading to two specific hypotheses: first, the appearance of [ʁ] only tokens should co-occur with higher cluster correct scores, indicating that the child is at a later stage of cluster development than we observed for Participants 1102 and 5110; and, second, the appearance of these tokens should be associated with targets that have a flat sonority profile (i.e., /fʁ/, /vʁ/).

Table 6.2 shows that there were 12 instances of [ʁ] only tokens at time 1, and 8 instances of this output pattern at time 2. Three children produced [ʁ] only tokens at time 1. Participant 4108 produced 9 correct clusters, 5 simplified clusters, and 1 [ʁ] only token, the latter in place of the /vʁ/ in *chevreuil*. At time 2 this child produced 11 correct clusters and no [ʁ] only tokens. Participant 6111 produced 11 correct clusters and 4 reduced clusters, of which 2 were [ʁ] only tokens, specifically for the words *batterie* and *citron*. One of these [ʁ] only tokens reappeared at time 2, in the word *citron*. Participant 6113 produced 5 correct clusters, 1 null onset, and 9 [ʁ] only tokens. Of these 9 [ʁ] only tokens, only 3 involved a fricative in the C1 position; the remaining cases of deleted stops in C1 position were in the unstressed syllable or the word final syllable. The only instance that remained at time 2 was for the word *chevreuil*. Regarding the 8 instances of [ʁ] only tokens at time 2, we have addressed the 2 that were produced by Participants 6111 and 6113. Participants 3107 and 4107 produced 3 each of the remaining [ʁ] only tokens, and again these instances involved both stops and fricatives in the C1 position, with one of these occurring in a word initial stressed context.

With respect to Jongstra's proposal, it is clear that these children who reduced to the /ʁ/ in C2 position were at a much higher level of cluster development than those children who consistently reduced to the C1 segment: specifically, all of these children produced a large proportion of completely correct clusters which is consistent with the predictions of the "head" stage being a later stage of development than the "sonority" stage. On the other hand, our specific hypothesis that [ʁ] only tokens would be more likely to appear as a substitute for fricative + [ʁ] targets than for stop + [ʁ] targets was not supported. The assumption that fricative + [ʁ] clusters are closer in sonority than stop + [ʁ] clusters was well motivated: greater sonority distance typically predicts greater accuracy in cluster production (Yavaş & McLeod, 2010), and Figure 6.1B shows lower production accuracy on average for the fricative + [ʁ] targets than for stop + [ʁ] targets. However, the distance may be close enough in both cases to create ambiguity about the identity of the head in the input, especially given the uncertain status of /ʁ/ in Québec French. Therefore, variable outcomes for these clusters may not be surprising: if the child represents this phoneme as a fricative, stop + [ʁ] and fricative + [ʁ] targets may be close enough in sonority profile to trigger confusion about the identity of the head; if the child represents this phoneme as a glide, both types of targets may be equally protected from misrepresentation with an appendix. Even this explanation is not fully satisfying, however, because these children who produced [ʁ] only tokens also produced simplified clusters and in some cases glide only tokens (see Participant 4107 at time 2). If the children represent the /ʁ/ as a glide their clusters should be even less vulnerable to representation with the appendix structure. Furthermore, in relation to Jongstra's proposal—that there is no clear developmental progression from stop only to [ʁ] only tokens—in some cases this occurred but in others the child changed a correct stop + [ʁ] production to an [ʁ] only token. Our sense is that there are other phonetic and phonological factors at play in the particular instances of [ʁ] only tokens that we described. Given the likelihood of occurrence in unstressed syllables or word internal contexts there may be issues with perceptual salience that play a role, and it is also possible that the stop in words such as *batterie* and *citron* is syllabified as a word internal coda. In a prior report, word internal codas were deleted as frequently as 10% of the time by francophone children with speech delay although, in general, clusters were much more vulnerable to deletion (Brosseau-Lapré & Rvachew, 2014).

Even in the word initial position of single-syllable words there may be individual differences in the perceptual salience of the /ʁ/ phoneme based on the child's ability to produce the phoneme. In other words, following Vihman's hypothesized "articulatory filter" (Vihman, DePaolis, & Keren-Portnoy, 2009), children who have recently learned to produce this phone may subsequently develop a heightened perceptual awareness of /ʁ/ in the input. Those children who did not produce this phoneme appeared to be unaware of the phoneme and prosodified the C1 segment as the head of the onset. Those children who produced the /ʁ/ phoneme some of the time may be especially aware of the phoneme and have difficulty working out the acoustic-phonetic details of the abutting stop or fricative. In principle, this hypothesis could be explored by examining patterns of coalescence in the data. According to this proposal, spreading of Dorsal to the C1 consonant should not occur if the child never produces /ʁ/ in the C2 position (although spreading from /w/ in this position may occur for those children who consistently substitute [w] for /ʁ/). In our sample a complete absence of productive phonological knowledge of /ʁ/ was rare, but we will describe patterns of coalescence in the data set in any case.

Table 6.3 identifies the target words that were subject to Dorsal spreading and provides some details about the resulting output forms. Overall, the children produced 27 tokens that suggest Dorsal spreading within the onset for Coronal targets and 7 instances of this pattern for Labial targets at time 1. At time 2, there were 31 instances of this pattern involving Coronal targets and 5 instances involving Labial targets. At both time points, this pattern was limited to the words *dragon*, *trophée*, *citron*, and *batterie* among the Coronal targets; the words *fromage* and *brochette* were sometimes subject to Dorsal spreading despite the target C1 specified for Labial place; one instance of Dorsal spreading involving the word *bras* occurred. These exemplars of Dorsal spreading were produced by 12 children at time 1 and 17 children at time 2; of these, 15 produced instances of spreading during both probe assessments, 3 produced a few exemplars at time 1 but none at time 2, and 4 were observed to produce spreading at time 2 only. This left only three children who did not produce an instance of Dorsal spreading at either time point.

The children who produced Dorsal forms in place of Coronal and/or Labial targets at both time points, time 1 only, time 2 only, or not at all were remarkably similar with respect to their error patterns (with two exceptions to be discussed further below). These children produced a mix of obstruent + [ʁ], obstruent + glide, and obstruent only forms in their output. The production of an [ʁ] only token was somewhat less

Table 6.3 Counts of Output Forms That Represent Dorsal Spreading by Target Word and Probe Time

Child's Production	Target Word						
	dragon	*trophée*	*citron*	*batterie*	*fromage*	*brochette*	*bras*
Time 1 Probe Assessment							
g	3						
k	1	1		1	1		
gʁ	5					1	
kʁ	1	3	6	2	2	1	
gw					1		
kw		1	1	1	2		
Time 2 Probe Assessment							
g	3						
k		1	1	2	1		
gʁ	6				1	1	1
kʁ		5	4	6	1		
gw							
kw		1	1	1			

common but was observed in the output forms of 5 children as detailed above; in these children, knowledge of /ʁ/ is obvious, and thus Dorsal spreading to the obstruent in the C1 position is uncontroversial regardless of whether the C2 segment was produced correctly or produced as a glide.

The outliers in the sample included one child who produced obstruent + [ʁ] forms exclusively and two children who reduced targets to a single stop consonant at both time points. The rare occurrence of the former pattern (consistent matching of the obstruent + [ʁ] target) was of course due to selection bias since children with cluster reduction were more likely to be selected for inclusion in the study and were more likely to be treated for remediation of /ʁ/-cluster errors. The rare occurrence of the latter pattern (consistent reduction of the cluster) was likely due to the age of the children. The fact that two children evidenced a Dorsal output form in place of a Coronal target despite never producing an [ʁ] in their inventory was unexpected, however; inspection of the data reveals that this pattern occurred for the word *dragon* in these cases (see Participant 5110 at time 1 and Participant 1102 at time 2). In both instances it is likely that Dorsal spread from the /g/ in the second syllable of the target /dʁagɔ̃/. The only exception in the entire data set to our expectation that Dorsal spreading would not occur unless the child had knowledge of /ʁ/ was the production of the onset in the word *trophée* as [k] by Participant 5110. This child produced a single simplified cluster at time 1 (/bʁ/ → [bw]) and began to produce /ʁ/ 6 weeks later upon follow-up testing; therefore, this production might be an indication of emerging awareness of the /ʁ/ and/or the C2 segment position, especially after 6 weeks of intervention. On the other hand, it could be an articulatory accident or transcription error.

SUMMARY AND CONCLUSIONS

These data suggest a developmental progression in the acquisition of /ʁ/-clusters by francophone children that mirrors findings reported for other language groups and suggests that perceptual and articulatory phonetic factors underpin aspects of the children's accumulating phonological knowledge as they move toward increasingly accurate speech output. We consider first the surface characteristics of the children's productions in relation to what is generally reported for cluster development (McLeod, Van Doorn, & Reed, 2001b). First, our data do give the impression that cluster reduction is an early stage of cluster development given that a small number of children consistently reduced clusters to the obstruent segment in C1 position whereas the remaining children produced a variety of realizations including reduced, simplified, and correct tokens of the target cluster. A clear sense of the expected progression from reduced to simplified to correct exemplars of the clusters was not observed, possibly because these children were receiving intervention to promote accurate production of the cluster. Progression to mastery of the cluster at time 2 was better predicted by the presence of /ʁ/ in the inventory than the number of simplification versus reduction errors at time 1. The considerable degree of individual variation and "reversals and revisions" that McLeod et al. describe for English was certainly notable in our sample of children speaking Québec French.

Turning to phonological development, and in particular in relation to Jongstra's (2003) proposal based on observations of Dutch-speaking children, we again observe partial concordance with previous findings. First, a few children clearly appeared to correspond to the "sonority" stage, prosodifying the clusters with only one segment, in this case the least sonorant option from the input. Progression from the "sonority" stage to a "head" stage of cluster development also seems to be attested. Note, for example, Participant 4107, who reduced the clusters in *fromage*, *dragon*, *brochette*, and *trophée* to a single consonant at time 1 and time 2: at time 1 these clusters were realized as [f], [d], [b], and [t] respectively, whereas at time 2 they were produced as [ʁ], [ʁ], [ʁ], and [kʁ]. The surprise in these data, however, was that this pattern was not restricted to items involving a fricative consonant in the C1 position in the input. Therefore, it seems that the ambiguous status of the Québec French [ʁ], being uncertainly classified as a fricative or an approximant, leads to a situation wherein children may prosodify stops and fricatives in C1 position as an appendix. The fact that [ps] clusters occur in the input may encourage this strategy in the early stages of cluster acquisition. This misrepresentation of the [ʁ]-cluster was found to be particularly likely to occur in /$^{cc}\sigma\sigma$/ words (i.e., unstressed syllables) and sometimes in /$\sigma^{cc}\sigma$/ words but almost never in /$^{cc}\sigma$/ words. Therefore, perceptual salience and access to the acoustic-perceptual cues that define the C1 and C2 targets in these words may be an important factor in the acquisition of these clusters in French. This conclusion is reinforced by the finding that all error types, including reduction, simplification, and coalescence, were more frequent in the /$^{cc}\sigma\sigma$/ words.

Our conclusion that perceptual salience may be an important explanatory factor in the acquisition of [ʁ]-clusters in Québec French is offered with some caution given the many drawbacks of the study reported here. The data were not collected for the purpose of testing this hypothesis, and the word list that we used was not systematically designed to sample the relevant data. The children were drawn from a fairly narrow age range and were receiving treatment for remediation of their cluster errors during the course of the study. There is no reliable information about their ability to perceive the [ʁ] phoneme or [ʁ]-clusters. However, we hope that the raw data supplied in Appendix B and the hypothesis put forward here will stimulate creation of the necessary research tools, properly designed for Québec French, and further investigation of cluster acquisition in this population using longitudinal designs.

ACKNOWLEDGMENTS

We thank the children and their parents who participated in the research project, as well as the speech-language pathologists from the Montréal Children's Hospital who referred them to the project. The authors would like to acknowledge the numerous research assistants and student volunteers who assisted with data collection and processing: Tara Commandeur, Joelle Chagnon, Elizabeth Christe, Catherine Clémence, Raphaelle Curis, Claudine Joncas, Annie Ladouceur, Patrizia Mazzocca, Rachel Morasse, Mahchid Namazzi, Stéphanie Arcand, Geneviève Beauregard-Paultre, Elisa Bucarel, Hannah Jacobs, Annie Jacques, Amanda Langdon, Marianne Paul, Daniel Phelan, Anit Saini, and Hope Valeriote. These data arise from the project Essai Clinique sur les Interventions Phonologique, which was supported by a Standard

Research Grant to the first author from the Social Sciences and Humanities Research Council of Canada and Bourse de formation de doctorat to the second author from the Fonds de la recherche en santé. We are also indebted to the Montréal Children's Hospital and the Centre for Research on Brain, Language and Music for the use of their facilities.

REFERENCES

Bérubé, D., Bernhardt, B., & Stemberger, J. P. (2013). Un test de phonologie du Français: Construction et utilisation. *Canadian Journal of Speech-Language Pathology and Audiology, 37*(1), 26–40.

Brosseau-Lapré, F., & Rvachew, S. (2014). Cross-linguistic comparison of speech errors produced by English- and French-speaking preschool age children with developmental phonological disorders. *International Journal of Speech-Language Pathology, 16,* 98–108.

Coté, M.-H. (2004). Consonant cluster simplification in Québec French. *Probus, 16,* 151–201.

Dell, F. O. (1995). Consonant clusters and phonological syllables in French. *Lingua, 95,* 5–26.

Dunn, L. M., Theriault-Whalen, C. M., & Dunn, L. M. (1993). *Echelle de Vocabulaire en Images Peabody*. Toronto: Psycan.

Echols, C. H. (1993). A perceptually-based model of children's earliest productions. *Cognition, 46,* 245–296.

Fant, G., Kruckenberg, A., & Nord, L. (1991). Durational correlates of stress in Swedish, French and English. *Journal of Phonetics, 19,* 351–365.

Fikkert, P., & de Hoop, H. (2009). Language acquisition in optimality theory. *Linguistics, 47,* 311–357.

Friesner, M. (2010). Une prononciation "tsipéquement" québécoise? La diffusion de deux aspects stéréotypés du français canadien. *Canadian Journal of Linguistics, 55*(1), 27–53.

Jongstra, W. (2003). Variable and stable clusters: Variation in the realization of consonant clusters. *Canadian Journal of Linguistics, 48,* 265–288.

Jun, S.-A., & Fougeron, C. (2002). Realizations of accentual phrase in French intonation. *Probus, 14,* 147–172.

Kaufman, A. S., & Kaufman, N. L. (2004). *Kaufman Brief Intelligence Test* (2nd ed.). Circle Pines, MN: American Guidance Service.

Kehoe, M. M., Hilaire-Debove, G., Demuth, K., & Lleó, C. (2008). The structure of branching onsets and rising diphthongs: Evidence from the acquisition of French and Spanish. *Language Acquisition, 15*(1), 5–57. doi: 10.1080/10489220701774229

MacLeod, A. A. N., Sutton, A., Trudeau, N., & Thordardottir, E. (2011). The acquisition of consonants in Québec French: A cross-sectional study of preschool aged children. *International Journal of Speech-Language Pathology, 13*, 93–109.

Martin, P. (1996). *Éléments de phonétique avec applications au français*. Québec: Les presses de l'université Laval.

McLeod, S., Van Doorn, J., & Reed, V. A. (2001a). Consonant cluster development in two-year-olds: General trends and individual difference. *Journal of Speech, Language, and Hearing Research, 44*, 1144–1171.

McLeod, S., Van Doorn, J., & Reed, V. A. (2001b). Normal acquisition of consonant clusters. *American Journal of Speech-Language Pathology, 10*, 99–110.

Ménard, L., & Thibeault, M. (2009). Developpement de la parole et émergence de la structure prosodique chez l'enfant: Une étude de l'accent d'emphase en français. *Canadian Journal of Linguistics, 54*, 117–136.

Paul, M. (2009). *Predictors of consonant development and the development of a test of French phonology*. M.Sc., McGill University, Montréal, Québec.

Paul, M., & Rvachew, S. (2008). Test Francophone de Phonologie. McGill University. www.medicine.mcgill.ca/srvachew/

Rose, Y. (2000). *Headedness and prosodic licensing in the L1 acquisition of phonology*. Unpublished Ph.D. Dissertation, McGill University, Montréal, Québec.

Rose, Y., & dos Santos, C. (2010). Stress domain effects in French phonology and development. In K. Arregi, Z. Fagyal, S. Montrul, & A. Tremblay (Eds.), *Papers from the 38th Linguistic Symposium on Romance Languages* (pp. 89–104). Amsterdam: John Benjamins.

Rose, Y., & Wauquier-Gravelines, S. (2007). French speech acquisition. In S. McLeod (Ed.), *The International Guide to Speech Acquisition* (pp. 364–384). Clifton Park, NY: Thomson Delmar Learning.

Rvachew, S., & Brosseau-Lapré, F. (2012). *Developmental Phonological Disorders: Foundations of Clinical Practice*. San Diego, CA: Plural Publishing.

Rvachew, S., Marquis, A., Brosseau-Lapré, F., Royle, P., Paul, M., & Gonnerman, L. M. (2013). Speech articulation performance of Francophone children in the early school years: Norming of the *Test de Dépistage Francophone de Phonologie*. *Clinical Linguistics & Phonetics, 27*(12), 950–968.

Sankoff, G., & Blondeau, H. (2007). Language change across the lifespan: /r/ in Montreal French. *Language, 83*, 560–588.

Smit, A. B. (1993). Phonological error distributions in the Iowa-Nebraska Articulation Norms Project: Consonant singletons. *Journal of Speech, Language, and Hearing Research, 36*, 533–547.

Snow, D. (1998). A prominence account of syllable reduction in early speech development: The child's prosodic phonology of tiger and giraffe. *Journal of Speech, Language & Hearing Research, 41*, 1171–1184.

Vihman, M. M. (2006). *Phonological templates in early words: A cross-linguistic study.* Paper presented at the 10th Conference on Laboratory Phonology, Paris, France, June 29–July 1.

Vihman, M. M., DePaolis, R. A., & Keren-Portnoy, T. (2009). Babbling and words: A dynamic systems perspective on phonological development. In E. L. Bavin (Ed.), *The Cambridge Handbook of Child Language* (pp. 163–182). Cambridge: Cambridge University Press.

Wauquier, S., & Yamaguchi, N. (2014). Templates in French. In M. Vihman & T. Keren-Portnoy (Eds.), *The Emergence of Phonology: Whole-Word Approaches and Cross-Linguistic Evidence* (pp. 317–342). Cambridge, UK: Cambridge University Press.

Yavaş, M., & McLeod, S. (2010). Acquisition of /s/ clusters in English-speaking children with phonological disorders. *Clinical Linguistics & Phonetics, 34,* 177–187.

APPENDIX

Appendix A Treatment Targets by Participant

Participant	Target 1	Target 2	Target 3
1102	Onset:[+continuant]	Branching onset:/ʁ/	Glide nucleus
1109	Onset:[+continuant]	Branching onset:/ʁ/	Glide nucleus
1111	Segment: /l/	Branching onset:/ʁ/	
2104	Segment: /ʃ/	Branching onset:/ʁ/	
2108	Segment: /l/	Segment: /ʃ/	Branching onset:/ʁ/
3104	Segment: /ʃ/	Coda:Nasal	Branching onset:/ʁ/
3107	Onset:Dorsal	Segment: /s/	Branching onset:/ʁ/
3111	Segment: /ʃ/	Word internal coda	Branching onset:/ʁ/
3112	Segment: /ʃ/	Segment: /s/	Branching onset:/ʁ/
3113	Segment: /ʃ/	Word internal coda	Branching onset:/ʁ/
4101	Segment: /l/	Branching onset:/ʁ/	Multisyllable words
4102	Segment: /ʃ/	Branching onset:/ʁ/	Word internal coda
4103	Segment: /s/	Word internal coda	Branching onset:/ʁ/
4107	Onset:[+continuant]	Branching onset:/ʁ/	Word internal coda
4108	Onset:[+continuant]	Branching onset:/ʁ/	Multisyllable words
5105	Word internal coda	Branching onset:/ʁ/	Segment: /ʃ/
5110	Branching onset:/ʁ/	Word internal coda	Multisyllable words
6101	Word internal coda	Branching onset:/ʁ/	Multisyllable words
6110	Segment: /ʃ/	Word internal coda	Branching onset:/ʁ/
6111	Segment: /ʃ/	Glide nucleus	Branching onset:/ʁ/
6113	Branching onset:/ʁ/	Word internal coda	Multisyllable words

APPENDIX B

Table A.1 Cluster Realizations by Participant and Word at Time 1

Participants	bras bʁa	front fʁɔ̃	crêpes kʁɛp	frites fʁit	griffes gʁif	cravate kʁavat	fromage fʁɔmaʒ	dragon dʁagɔ̃	brochette bʁɔʃɛt	trophée tʁɔfe	écran ekʁɑ̃	citron sitʁɔ̃	micro mikʁo	batterie batʁi	chevreuil ʃəvʁœj
1102	b	f	k	f	g	k	f	d	b	t	k	t	k	t	v
1109	bw	t	t	f	gr	t	fw	dʁ	bw	t	kʁ	t	kʁ	t	v
1111	bʁ	fʁ	kʁ	fʁ	gʁ	k	fʁ	d	bʁ	tʁ	kʁ	tʁ	kʁ	tʁ	vʁ
2104	bʁ	fl	k ʁ	fw	kl	k	n	n	bʁ	tw	kʁ	tʁ	tʁ	tʁ	vj
2108	b	fj	kj	fj	g	kj	fʁ	dj	bj	tw	kj	kw	kw	tw	vj
3104	bw	fw	kʁ	fw	g	k	s	g	b	k	k	kʁ	kw	k	v
3107	dʁ	p	kʁ	fʁ	gʁ	k	k	gʁ	b	t	kʁ	kʁ	kʁ	t	v
3111	bʁ	fʁ	kʁ	fʁ	gʁ	kʁ	pʁ	dʁ	bʁ	kʁ	kʁ	kʁ	kʁ	kʁ	vʁ
3112	bw	fʁ	kʁ	bw	gʁ	t	kʁ	d	bw	tʁ	kʁ	tw	kʁ	gw	vʁ
3113	bʁ	f	kʁ	fw	gʁ	k	s	gʁ	gʁ	tʁ	kʁ	tʁ	kʁ	tʁ	vʁ
4101	bʁ	fʁ	kw	fw	gw	kʁ	kw	g	bʁ	kw	kʁ	tʁ	kw	kw	v
4102	bw	fʁ	kw	fw	gʁ	k	ʃ	k	bʁ	t	k	tʁ	k	t	v
4103	bʁ	fʁ	kʁ	fʁ	gʁ	kʁ	fʁ	gʁ	fʁ	t	fʁ	kʁ	kʁ	tʁ	vʁ
4107	bw	fʁ	kʁ	fw	g	kw	f	d	b	t	kʁ	kʁ	kw	tʁ	vw
4108	bw	fw	kʁ	fw	gʁ	kʁ	kw	kʁ	bw	kʁ	t	tʁ	kʁ	kʁ	ʁ
5105	bʁ	m	kʁ	fʁ	kʁ	k	kʁ	gʁ	kʁ	tʁ	t	tʁ	tʁ	ʁtʃ	ʁtʃ
5110	b	f	k	f	d	g	f	g	b	t	t	t	k	t	v
6101	bʁ	fj	kj	f	gj	kʁ	f	d	bw	t	kj	tj	kj	t	vj
6110	bʁ	f	kw	f	g	k	f	d	b	t	kʁ	tj	k	t	v
6111	bʁ	fʁ	kʁ	fʁ	g	kʁ	fʁ	gʁ	bʁ	kʁ	kʁ	ʁ	tʁ	ʁ	v
6113	bʁ	ʁ	kʁ	ʁ	gʁ	ʁ	Ø	dʁ	ʁ	ʁ	ʁ	ʁ	ʁ	tʁ	ʁ

Table A.2 Cluster Realizations by Participant and Word at Time 2

Participants	bras bʁa	front fʁɔ̃	crêpes kʁɛp	frites fʁit	griffes gʁif	cravate kʁavat	fromage fʁɔmaʒ	dragon dʁagɔ̃	brochette bʁɔʃɛt	trophée tʁɔfe	écran ekʁɑ̃	citron sitʁɔ̃	micro mikʁo	batterie batʁi	chevreuil ʃəvʁœj
1102	b	f	k	f	g	k	f	g	b	t	k	k	k	k	v
1109	bʁ	fʁ	kʁ	fʁ	gʁ	kʁ	fʁ	gʁ	bʁ	tʁ	kʁ	tʁ	kʁ	tʁ	vʁ
1111	bʁ	fʁ	kʁ	fʁ	gʁ	kʁ	fʁ	dʁ	bʁ	tʁ	kʁ	tʁ	kʁ	tʁ	vʁ
2104	bʁ	fʁ	kw	fʁ	gʁ	n	fʁ	l	bʁ	tʁ	kʁ	tʁ	tʁ	t	vl
2108	bj	fj	kj	fj	gj	kj	fʁ	dj	bj	kw	kw	kw	kw	kw	Ø
3104	m	fw	k	fw	gʁ	k	fw	g	b	kʁ	kʁ	kʁ	kʁ	kʁ	v
3107	gʁ	ʁ	ʁ	v	gʁ	t	ʃʁ	ʁ	f	t	k	tʁ	kʁ	tʁ	v
3111	bʁ	fʁ	kʁ	fʁ	gʁ	kʁ	pʁ	dʁ	bʁ	kʁ	kʁ	kʁ	kʁ	kʁ	vʁ
3112	bʁ	fʁ	kʁ	fʁ	gʁ	kʁ	k	dʁ	bʁ	Ø	kʁ	tʁ	kʁ	tʁ	v
3113	bʁ	f	kʁ	fʁ	gʁ	kʁ	fʁ	dl	bʁ	tʁ	kj	tʁ	kj	tʁ	vʁ
4101	bʁ	fʁ	kʁ	fʁ	gʁ	kʁ	fʁ	gʁ	fʁ	fʁ	kʁ	tʁ	kʁ	k	v
4102	bw	fʁ	kʁ	fw	kw	kʁ	fʁ	d	b	t	kʁ	tʁ	k	tw	v
4103	bʁ	fʁ	kʁ	fʁ	gʁ	kʁ	fʁ	gʁ	bʁ	kʁ	kʁ	tʁ	tʁ	t	v
4107	w	fʁ	kʁ	w	w	kʁ	ʁ	ʁ	ʁ	kʁ	kʁ	kʁ	kʁ	kʁ	v
4108	bʁ	f	kʁ	fʁ	gʁ	kʁ	kʁ	gʁ	bʁ	f	kʁ	kʁ	tʁ	kʁ	v
5105	bʁ	fʁ	kʁ	fʁ	gʁ	kʁ	f	gʁ	gʁ	kʁ	kʁ	tʁ	tʁ	kʁ	v
5110	b	f	k	f	g	k	f	g	b	k	k	t	k	t	v
6101	bʁ	fj	pɐʁ	ʁʁ	gl	kaʁ	g	g	b	t	kl	ts	kj	t	fj
6110	bʁ	fʁ	kʁ	fʁ	gʁ	kʁ	fʁ	dʁ	bʁ	tʁ	kʁ	kʁ	kʁ	tʁ	v
6111	bʁ	fʁ	kʁ	fʁ	gʁ	kʁ	fʁ	gʁ	bʁ	tʁ	kʁ	ʁ	tʁ	tʁ	vj
6113	bʁ	fʁ	kʁ	fʁ	gʁ	k	fʁ	gʁ	pʁ	b	kʁ	tʁ	kʁ	kʁ	ʁ

7

CHILDREN'S INCIPIENT CONSPIRACIES

**Daniel A. Dinnsen, Judith A. Gierut, and
Michele L. Morrisette**

The phonological error pattern(s) of a young child (normal or disordered) might be judged 'unusual' on any one of a number of counts. For one, the error pattern might be unique or rare, i.e. either not occurring or rarely occurring in the phonologies of other children or of other fully developed languages (e.g. Leonard & Brown, 1984). Alternatively, the error pattern could be a common phenomenon in children's sound systems, but it might otherwise be unexpected based on well-established principles of language (e.g. Dinnsen & Farris-Trimble, 2008b; Goad, 1997). Additionally, an error pattern might appear to be unusual because it has been obscured in some way by another interacting phonological process (e.g. Barlow, 2007). Finally, for children with a phonological disorder, an error pattern might be judged unusual based on its response to clinical intervention, in particular, its resistance to remediation (e.g. Dinnsen, 2008).

The available accounts of unusual error patterns have yielded little in the way of a common thread that could tie them together. An understandable limitation of these accounts is their focus on the children's presenting phonology after the unusual error pattern emerged. There is, however, a promising alternative that has not yet been pursued, namely a longitudinal examination of the children's earlier stages of phonological development leading up to the emergence of the seemingly unusual error pattern. Toward this end, this chapter attempts to discover the source of the problem by focusing on the natural emergence of the 's > θ > f chain shift', which, while commonly occurring, is unusual in at least two respects: First, it is known to be especially resistant to clinical intervention, either yielding anomalous results or requiring a non-conventional treatment protocol (e.g. Dinnsen & Barlow, 1998; Gierut & Champion, 1999; Morrisette & Gierut, 2008). Second, the chain shift involves two seemingly unrelated processes that interact with one another in a way that obscures the generalization behind one of those processes. More specifically, one part of the chain shift involves a process of Labialization, replacing interdental fricatives with a labial fricative (e.g. 'thumb' realized as [fʌm]). The other process in the chain shift, Dentalization, replaces grooved coronal fricatives with an interdental fricative (e.g. 'soup' realized as [θup]). Importantly, the interdental fricatives that are produced by the Dentalization process do not undergo Labialization (i.e. 'soup' is not realized as *[fup]). This apparent exception to Labialization renders the process opaque (i.e. Labialization does not result in a surface-true generalization). Our analyses trace the early series of phonological steps that a child took along the path before and after arriving at this chain shift. The results reveal an unexpected source for this troublesome error pattern, namely a 'conspiracy' to avoid coronal fricatives. Conspiracies have long been known to occur in fully developed languages and are acknowledged to pose significant problems for rule-based theories of phonology (e.g. Kiparsky, 1976; Kisseberth, 1970). However, it is only recently that conspiracies have begun to come to light in young children's developing phonologies (e.g. Barlow, 1997; Dinnsen, 2011; Dinnsen & Farris-Trimble, 2008a; Łukaszewicz, 2007; Pater & Barlow, 2003). These recent reports of children's incipient conspiracies raise questions about how they might compare to conspiracies in fully developed languages and how they evolve with or without clinical intervention. Typical conspiracies in fully developed languages involve multiple phonological processes that work together to effect different repairs in response to one and the same problem. As we will see, connecting this chain shift with a conspiracy is important on both clinical and theoretical grounds, largely because it identifies a common source for seemingly different problems and elucidates the language-specific and universal properties that underlie those patterns.

The chapter is organized as follows: In the next section ('The Life-Cycle of a Conspiracy'), we report the results from a longitudinal study, tracing the developmental path of the conspiracy leading to the chain shift and beyond. Adopting Optimality Theory (e.g. Prince & Smolensky, 1993/2004) for its advantages in characterizing acquisition and especially conspiracies, we then go on to formulate an account of the developmental facts, making explicit reference to the universal and language-specific factors behind the various error patterns. After that, we consider the clinical implications of our findings. The chapter concludes with a brief summary.

THE LIFE-CYCLE OF A CONSPIRACY

The case study of a child with a phonological delay, Child 181 (female, age 4;1 to 4;6), was selected to illustrate an early conspiracy that subsequently evolved into the $s > \theta > f$ chain shift. These data were drawn from the Developmental Phonology Archive of the Learnability Project at Indiana University (Gierut, 2008b). As with the other children in the archive, this child was typically developing in all respects, except for evidence of a phonological delay. Also, as part of a larger experimental study (not related to conspiracies or the error patterns considered here), this child participated in a clinical treatment experiment that was designed to suppress her Gliding error pattern by teaching her a liquid consonant for her glide substitutes. For details about the structure of these treatment experiments, see Gierut (2008a). The larger experimental study called for each child's entire phonology to be reassessed at multiple pre-established intervals during and following treatment, using the same extensive word list that had been used to establish the pre-treatment phonology. The words on this list were never used as treatment stimuli. The various sampling intervals afforded an opportunity to observe and document changes in the child's phonology over time. The longitudinal analyses for this child identified four distinct stages of development, two of which preceded the introduction of the chain shift and one of which followed the chain shift.

A conspiracy to avoid coronal fricatives can be instantiated in different ways within and across children and at one or more points in time. The first sampling interval for Child 181 revealed one instance of the conspiracy against coronal fricatives by invoking a single, uniform repair, namely Stopping, which had the effect of excluding all coronal fricatives from the phonetic inventory. The data in (1a) and (1b) show that both grooved and interdental coronal fricatives were repaired in the same way, being replaced by coronal stops. The forms in (1c) show that Stopping was limited to coronal fricatives, given that labial fricatives occurred in the phonetic inventory and were produced target-appropriately. Stated differently, labial fricatives did not undergo Stopping, nor did they serve as repairs for illicit coronal fricatives.

(1) Stage 1 (age 4;1)

a. Grooved coronal fricatives replaced by coronal stops (Stopping)[1]

    [tup] 'soup'   [toʊp] 'soap'

    [bʌti] 'bus-i'   [aɪt] 'ice'

b. Interdental fricatives replaced by coronal stops (Stopping)

    [tʌti] 'thirsty'   [deɪʔnu] 'thank you'

    [titi] 'teeth-i'   [wit] 'wreath'

c. Labial fricatives produced target-appropriately

    [fʊt] 'foot'   [feɪ] 'face'

    [faɪjʊ] 'fire'   [fɪht] 'fish'

While this child employed Stopping for all coronal fricatives at the first interval available to us, her phonology changed in a significant way at the next sampling interval, three months later. That is, part of the Stopping process was suppressed, with interdental fricatives being produced instead as labial fricatives by a process of Labialization, as shown in (2b). Target grooved coronal fricatives continued to be produced as stops at that point in time (2a). Importantly, all coronal fricatives continued to be produced in error, but this instance of the conspiracy manifested itself by two different repairs, Labialization and Stopping. Despite the introduction of a new error pattern for interdental fricatives, Labialization can be seen as a positive step forward because at least a fricative served as the substitute for another target fricative. This change emerged naturally, with no apparent connection to the child's treatment (which had been directed at her Gliding process).

(2) Stage 2 (age 4;4)

a. Grooved coronal fricatives produced as coronal stops (Stopping)

    [tup] 'soup'   [toʊp] 'soap'

    [duti] 'juicy'   [aɪti] 'icy'

b. Interdental fricatives realized as labial fricatives (Labialization; Stopping partially suppressed)

    [fʌm] 'thumb'   [fʌndʊ] 'thunder'

    [wifi] 'wreath-i'   [maʊf] 'mouth'

c. Labial fricatives produced target-appropriately

    [fʊt] 'foot'   [naɪfi] 'knife-i'

    [wʊfi] 'roof-i'   [wæf] 'laugh'

Approximately one month later, the child's phonology changed yet again, introducing the chain shift, as shown in (3). More specifically, the remaining part of the Stopping process affecting grooved coronal fricatives was suppressed and was supplanted by a different error pattern, namely Dentalization of grooved coronal fricatives (3a). Labialization of target interdentals persisted (3b). Importantly, interdentals derived from Dentalization did not undergo Labialization. This rendered the Labialization process opaque. Despite the fact that a coronal fricative was produced as a substitute for another coronal fricative, it remained true that all target coronal fricatives were still produced in error, consistent with the conspiracy to avoid coronal fricatives. Also, despite the clinical challenge posed by a chain shift, this development can also be seen as a positive step forward in that two different fricatives served as substitutes for the two types of coronal fricatives. The child's phonology was, in some sense, moving closer to the target phonology.

(3) Stage 3 (age 4;5)

a. Grooved coronal fricatives replaced by interdental fricatives (Dentalization; Stopping suppressed)

[θup] 'soup'	[θænə] 'Santa'
[beɪθba] 'baseball'	[mauθ] 'mouse'

b. Interdental fricatives replaced by labial fricatives (Labialization)

[fʌm] 'thumb'	[fʌndə] 'thunder'
[tifi] 'teeth-i'	[tuf] 'tooth'

c. Labial fricatives produced target-appropriately

[faɪv] 'five'	[læfin] 'laughing'
[ɛʊfɪnt] 'elephant'	[lif] 'leaf'

Throughout the above three sampling intervals, the error patterns targeting coronal fricatives varied in their repairs. The consistent result was that all coronal fricatives were produced in error, as might be expected of a conspiracy. The one anomaly for general conceptions of conspiracies was the attendant opacity that goes along with any chain shift. Conspiracies in fully developed languages have generally been thought to result in transparent generalizations, i.e. generalizations that are surface-true (e.g. Kiparsky, 1976). The opacity evident in Stage 3 is certainly in contrast to the transparency of the generalizations of Stage 1 and Stage 2. While opacity might not be an expected property of conspiracies, we will show in the next section that opacity is a natural consequence of this and possibly other incipient conspiracies, at least when viewed from the perspective of Optimality Theory (henceforth OT).

The pre-established sampling schedule of the study afforded one final opportunity to examine Child 181's phonology after the chain shift had emerged. That is, approximately one month after treatment ceased on the unrelated Gliding error pattern, the Dentalization process appeared to be suppressed, with grooved coronal fricatives being produced target-appropriately (4a). However, Labialization of interdental fricatives persisted (4b). With the loss of Dentalization, the Labialization process was no longer opaque, and the correct production of the grooved fricatives suggested that the chain shift (and the conspiracy) had been at least partially eradicated. However, we will see shortly that these correct productions cannot necessarily be taken as evidence that a process has truly been suppressed.

(4) Stage 4 (age 4;6)

   a. Grooved coronal fricatives produced target-appropriately (Dentalization seemingly suppressed)

[sat] 'sock'	[sænə] 'Santa'
[dʒusi] 'juicy'	[aɪs] 'ice'

   b. Interdental fricatives produced as labial fricatives (Labialization)

[fʌm] 'thumb'	[fʌndʊ] 'thunder'
[maʊfi] 'mouth-i'	[wif] 'wreath'

   c. Labial fricatives produced target-appropriately

[faɪjʊ] 'fire'	[lifi] 'leaf-i'
[læf] 'laugh'	[naɪf] 'knife'

As we reflect on these facts, it should be noted that similar phonologies corresponding to each of the above stages were also independently attested in a related cross-sectional study of the pre-treatment phonologies of 160 young children with phonological delays (Dinnsen, Green, Gierut, & Morrisette, 2011). That is, many (but certainly not all) of the other children from that study were found to exhibit the processes of Stopping, Labialization, and/or Dentalization alone or in combination as described above. The longitudinal results presented here have the added advantage of revealing the natural progression and unfolding of the conspiracy against coronal fricatives. The theoretical challenge now is to arrive at an account that captures the generalization behind these various error patterns, in both their cross-sectional and longitudinal manifestations.

THE OPTIMALITY THEORETIC ACCOUNT

We adopt here the constraint-based framework of OT in an effort to provide a unified account of this child's conspiracy with its various longitudinal instantiations, including the troublesome 's > θ > f' chain shift. This framework enjoys well-documented advantages not available in other approaches in the characterization of conspiracies and acquisition. Additionally, OT makes a number of substantive claims about the universal and language-specific properties of grammar that account for phonological phenomena. For example, while there are no universal or language-specific rules within OT, violable constraints are employed instead, and those constraints are presumed to be universal. On the other hand, the ranking of the constraints (i.e. the constraint hierarchy) is determined largely on language-specific grounds. Constraints are of two types, i.e. markedness and faithfulness, and they often conflict in their demands. Conflict is resolved by ranking the constraints. Markedness constraints refer exclusively to properties of output representations, without regard to the input (or underlying) representations, and assign violations to marked structures in potential output candidates. Faithfulness constraints, on the other hand, refer to a correspondence relation between input (underlying) and output representations, demanding identity between the two and assigning violations to output candidates that differ from the input. The output candidate that best satisfies the constraint hierarchy (i.e. the candidate that incurs the least serious violations) is selected as optimal (i.e. the winner).

OT makes a number of other assumptions that have special significance for acquisition and learning. For one, it is assumed that markedness constraints outrank faithfulness constraints by default in the initial-state (e.g. Smolensky, 1996). This accounts for children's predisposition for production errors in early phonological development. To eliminate those errors, it is then left to the child to demote the relevant markedness constraints below the critical faithfulness constraints based on positive evidence from the target language. Several different formal learning algorithms have been put forward (e.g. Prince & Tesar, 2004, and references therein), but the basic idea is that a constraint that had favored the previous winner must now be demoted just below the highest ranked constraint (markedness or faithfulness) that the previous winner violated. Related to this point is the further assumption that faithfulness constraints remain ranked as low as possible throughout the acquisition process. We will see below how these various points are implemented. Finally, OT maintains via 'Richness of the Base' that there can be no language-specific restrictions on input representations (e.g. Smolensky, 1996). This is a significant departure from earlier theories of phonology, but the consequence for accounts of acquisition is that we, as analysts, must allow for the possibility that children have internalized richly specified underlying representations, essentially as rich as target (underlying) representations. This shifts the analytical burden entirely to the constraint hierarchy to derive the observed output no matter what might be assumed about the child's underlying representations.

The constraints that are most relevant to the characterization of this child's error patterns are given in (5) with their definitions. The markedness constraints in (5a) belong to a family of constraints disfavoring different subclasses of fricatives, and each is independently necessary on typological grounds (e.g. Dinnsen, Dow, Gierut, Morrisette, & Green, 2013). The faithfulness constraints in (5b) are antagonistic to the markedness constraints and make reference to features that are implicated in the various repairs that were documented in the previous section. For example, Stopping results in a violation of ID[cont] because it entails a change in the feature [continuant] when an input fricative changes to a stop in the output. Similarly, ID[pl] incurs a violation as a result of Labialization when an interdental fricative changes from a coronal to a labial fricative. Dentalization entails a violation of ID[grv] when a grooved coronal fricative /s/ changes to a non-grooved interdental fricative [θ]. Finally, the locally conjoined constraint, LC, is a special type of faithfulness constraint that is most relevant to the characterization of chain shifts (e.g. Dinnsen & Barlow, 1998; Morrisette & Gierut, 2008). This particular constraint conjoins the two faithfulness constraints ID[pl] and ID[grv] in the local domain of a single segment and is violated if and only if both of the individual conjuncts are violated. Consequently, a change from an input /s/ to an output [f] would violate LC because a [+grooved] coronal segment has changed to a [−grooved] labial segment. An important metacondition of the theory is that locally conjoined constraints such as LC must be ranked above their individual conjuncts in all constraint hierarchies.

(5) Constraints

a. Markedness
*f: Labial fricatives are banned
*θ: Interdental fricatives are banned
*s: Grooved coronal fricatives are banned
b. Faithfulness
ID[cont]: Corresponding input and output segments must have the same specification for the feature [continuant]
ID[pl]: Corresponding input and output segments must have the same primary place feature
ID[grv]: Corresponding input and output segments must have the same specification for the feature [grooved]
LC: Local conjunction of ID[pl] and ID[grv] in the domain of the same segment

We turn now to the specifics of our longitudinal account leading to and following from the s > θ > f chain shift. At the first observation point (Stage 1), Child 181 employed Stopping to eliminate all coronal fricatives. The required ranking of constraints is given in (6). Note first that the markedness constraints against coronal fricatives are undominated. This is consistent with the default ranking of markedness over faithfulness and conforms to standard schemata for conspiracies, namely one or more markedness constraints ranked over two or more crucially ranked faithfulness constraints. Note, too, that the markedness constraint against labial fricatives (*f) has already been demoted to reflect the fact that labial fricatives were produced target-appropriately. Finally, because Stopping appears to be the default repair for coronal fricatives, ID[cont] must be ranked relatively low among the faithfulness constraints in the initial-state.

(6) Stage 1 (Stopping)
*s, *θ >> LC >> ID[pl] >> ID[cont] >> *f >> ID[grv]

The tableaux in (7) and (8) for 'soup'- and 'thumb'-words, respectively, show how the most likely competing output candidates are evaluated by these constraints with the hierarchy in (6). In both tableaux, candidates (a) and (b) with coronal fricatives are eliminated immediately due to their violations of the undominated markedness constraints. Additionally, in (7), candidate (c) with a labial fricative incurs a fatal violation of LC due to its changes in two features, namely place (from coronal to labial) and from [+grooved] to [−grooved]. Consequently, even though the candidate with a stop (7d) violates ID[cont], it is selected as optimal because all other competitors have been eliminated by higher ranked constraints.[2]

(7) Stopping of grooved fricatives

/sup/	*s	*θ	LC	ID[pl]	ID[cont]	*f	ID[grv]
a. sup	*!						
b. θup		*!					*
c. fup			*!	*		*	*
d. ☞ tup					*		

The only real difference of note in (8) is that candidate (c), which represents a change from a non-grooved coronal fricative to a non-grooved labial fricative, is eliminated due to its violation of ID[pl] (rather than

LC, as was observed in (7c)). It is this fact that provides the ranking argument for ID[pl] outranking ID[cont].

(8) Stopping of interdental fricatives

/θʌm/		*s	*θ	LC	ID[pl]	ID[cont]	*f	ID[grv]
a.	sʌm	*!						*
b.	θʌm		*!					
c.	fʌm				*!		*	
d. ☞	tʌm					*		

As for the change from Stage 1 to Stage 2, recall that Stopping was partially suppressed, giving way to the introduction of Labialization as the repair for the ban on interdental fricatives. This called for a minimal change in the constraint hierarchy, specifically the demotion of ID[pl] below ID[cont], capturing the generalization that the preservation of manner was more important than preservation of place, at least for target interdentals. The new hierarchy is given in (9). This reranking was presumably motivated by the child's observation that target interdentals differed from stops and were in fact fricatives. The place specification of those fricatives was apparently a less salient property.

(9) Stage 2 (Stopping and Labialization)
*s, *θ >> LC >> ID[cont] >> ID[pl] >> *f >> ID[grv]

This reranking of the constraints did not impact Stopping of grooved coronal fricatives, as can be seen in (10).

(10) Stopping of grooved coronal fricatives

/sup/		*s	*θ	LC	ID[cont]	ID[pl]	*f	ID[grv]
a.	sup	*!						
b.	θup		*!					*
c.	fup			*!		*	*	*
d. ☞	tup				*			

The new hierarchy in (9) did, however, result in a different repair for interdental fricatives, as illustrated in (11). The higher ranking of ID[cont] assigned a fatal violation to the previous winner, candidate (11d), yielding candidate (11c) with a labial fricative as the new winner.

(11) Labialization of interdental fricatives

/θʌm/	*s	*θ	LC	ID[cont]	ID[pl]	*f	ID[grv]
a. sʌm	*!						*
b. θʌm		*!					
c. ☞ fʌm					*	*	
d. tʌm				*!			

The change from Stage 2 to Stage 3 involved the further suppression of Stopping and the introduction of Dentalization as the new repair for grooved coronal fricatives. That, combined with the persistence of Labialization, resulted in the emergence of the s > θ > f chain shift. In optimality theoretic terms, this would come about from a minimal change in the hierarchy, specifically the demotion of *θ below ID[cont]. This demotion would presumably follow from the child's recognition that target grooved fricatives differ from stops and other fricatives by being specified phonetically as a [+continuant] coronal. The grooved nature of those target fricatives remained a prohibited property of pronunciation. The new hierarchy is given in (12). The lower ranking of *θ reflects the fact that interdentals can now occur, although not as realizations of target interdentals. Note nevertheless that *θ remains active, as evidenced by the fatal violation that it assesses in the tableau for 'thumb'-words in (14).

(12) Stage 3 (Dentalization and Labialization)
*s >> LC >> ID[cont] >> *θ >> ID[pl] >> *f >> ID[grv]

The effect of the new hierarchy in (12) is most evident in the tableau in (13) for 'soup'-words. By demoting *θ below ID[cont], the previous winner, with a stop (13d), is eliminated due to its fatal violation of ID[cont], which allows the Dentalization candidate (13b) to be selected as optimal (even though it violates the newly demoted and lower ranked constraint *θ).

(13) Dentalization of grooved coronal fricatives

/sup/	*s	LC	ID[cont]	*θ	ID[pl]	*f	ID[grv]
a. sup	*!						
b. ☞ θup				*			*
c. fup		*!			*	*	*
d. tup			*!				

The new ranking in (12) does not change the Labialization repair for target interdentals, as shown in (14). The markedness constraints banning coronal fricatives continue to actively eliminate candidates (14a) and (14b), and the persistent ranking of ID[cont] over ID[pl] eliminates the stop candidate (14d) in favor of candidate (14c) with a labial fricative.

(14) Labialization of interdental fricatives

/θʌm/	*s	LC	ID[cont]	*θ	ID[pl]	*f	ID[grv]
a. sʌm	*!						*
b. θʌm				*!			
c. ☞ fʌm					*	*	
d. tʌm			*!				

Finally, the change from Stage 3 to Stage 4 resulted in the apparent suppression of Dentalization with concomitant target-appropriate realizations of grooved coronal fricatives. The other error pattern, Labialization, persisted. Again, these facts entailed a minimal change in the hierarchy, this time with *s being demoted below the highest ranked constraint that the previous winner violated, namely below *θ. The new ranking is spelled out in (15). The demotion of *s was presumably motivated by the child's recognition that grooved coronal fricatives could occur in faithful correspondence with target inputs.

(15) Stage 4 (Target-appropriate realizations of grooved fricatives and Labialization)

LC >> ID[cont] >> *θ >> *s >> ID[pl] >> *f >> ID[grv]

The effect of the new ranking is most evident in the tableau for 'soup'-words in (16). The Dentalization candidate (16b) now incurs a fatal violation of *θ. All other competitors, except for the new optimal candidate (16a) with the grooved coronal fricative, are eliminated by the highly ranked faithfulness constraints.

(16) Target-appropriate realizations of grooved coronal fricatives

/sup/	LC	ID[cont]	*θ	*s	ID[pl]	*f	ID[grv]
a. ☞ sup				*			
b. θup			*!				*
c. fup	*!				*	*	*
d. tup		*!					

As for 'thumb'-words, note that the demoted constraint *θ remains the highest ranked markedness constraint and is still active, assessing a fatal violation to the faithful candidate (17b). Even the lower ranked markedness constraint *s is active, eliminating candidate (17a), and, of course, the stop candidate (17d) is also eliminated by its fatal violation of highly ranked ID[cont]. The remaining Labialization candidate (17c) is thus selected as optimal, violating only lower ranked ID[pl] and, of course, *f.

(17) Labialization of interdental fricatives

/θʌm/	LC	ID[cont]	*θ	*s	ID[pl]	*f	ID[grv]
a. sʌm				*!			*
b. θʌm			*!				
c. ☞ fʌm					*	*	
d. tʌm		*!					

Our optimality theoretic account of the longitudinal facts reveals a unified and persistent force behind the various error patterns at the different points in time, namely a conspiracy to avoid coronal fricatives. The conspiracy was driven by the two universal markedness constraints, *s and *θ, both of which remained active throughout all four stages (even when grooved coronal fricatives were being produced target-appropriately). The chain shift was shown to follow naturally from the minimal and principled demotion of constraints based on positive evidence that was readily observable in the target language. As we will see in the next section, our OT account also begins to offer some insight into why this chain shift has been so problematic in clinical treatment studies.

CLINICAL IMPLICATIONS

Several points of clinical relevance emerge from our OT account of the troublesome chain shift as an instance of a conspiracy. One important observation relates to the constraint hierarchy in (15) for Stage 4, when grooved coronal fricatives were produced target-appropriately and Labialization persisted. More specifically, note that *θ was ranked above *s and that both markedness constraints were ranked high enough to actively eliminate some competing output candidates. If Labialization were to be suppressed either naturally or as a result of additional treatment, *θ would have to be demoted below

ID[pl], yielding the hierarchy in (18). While this would have the desired effect of eliminating Labialization, as demonstrated in (19), it would also have the unwelcome consequence of re-introducing the seemingly suppressed error pattern of Dentalization, as shown in (20).

(18) Predicted Regression Stage

LC >> ID[cont] >> *s >> ID[pl] >> *θ, *f >> ID[grv]

(19) Labialization suppressed

/θʌm/	LC	ID[cont]	*s	ID[pl]	*θ	*f	ID[grv]
a.　　sʌm			*!				*
b. ☞ θʌm					*		
c.　　fʌm			*!			*	
d.　　tʌm		*!					

(20) Dentalization of grooved coronal fricatives (regression)

/sup/	LC	ID[cont]	*s	ID[pl]	*θ	*f	ID[grv]
a.　　sup			*!				
b. ☞ θup					*		*
c.　　fup	*!			*		*	*
d.　　tup		*!					

These extended longitudinal predictions find support in the treatment-induced results from Gierut (1998) for Child LP33 (male, age 5;7), who presented with a phonology similar to that of Child 181 at Stage 4 (i.e. the hierarchy in (15)). This child was taught an interdental fricative with the intent of suppressing Labialization. While Child LP33 learned the treated sound, suppressing Labialization, he also regressed at that point in time by introducing Dentalization of grooved coronal fricatives. Apparently, the process of Dentalization had not really been fully suppressed at that earlier point in time. For a child like LP33 who might arrive at the hierarchy in (18) naturally or after treatment on Labialization, one or more rounds of treatment aimed at the demotion of *s below ID[grv] would likely be necessary to truly suppress Dentalization. These findings underscore the clinical importance of not taking target-appropriate realizations of a sound as evidence that the problem has been resolved.

These findings also offer a theoretical explanation for why some treatments aimed at the eradication of the s > θ > f chain shift have been more effective than others. On the one hand, those treatment studies that have attacked the chain shift by focusing on the suppression of either Labialization or Dentalization (but not both) have met with little or no success (e.g. Dinnsen & Barlow, 1998; Gierut & Champion, 1999). The limitation of those efforts can be attributed to the fact that one and only one markedness constraint was being targeted for demotion. Moreover, because demotion is minimal, those minimal changes in the rankings of constraints can, as we saw above, yield hierarchies that pose new problems and that may not represent target end-state grammars. On the other hand, the Morrisette and Gierut (2008) experimental treatment study employed a novel protocol that was more effective, targeting both parts of the chain shift by teaching minimal triplets of non-words that began with /s/, /θ/, and /f/. The relative success of this protocol can be attributed to the fact that both markedness constraints driving the conspiracy to avoid coronal fricatives were being demoted simultaneously, forcing their demotion below antagonistic faithfulness constraints, i.e. *θ below ID[pl] and *s below ID[grv].

While the Morrisette and Gierut (2008) treatment protocol was designed to eradicate specifically the s > θ > f chain shift, we hypothesize that it should be equally effective in eradicating any or all of the error patterns associated with this conspiracy no matter which of the above stages might serve as the presenting phonology. This includes any of the four stages from Child 181 and the fifth Regression Stage from Child LP33. The rationale behind this conjecture is that each of the above stages is simply a particular instance of the larger conspiracy to avoid coronal fricatives, and effectively foiling the conspiracy appears to depend on the simultaneous demotion of the two markedness constraints driving the conspiracy (i.e. *s and *θ). The novelty of this hypothesis and its potential impact call out for clinical validation through future experimental treatment studies aimed at the eradication of this and other conspiracies.

CONCLUSION

This chapter attempted to get at the problem of unusual error patterns by appealing to OT for the analysis of the stages of phonological development that preceded and followed the emergence of the troublesome s > θ > f chain shift. Longitudinal evidence was presented that traced the chain shift back to a larger, persistent conspiracy to avoid coronal fricatives. OT afforded an account of the different manifestations of the conspiracy, offering an explanation for the natural emergence of the chain shift, its clinical recalcitrance, and its attendant opacity. These explanations relied on both language-specific and universal properties of grammar as spelled out by the theory. More specifically, the earliest observed stages of the unusual error pattern were shown to follow from the default ranking of markedness constraints over faithfulness constraints. Those constraints were, moreover, presumed to be universal. The developmental progression from the initial-state to the unusual error pattern and beyond was attributed to the reranking of constraints, and it was language-specific evidence that motivated each of the constraint rerankings. The various peculiarities associated with this chain shift were shown to be a natural, expected consequence of algorithmic learning.

Connecting this chain shift with a conspiracy is important on both clinical and theoretical grounds. Clinically, a common, unified source was identified for seemingly unrelated processes. Also, the predictable nature of the developmental path preceding and following this chain shift should be useful for diagnostic purposes and for the projection of learning. On the theoretical front, the unusualness of this particular chain shift and its connection with a conspiracy suggest that there might be some value in examining other chain shifts and/or unusual error patterns for possible origins in a conspiracy. The fruitfulness of this prospect is supported by the recent discovery of other incipient conspiracies with similar properties. For example, some children's conspiracies have been found to involve several processes that work together to avoid place and/or manner contrasts in word-initial position (e.g. Dinnsen, 2011; Dinnsen & Farris-Trimble, 2008a). Interestingly, those conspiracies happened to include a process of Consonant Harmony, which, while commonly occurring in children's phonologies, involves non-local assimilation and is unusual in that regard compared to the local assimilation that occurs in fully developed languages (e.g. Goad, 1997). Additionally, the merger of contrasts word-initially, while common in children's phonologies, is rare in fully developed languages (e.g. Dinnsen & Farris-Trimble, 2008b). The similarities of these conspiracies to the case at hand are even more striking in the particular conspiracy identified by Dinnsen and Farris-Trimble (2008a), which included an opacity-producing chain shift. Finally, the default ranking of markedness over faithfulness supplies one of the essential ingredients of a conspiracy, making children's grammars an especially promising venue for the investigation of incipient conspiracies. Those conspiracies might, in turn, serve as the seeds of other seemingly unusual error patterns.

ACKNOWLEDGMENTS

Research reported in this publication was supported by the National Institute on Deafness and Other Communication Disorders of the National Institutes of Health under Award Number R01DC001694. The content is solely the responsibility of the authors and does not necessarily represent the official views of the National Institutes of Health. We are most grateful to Jessica Barlow, Darcy Rose, and the members of the Learnability Project at Indiana University for their comments and assistance in the preparation of this paper.

NOTES

1. Throughout, illustrations for the error patterns involving grooved coronal fricatives will be limited to the anterior set /s, z/. It should, however, be noted that the non-anterior grooved fricatives /ʃ, ʒ/ were also excluded from the child's phonetic inventory. We do not consider further the behavior of this latter set of fricatives given the voiced cognate's low token frequency of occurrence relative to other fricatives in English and its distributional asymmetries.

2. It is assumed throughout that stop substitutes for input fricatives do not incur a violation of ID[grv] because stops are inherently (universally) underspecified for the feature [grooved]. Fricatives alone license the feature [grooved].

REFERENCES

Barlow, J. A. (1997). *A Constraint-Based Account of Syllable Onsets: Evidence from Developing Systems* (Unpublished doctoral dissertation). Indiana University, Bloomington, IN.

Barlow, J. A. (2007). Grandfather effects: A longitudinal case study of the phonological acquisition of intervocalic consonants in English. *Language Acquisition 14,* 121–164.

Dinnsen, D. A. (2008). Recalcitrant error patterns. In D. A. Dinnsen & J. A. Gierut (Eds.), *Optimality Theory, phonological acquisition and disorders* (pp. 247–276). London: Equinox.

Dinnsen, D. A. (2011). On the unity of children's phonological error patterns: Distinguishing symptoms from the problem. *Clinical Linguistics and Phonetics 25,* 968–974.

Dinnsen, D. A., & Barlow, J. A. (1998). On the characterization of a chain shift in normal and delayed phonological acquisition. *Journal of Child Language 25,* 61–94.

Dinnsen, D. A., Dow, M. C., Gierut, J. A., Morrisette, M. L., & Green, C. R. (2013). The coronal fricative problem. *Lingua 131,* 151–178.

Dinnsen, D. A., & Farris-Trimble, A. W. (2008a). An opacity-tolerant conspiracy in phonological acquisition. In A. W. Farris-Trimble & D. A. Dinnsen (Eds.), *Indiana University Working Papers in Linguistics: Vol. 6. Phonological opacity effects in Optimality Theory.* (pp. 99–118). Bloomington, IN: Indiana University Linguistics Club Publications.

Dinnsen, D. A., & Farris-Trimble, A. W. (2008b). The prominence paradox. In D. A. Dinnsen & J. A. Gierut (Eds.), *Optimality Theory, phonological acquisition and disorders* (pp. 277–308). London: Equinox.

Dinnsen, D. A., Green, C. R., Gierut, J. A., & Morrisette, M. L. (2011). On the anatomy of a chain shift. *Journal of Linguistics 47,* 275–299.

Gierut, J. A. (1998). Production, conceptualization and change in distinctive featural categories. *Journal of Child Language 25,* 321–342.

Gierut, J. A. (2008a). Fundamentals of experimental design and treatment. In D. A. Dinnsen & J. A. Gierut (Eds.), *Optimality Theory, phonological acquisition and disorders* (pp. 93–118). London: Equinox.

Gierut, J. A. (2008b). Phonological disorders and the Developmental Phonology Archive. In D. A. Dinnsen & J. A. Gierut (Eds.), *Optimality Theory, phonological acquisition and disorders* (pp. 37–92). London: Equinox.

Gierut, J. A., & Champion, A. H. (1999). Interacting error patterns and their resistance to treatment. *Clinical Linguistics & Phonetics 13,* 421–431.

Goad, H. (1997). Consonant harmony in child language: An Optimality Theoretic account. In S. J. Hannahs & M. Young-Scholten (Eds.), *Focus on phonological acquisition* (pp. 113–142). Philadelphia: John Benjamins.

Kiparsky, P. (1976). Abstractness, opacity and global rules. In A. Koutsoudas (Ed.), *The application and ordering of grammatical rules* (pp. 160–186). The Hague: Mouton.

Kisseberth, C. W. (1970). On the functional unity of phonological rules. *Linguistic Inquiry 1,* 291–306.

Leonard, L. B., & Brown, B. L. (1984). Nature and boundaries of phonologic categories: A case study of an unusual phonologic pattern in a language-impaired child. *Journal of Speech and Hearing Disorders 49,* 419–428.

Łukaszewicz, B. (2007). Reduction in syllable onsets in the acquisition of Polish: Deletion, coalescence, metathesis and gemination. *Journal of Child Language 34,* 53–82.

Morrisette, M. L., & Gierut, J. A. (2008). Innovations in the treatment of chain shifts. In D. A. Dinnsen & J. A. Gierut (Eds.), *Optimality Theory, phonological acquisition and disorders* (pp. 205–220). London: Equinox.

Pater, J., & Barlow, J. A. (2003). Constraint conflict in cluster reduction. *Journal of Child Language 30,* 487–526.

Prince, A., & Smolensky, P. (1993/2004). *Optimality Theory: Constraint interaction in generative grammar*. Malden, MA: Blackwell.

Prince, A., & Tesar, B. (2004). Learning phonotactic distributions. In R. Kager, J. Pater, & W. Zonneveld (Eds.), *Constraints in phonological acquisition* (pp. 245–291). Cambridge, UK: Cambridge University Press.

Smolensky, P. (1996). The initial state and "Richness of the Base" in Optimality Theory. Rutgers Optimality Archive, ROA-154.

8

WHEN PLACE DOES NOT FALL INTO PLACE
A Case Study of a Child with Diverse Linguistic Input

Margaret Kehoe

The aim of this chapter is to contrast two opposing approaches in phonological acquisition: *Universal Grammar* versus the *Language-Specific* Hypothesis. The Universal Grammar Hypothesis predicts that children start off by producing unmarked sound patterns, whereas the Language-Specific Hypothesis predicts that children initially produce those sound patterns which are the most frequent. As noted by Zamuner (2003), it is often difficult to contrast these two hypotheses because those sound patterns that are unmarked cross-linguistically are often the ones that are most frequent in a given language. Nevertheless, her study of coda acquisition in English indicated that children acquired codas that were frequent but also marked (e.g., dorsal /k/ and labial /m/), suggesting that frequency plays the decisive role (see also Zamuner, Gerken, & Hammond, 2005). Generative or Universal Grammar approaches to phonological acquisition do not exclude the role of frequency in influencing the course of development, but it is not seen to be the driving force (Rose & Brittain, 2011). Rather, development is characterized by emerging complexity in grammatical structure.

These two approaches will be contrasted when examining the productions of Max, an internationally adopted trilingual child, who displays protracted phonological development. Max is an interesting test case for the role of language input in shaping early phonological development, since Max's early input was both impoverished and diverse. He spent his first 1;8 years in an orphanage in Thailand, and, following adoption, he was exposed simultaneously to three languages (English, German, and French).[1] When faced with constructing a phonological system at 1;8, he was unable to rely on a dense data-base of phonological input in his target languages; such a data-base has usually already accrued during the first 12 months of an infant's life. Instead, he needed to acquire his phonological system "on-line". We will observe that many of Max's phonological patterns are suggestive of fragile phonological representations, possibly due to his early input conditions.

We focus on three independent but interconnected aspects of Max's phonology: his CV forms, his acquisition of velars, and his production of consonant clusters with respect to Place of Articulation (PoA). These processes are interconnected because they all pertain to restrictions on the realization of PoA within the word. Early in development, Max was dominant in English, and we consider mainly his English productions. Later in development, we consider his French and German productions as well. We will observe that Max's early speech is characterized by a U-shaped pattern of development, in which, after a period of producing codas and velar consonants, Max's production of these structures and segments declines. These changes cannot be accounted for by frequency but are consistent with the emergence of unmarked forms. At a later period, Max's cluster reduction patterns are consistent with place-determined onset reduction: Max selects the labial element of the cluster (*truck* → [wʌk]) (Pater & Barlow, 2003). This pattern, which is closely tied to Max's analysis of English /r/ as labial, applies to his English but not to his French and German words. Thus, we observe language-specific differences which are related to a grammatical rather than a frequency analysis.

While a case study is not an ideal empirical base to make generalizations on theoretical approaches, it will be seen that Max's pattern of acquisition in all three areas of phonology provides support for grammatical organization in a way that cannot easily be accounted for by frequency alone. Nevertheless, Max's diverse input conditions at the onset of phonological acquisition may have led to his protracted phonological patterns. In addition, the high frequency of certain PoA input patterns may have contributed to his preferred PoA output patterns (Fikkert & Levelt, 2008). Thus, we loosen the polemic between universal and input-based accounts by drawing attention to the fact that both approaches may explain different aspects of his acquisition.

The following section, "Literature Background," provides an overview of theoretical approaches within the field of phonological acquisition that are relevant to explaining Max's data. The first part of this section discusses the use of whole-word templates and the representation of PoA in children's early word forms; the second part discusses the importance of PoA with respect to two phonological processes:

positional velar fronting and cluster reduction. The final part of this section discusses phonological acquisition in internationally adopted children. The sections "Method" and "Results" present the data-base and results. In the final section, "Discussion," the data are interpreted in light of the Universal Grammar versus Language-Specific Grammar Hypothesis approaches.

LITERATURE BACKGROUND

Whole-Word Templates and the Representation of Place

During the last four decades, many child language researchers have observed that children's first words take the form of whole-word patterns or templates (Ferguson & Farwell, 1975; Macken, 1979; Menn, 1983; Waterson, 1971). A classic and often cited example is Waterson's (1971) son P, aged 1;6, who produced words such as *another, finger, Randall,* and *window* with a similar output pattern, namely, a CVCV form in which both consonants were nasals (e.g., [ɲaɲa], [ɲeːɲeː], [ɲɪːɲɪ], [ɲaɲø]). P appeared to focus on certain salient features of the target words (e.g., the presence of nasal consonants) and reproduce them using his own established articulatory patterns.

Vihman and colleagues formalized these observations in an approach called Radical Template Phonology (Velleman & Vihman, 2002; Vihman, 2002, 2010; Vihman & Croft, 2007; Vihman & Velleman, 2000). Their account of templates aligns with a usage-based approach to phonological acquisition, in which phonological organization first takes the form of analogically derived templates and only later sees the emergence of phonological categories. According to Vihman, templates are "inductive generalizations" based on two factors: (1) the child's individual motor preferences, which stem from pre-linguistic vocal practice (or babbling), and (2) implicit knowledge of the ambient language which is derived over the course of the first year. As will be observed later, Max's early phonology is characterized by whole-word templates; however, the influence of pre-linguistic vocal practice and ambient language knowledge will remain difficult to quantify in his case.

More recently, certain aspects of word-based phonology have been reinterpreted within the generative linguistic tradition by Fikkert and Levelt (2008). Focusing on the acquisition of PoA features, they propose that children's early consonant harmony templates can be explained in terms of developing phonological representations. Because their approach is relevant to the analysis of Max's data, we describe their findings in detail.

Fikkert and Levelt (2008) documented several stages in the acquisition of PoA features based on analyses of Dutch-speaking children's productions. At the first stage, both consonants share PoA (e.g., $C_1 = C_2$), and there are strong restrictions on the association between consonants and vowels: labial consonants (P) appear with round vowels (O) (e.g., PO(P)); coronal consonants (T) appear with front vowels (I) (e.g., TI(T)); velar consonants (K) appear with dorsal vowels (O) (e.g., KO(K)); and all consonants may appear with low vowels (A), which appear to have a neutral status, being neither front nor back nor round (e.g., PA(P), TA(T), KA(K)). At the second stage, both consonants share their PoA; however, the vowel can be different from the consonant; that is, front vowels can appear with labial consonants and round vowels can appear with coronal consonants (e.g., PI(P) and (TO(T)). At later stages, consonants can vary in PoA but in a restrictive fashion: at first C_1 is labial and C_2 is coronal, and, later, final velars are allowed.

According to Fikkert and Levelt (2008), children's initial patterns are consistent with a stage in which PoA is defined on the entire word. They refer to this as the "one word, one feature" stage. Later patterns are consistent with the segmentation of the word and with the individual representation of place for consonants and vowels; however, certain PoA restrictions may still apply: labials are preferred at the left of the word, and dorsals are avoided in this position. Importantly, Fikkert and Levelt (2008) do not deny that frequency plays a role. Once children have segmentalized their words, input frequency may play a role in determining which particular PoA combinations are observed. PVT forms (i.e., labial followed by coronal place) may occur early because they are frequent in the input. Indeed, Fikkert and Levelt (2008) distinguish between universal and emergent markedness constraints, with the former being present from the beginning, the latter emerging once children make generalizations across their lexicons. According to them, the emergence of PoA constraints such as [labial] (labial left) and *[dorsal] (no initial dorsals) is dependent on the distribution of PoA patterns in the ambient language.

Preferences for labial-coronal sequences or labial-first patterns have been often remarked on in the phonological acquisition literature (Davis, MacNeilage, & Matyear, 2002; Macken, 1979; Stoel-Gammon, 1998; Velleman, 1996). Davis et al. (2002) view these preferences as a self-organizational consequence of several factors: biomechanical, motor, and cognitive. This view emphasizes the motoric ease of labials and the demands placed on the child when initiating an action sequence, which implicates the lexicon and the motor system: variegated sequences may be easier to produce when they start with labials.

Later Phonological Processes

Later on in phonological development, children's productions are no longer characterized by whole-word templates but by systematic error patterns or processes. We consider two processes that are present in the speech of Max: positional velar fronting and place-determined cluster reduction. Interestingly, both processes lead to the avoidance of dorsals and to the favoring of labials in word-initial position, a situation which is reminiscent of the PoA restrictions observed in children's early word forms.

Positional Velar Fronting

A well documented error pattern in children's early speech is the substitution of velar stops by coronal ones. Although some children may substitute all velar stops with coronals, a positional variant of this process is frequently attested in which the velar surfaces in word-final position or in word-medial position preceding an unstressed syllable, and is replaced by a coronal in word-initial position or in word-medial position preceding a stressed syllable (Inkelas & Rose, 2008; McAllister Byun, 2012; Stoel-Gammon, 1996). Productions from Ben, a phonologically disordered English-speaking child, are shown in (1).

(1) Examples of positional velar fronting from Ben, aged 4;3 (adapted from McAllister Byun, 2012, p. 1044)
   a. Word-initial *can* [dɛn]
   b. Word-final *look* [wʊk]
   c. Word-medial preceding a stressed vowel *because* [biˈdʌs]
   d. Word-medial preceding an unstressed vowel *bucket* [ˈbakat]

One puzzling aspect of positional velar fronting is that the velar-coronal contrast is realized in prosodically weak positions (e.g., word-finally or preceding unstressed syllables) and is neutralized in prosodically strong positions (e.g., word-initially or preceding stressed syllables). The reverse tends to happen in adult languages: segmental contrasts are neutralized in prosodically weak positions (Inkelas & Rose, 2008; Marshall & Chiat, 2003; McAllister Byun, 2012). This has led authors to posit motor control limitations as the basis of these processes (Inkelas & Rose, 2008; McAllister Byun, 2012). In this chapter, we focus on velar fronting in terms of PoA restrictions and not on its possible speech-motor basis.

Place-Determined Cluster Reduction

Another frequent process in child speech is cluster reduction. When children attempt word-initial obstruent + liquid (OL) consonant clusters, they often omit one of the consonants, typically the most sonorous segment as shown in (2).

(2) Reduction of OL clusters showing the effects of sonority (adapted from Barlow, 2001, p. 299)

grow	/gɹoʊ/	[go]	KR	3;6
blow	/bloʊ/	[bo]	KR	3;6

Not all children follow the sonority pattern, however. Children may select the most sonorant member of a cluster to favor the production of labials, as shown in the examples reported by Pater and Barlow (2003) in (3). It is assumed that /r/ is underlyingly labial in child speech.

(3) Reduction of OL clusters showing the preservation of labial segments (adapted from Pater & Barlow, 2003, p. 510)

drink	/drɪŋk/	[wɪk]	Julie	1;9
grapes	/greps/	[wips]	Julie	1;9

As we will observe, Max displays cluster reduction patterns in English that resemble the patterns described by Pater and Barlow (2003).

Phonological Acquisition in Internationally Adopted Children

There is a growing body of research on the phonological development of internationally adopted children (Glennen, 2007; Pollock & Price, 2005; Pollock, Price, & Fulmer, 2003). Interestingly, this research shows that delayed phonological development is not typical of the majority of children adopted under the age of 2 years. Glennen (2007) found that the 2-year-olds in her study, who were adopted from Eastern Europe (mean age of adoption = 1;4), had articulation scores within normal limits. Similarly, Pollock and Price (2005) reviewed several studies indicating that most of the children adopted from China as infants or toddlers performed at levels comparable to non-adopted children on phonological tests.

Given current models of phonological development, which emphasize implicit learning of ambient language input in the first year of life, one could wonder why delay is not more frequently observed in internationally adopted children. Current models also emphasize the importance of children's own vocalizations and production routines as precursors to early phonological patterns. Children's vocalizations could also be assumed to be reduced in the absence of caregiver input which reinforces word-like approximations (Goldstein, King, & West, 2003). Max has a protracted course of phonological development, which could arguably be related to his early input conditions (i.e., impoverished input and a change of language input). It could also be due to a functional phonological delay/disorder which is unrelated to his history as an adopted child. It would be speculative to determine the relative effects of one or the other. We present the current case study as one that offers potential information on phonological acquisition in the case of diverse linguistic input.

METHOD

Participant

Max spent the first 1;8 years of his life in a Thai orphanage. It was reported that the caregiver to child ratio in the orphanage was 1:8 (1 caregiver to 8 children). His medical report indicated that he was a healthy child with no physical or psychological concerns. His birth weight, APGAR score, and motor milestones were all normal. At the time of adoption, his caregiver indicated he could say [bababa] (no word referent) and [mʌm mʌm] (for food) but no other words. Following adoption, Max was exposed to English (from his mother) and German (from his father). Consistent exposure to French came at age 2;0 when Max spent 12–15 hours per week with a Maman-de-Jour. Following adoption, Max was silent for a one-month period in which he made no consonantal vocalizations and produced no words. He occasionally produced some high pitched vowel squeals.

Data-Base

Diary Study

Diary entries were kept on Max from age 1;9.07, when he produced his first word, through to age 4;10 years. The data were collected by his mother, a trained phonologist. During the initial stages of diary collection, an attempt was made to write down *all* words produced by Max on a given day, whereby words included both new and previously used words. Later on, once Max produced a large number of words on a given day, it is likely that certain words were missed, with a bias towards including new words or new phonetic forms of previously used words. The diary entry also noted down variable phonetic forms of a given word. That is, if Max produced the word *key* as [gi] and [di], both phonetic renditions were documented. However, the diary records did not keep account of the number of times Max produced the [gi] versus the [di] form in a given day. The diary also included notation as to whether the word was imitated or spontaneous, and whether it was a questionable form (i.e., a newly produced word which required verification). In the current study, all imitated and questionable forms were excluded.

The diary study documents all English productions heard by the mother, who was the source of English input for Max. It also includes German and French productions spoken by Max in the presence of his mother. German and French productions spoken when Max was alone with his father or Maman-de-Jour were not captured in the diary entries. Thus, the early diary entries are biased towards English, which was Max's dominant language at the earliest stages of phonological development.

Diary studies have been criticized for methodological reasons including the impossibility of conducting acoustic analysis or of verifying the phonetic transcription. We assume the viewpoint of Inkelas and Rose (2008), who point out that the field of phonological development was founded on diary studies and that diary studies may offer advantages which experimental studies do not, such as the dense longitudinal tracking of a child's phonological development.

Data Reduction

In order to examine the phonetic forms of Max's early words, all word types produced in a one-month period were identified. To simplify the analysis, a single output form for each word type was selected (see Keren-Portnoy, Majorano, & Vihman, 2009). If there was more than one output form, the most frequent form was selected. If there was no dominant form, the most target-like phonetic variant was chosen. On some occasions in the chapter, we also present information on the number of diary entries in a given month for a given word type. Diary entries provide an approximate measure of the frequency of production since frequently produced words appeared on a regular (daily) basis in the records. The data-base from 1;9 to 2;6 includes 368 word types and 4495 diary entries.

RESULTS

Following a general description of Max's early templates and PoA patterns, we examine his phonological data in more detail, focusing on (C)V forms, acquisition of velars, and the realization of consonant clusters with respect to place. The analysis of the first two aspects focuses on Max's English productions; the analysis of the third aspect includes French and German productions as well.

Early Templates and PoA Patterns

Max's acquisition of lexical types was unremarkable; by two years of age, he had acquired over 100 words (at 1;9, he had produced 6 word types; at 1;10, 16 words; at 1;11, 74 words; and at 2;0, 102 word types). Many aspects of his phonological development were also unremarkable. His early word forms were (C)V, (C)VC, and (C)VCV, and his phonetic inventory consisted of stops [p/b, t/d, k/g], nasals [m, n], semivowels [w, j], and the fricatives [ʃ, ç], similar to the word forms and phonetic inventories of a wide range of young English-speaking children (Stoel-Gammon & Dunn, 1985). His (C)VC and (C)VCV forms were templatic, often restricted to consistent phonetic shapes. At age 1;10–1;11, his frequent templates included a final sibilant <V>C_{sib}> template (e.g., *fish* [ɪʃ], *juice* [ɪç], *light* [aɪç]), a velar <$C_{velar}VC_{velar}$> template, (e.g., *egg* [gæg], *gate* [gæg], *yoghurt* [gɛk]), and a nasal template <$C_{nasal}VC_{nasal}$> (e.g., *mouse* [mʌm], *man* [mam], *nose* [nan]).

With respect to PoA restrictions, Max produced bilabial and coronal consonants with low vowels in the first month of word onset (e.g., *car* [daː] 1;9.07, *duck* [dʌ] 1;9.16, *daddy* [dæ] 1;9.28, *bus* [bʌ] 1;9.29), but already in his second month, he was able to produce velars in combination with front vowels (e.g., *dog* [gɛg] 1;10.18, *yoghurt* [gɛk] 1;10.18, *key* [gi] 1;10.25), indicating that he was beyond the consonant-vowel restrictions of Fikkert and Levelt's (2008) first stage of acquisition.[2] By the fourth month, he produced consonants with all vowel combinations (TA, TI, TO, PA, PI, PO, KA, KI, and KO); however, CVC and CVCV forms were generally restricted to one single consonantal PoA and remained so for the first 9 months of word production. From 1;10 to 2;5, over 90% of his output forms consisted of a single consonantal PoA; only at 2;6 did this value drop down to 86%. Examples of CVC and CVCV forms consisting of a single PoA are given in (4).

(4) CVC and CVCV forms consisting of a single (consonantal) PoA produced by Max during the period 1;10 through 2;5

PVP		TVT		KVK	
sheep	[bip]	*knife*	[naɪn]	*pig*	[gʌg]
frog	[wɒb]	*dog*	[dɒd]	*gate*	[gɛk]
shampoo	[baˈbu]	*tiger*	[ˈdaɪdʌ]	*bicycle*	[ˈgægʌ]

At 2;5 to 2;6, we see the first evidence of PoA variegation in the form of PVT, as shown in (5). At this stage, a variety of different target forms (including target KVP, TVP, and KVT) were altered to PVT via processes such as metathesis (e.g., *climb* [baɪn], *soap* [wot]), cluster reduction (e.g., *green* [win]), and context insensitive substitutions (or possibly consonant harmony) (e.g., *kiss* [wɪs]).

(5) Place variegation in the form of PVT at 2;5–2;6

<wVn>		<bVt>		<wVç>	
green	[win]	book	[bʊtʰ]	kiss	[wɪç]
train	[wen]	bread	[bɛːtʰ]	racing	[weɪç]
flying	[waɪn]	bike	[baɪtʰ]		

Later PoA variegation came in the form of final velars, which started to appear as of 2;8–2;9 years (PVK: *bike* [baɪk], *playschool* [beɪguː]; TVK: *snake* [nek], *tricycle* [daɪgʊ]).

The Rise of (C)V Forms

Figure 8.1 illustrates the proportions of word shapes in Max's early words as of his second month of word production; in his first month, 1;9, he produced only 6 word types, all of which were (C)V. As can be seen, (C)VC and (C)VCV forms were present early on alongside (C)V forms, but they declined in frequency, giving rise to the predominance of (C)V forms at ages 2;0 through 2;4. For example, at 1;11, 53% of the output forms were (C)V (i.e., 39/74 types), whereas at 2;2, 86% of them were (164/190 types). Several target forms that were consistently produced as CVCV or (C)VC at 1;10–1;11 were produced later on as (C)V forms. Examples include *banana* (['nænʌ] → [na]), *flower* (['jaja] → [ja]), *fish* ([ɪç] → [i]), *arm* ([om] → [õ]), and *home* ([om] → [õ]). Only later in the analysis period (at age 2;6) did other word shapes start to take precedence over (C)V forms. Max's wholesale deletion of consonants is one way in which constraints on PoA sequences are satisfied.

To provide an example of Max's (C)V period, Table 8.1 displays the most common output form for 60 of the 147 word types in his lexicon at age 2;1.[3] The table shows CV forms arranged according to the PoA of consonants and vowels (e.g., TA, TO, TI, etc.). Single vowels were also frequent phonological forms, often arising from his ban on fricatives and the liquid /l/ (e.g., *seal* [i], *leaf* [i]). It can be observed that Max's phonological forms consisted of a limited range of consonant and vowel combinations, giving rise to numerous homophonous forms.

In sum, the analysis of Max's early data indicates (1) Max's (C)V word forms increased rather than decreased in frequency; (2) Max's

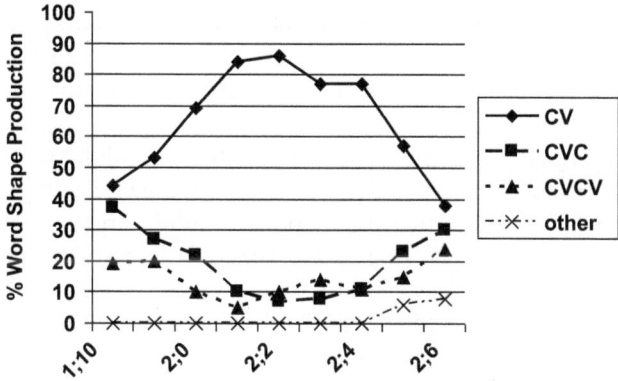

Figure 8.1 The percentage of lexical types realized as different word shapes in Max's speech during the period 1;10 to 2;6.

CVC and CVCV word forms were restricted to a single consonantal PoA; and (3) Max's first examples of variegated PoA forms were PVT, later followed by TVK and PVK forms.

The Decline of Velars and Their Reappearance

Velars were strongly present in Max's early word forms. Output forms containing initial velars represented 28% of his diary entries (16 out of 57 diary entries) at 1;10, and 19% at age 1;11 (92 out of 489 diary

Table 8.1 Max's most frequent (C)V output forms for lexical types at 2;1, organized according to the PoA of consonant and vowel

	T	P	K	Ø
A	cat [dæ?]	apple [pa]	cup [gʌ?]	hat [æ?]
	guitar [da]	basket [bʌ]	glasses [gʌ]	towel [a]
	scarf [da]	pasta [ba]	cloud [gaʊ]	eye [aɪ]
	truck [dʌ?]	butter [bʌ?]	cow [kaʊ]	light [aɪ]
	run [ra]	watch [wa]	cat [gæ]	house [aʊ]
O	carrot [do]	balloon [bu]	goose [gu]	tulip [u]
	goat [doʊ]	book [bu]	juice [gu]	home [õ]
	toe [doʊ]	ball [bɔ]	squirrel [gu]	hose [oʊ]
	door [dɔ]	broccoli [bɒ]	grape [gɒ]	olive [oʊ]
	nose [no]	helmet [mɔ]	hedgehog [gɒ]	arm [õ]
I	biscuit [di]	beard [bi]	cheese [gi]	seal [i]
	chick [dɪ?]	plate [beɪ]	geese [gi]	shoe [i]
	stick [dɪ?]	meat [mi?]	key [gi]	fish [i]
	bird [dɛ]	wheel [wi]	chick [gɪ?]	feet [i]
	feather [dɛ]	kiwi [wi]	biscuit [gi]	music [i]

entries).[4] It is important to note that output forms containing initial velars were not necessarily productions of target forms with initial velars. At 1;11, 41% of Max's KV(K) forms represented productions of adult targets containing /k, g/ in initial position (e.g., *key* [gi], *carrot* [gɒ], *gate* [gæg], *cup* [gʌ]); 41% represented productions of adult targets containing /k, g/ in non-initial position (e.g., *tiger* [gaɪgʌ], *truck* [gʌ], *biscuit* [gɪ]); and 17% represented productions of adult targets containing no /k, g/ (e.g., *cheese* [gɪ], *strawberry* [gɔ]). Progressively, initial velar output forms became less and less frequent (e.g., at 2;0, 13.5% (58/431 diary entries); at 2;2, 12.0% (75/603 diary entries); at 2;4, 3% (20/658 diary entries)) until by 2;6 they were present in only 2% of diary entries (14/766 diary entries). Words previously produced with velar consonants were replaced predominantly by coronal forms, as shown in (6). An interesting aspect of this velar extinction was that at 1;11 almost 60% (53/92 diary entries) of the initial velar forms were KI(K) forms, whereas at 2;6 the few velar forms which remained occurred with dorsal vowels; that is, they were KO(K) forms (e.g., *girl* [goʊ], *hedgehog* [gɒg]), containing the consonant-vowel restrictions often observed at the earliest stages of phonological acquisition (Fikkert & Levelt, 2008; Levelt, 1994; MacNeilage & Davis, 2000; Stoel-Gammon, 1996).

(6) Examples of phonetic forms indicating the gradual disappearance of velar consonants

	cat	*gate*	*cup*	*juice*
1;11	[kæ]	[gek]	[kʌ]	[gɪʃ]
2;1	[dæ]	[gek]	[gʌ?]	[gu]
2;3	[dæ]	[dek]	[bʌ?]	[gu]
2;5	[dʌ?]	[det]	[bʌ?]	[du]

When velars start to reappear, their variable presence takes the form of a positional velar fronting constraint. Figure 8.2 displays Max's percentage of correct production of velars in three positions: syllable-initial pre-tonic (which includes word-initial and medial pre-tonic, as in the words *cat* and *spaghetti*), syllable-final (word-final and word-medial syllable-final, as in the words *dog* and *doctor*), and medial post-tonic (as in the word *parking)*. As can be seen, velars start to be present in all three word positions at 2;9; however, by 3;0 velars are considerably more present in syllable-final and medial post-tonic positions than in syllable-initial position, an effect that becomes even stronger at 3;6.[5]

In sum, we observe: (1) Max starts off with a whole-word template that is characterized by initial (and final) velars and is associated with front, low, and dorsal vowels. This template gradually disappears, and

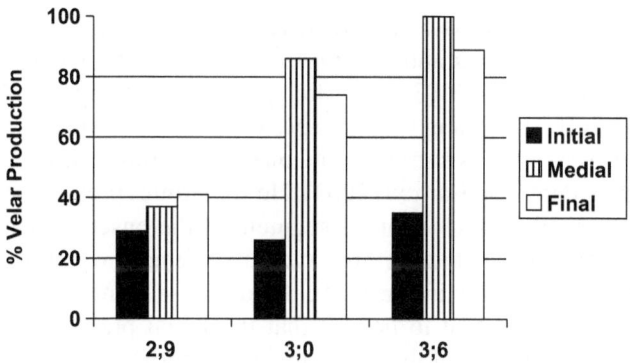

Figure 8.2 Percentage of correct realization of velars in syllable-initial pre-tonic (which includes word-initial and medial pre-tonic positions), syllable-final (word-final and word-medial syllable-final), and medial post-tonic positions. The data at 2;9 include diary entries from 2;8 to 2;10 (number of diary entries containing target velars in syllable-initial position = 78; syllable-final = 54, and medial = 19). The data at 3;0 include diary entries from 2;11 to 3;1 (number of diary entries containing target velars in syllable-initial position = 70, syllable-final = 55, and medial = 29). The data at 3;6 include diary entries from 3;5 to 3;7 (number of diary entries containing target velars in syllable-initial position = 46, syllable-final = 36, and medial = 21).

the few initial velar forms that remain are associated with dorsal vowels. (2) The reappearance of velars takes the form of a positional velar fronting constraint in which final and medial post-tonic velars are realized more accurately than syllable-initial velars.

Realization of Consonant Clusters and Labial-Left Constraint

At the end of the early period, input forms with final labials were transformed so that labials always appeared in initial position (e.g., *climb* [baɪm] 2;6.04, *cup* [bʌʔ] 2;5.14). We see the workings of a labial-left constraint in Max's phonology at later stages of development as well. Word-initial /Cw/ sequences in French and English were always reduced to the labial element, as seen in (7).

(7) Max's productions of word-initial consonant + [w] sequences in French (a) and English (b)[6]

a. *toi*	/twa/	[wa]	3;11.26	"you"
noir	/nwa/	[wa]	4;1.08	"black"
b. *quick*	/kwɪk/	[wɪk]	3;11.04	
koala	/kwalə/	[wawʌ]	3;11.04	

In English, Max's /Cr/ clusters were also reduced so that the labial element surfaced in initial position. As mentioned above, we assume that /r/ is represented as [+labial] in early child English as has been suggested by numerous authors (Gnanadesikan, 2004; Goad & Rose, 2004; Pater & Barlow, 2003). It is often produced with lip rounding and is realized as [w] by young English-speaking children. Max's pattern of segment preservation is similar to the place-determined onset selection described by Pater and Barlow (2003). He sometimes preserves the least and sometimes the most sonorous segment of the onset sequence. The main generalization is that he preserves the segment which is marked for [labial]. This results in /pr, br, tr, dr, kr, gr/ sequences surfacing as [p/b] and [w]. Important to note is that the labial presence is mainly confined to the left side of the word: in word-internal /tr, dr/ sequences, the labial doesn't surface (e.g., *petrol* ['bɛde], *Audry* ['ɔgi]). Reduction patterns of OL clusters are summarized in (8), and phonetic examples are given in (9).

(8) Reduction patterns of OL onset clusters in Max's phonology (3;0–3;9)

/Cr/ clusters		/Cl/ clusters	
Cluster	**Segment preserved**	**Cluster**	**Segment preserved**
pr	b	pl	b
br	b	bl	b
fr	w[7]	fl	w
tr	w		
dr	w		
kr	w[8]	kl	g
gr	w	gl	g

(9) Examples of reduction patterns in English
   /br, pr/   *bread* [bɛd], *broom* [bum], *pram* [ba:n], *present* [bɛʔn̩]
   /bl, pl/   *black* [bæk], *blue* [bu], *plane* [ben], *plug* [bʌg]
   /dr, tr/   *drink* [wɪŋk], *drive* [waɪv], *train* [wen], *tree* [wi]
   /fr, fl/   *French* [wɛnts], *frog* [wɒb], *flag* [wæg], *fly* [waɪ]
   /gr, kr/   *green* [win], *crane* [wen], *crabs* [wabz]
   /gl, kl/   *glue* [gu], *claw* [gɔ], *cleaning* [dinɪn]

When we examine Max's cluster reduction patterns in French and German, we see clear differences in the realization of coronal and dorsal /r/ clusters. They are realized as coronal or dorsal but never as labial, as shown in (10). The different preservation patterns result from the different place representations of /r/ in the target languages, /r/ being represented as [+dorsal] in French and German (see Rose, 2000, for French).

(10) Examples of reduction patterns in French and German
    Fr: /tr/   *train* [gɛ̃], *tres* [te], *trompette* [tɔ̃'pɛt], *citron* [si'tɔ̃]
    Ge: /dr/   *drin* [dɪn], *drei* [gaɪ]
    Fr: /gr, kr/   *grand* [gã], *grave* [gav], *gris* [gi], *crèpe* [gɛp]
    Ge: /gr, kr/   *gross* [gos], *krank* [kaŋk], *Krach* [kaχ]

Since we observed changing patterns in the presence of initial velars during the early developmental period, we also examine whether the labial preservation patterns for onset clusters are already present at the early stages. The most common output forms for the words *truck, train, drain, grass,* and *glasses* from their earliest appearance in the diary entries, namely, at 1;11 through 2;5, are given in (11).

(11) Max's realizations of the words *truck, drain, train, grass,* and *glasses* (each phonetic form represents the most frequent output pattern during a one-month period)

	truck	drain	train	grass	glasses
1;11	[gʌʔ]	[wʌb]	[wʌb]	no example	no example
2;0	[dʌʔ]	no example	[wob]	[ra]/[ga]	[gʌ]
2;1	[dʌʔ]	[wʌb]	[wʌb]	[ra]	[gʌ]
2;2	[gʌʔ]	[wo]	[wo]	[ra]	[gʌʔ]
2;3	[gʌʔ]	[wo]	[wo]	[ra]	[gʌʔ]
2;4	[wʌʔ]	[wiŋ]	[wo]	[wa]	[dʌʔ]
2;5	[wʌʔ]	no example	[wen]	[wa]	[dʌʔ]

What we can observe in the examples in (11) is the gradual takeover of the labial-initial pattern in Max's phonology. In the case of the words *train* and *drain*, they were produced as whole-word labial forms right from the beginning (e.g., PAP [wʌb] or PO [wo]), even though the target vowel was non-labial. Max appears to represent these words with a single labial feature, which is consistent with Fikkert and Levelt's (2008) "one word, one feature" stage. In their analysis, vowel place drives consonantal place, whereas consonantal place appears to drive vowel place in this instance. The target words *drain* and *train* contain no place specification (assuming that coronal is unspecified for place) with the exception of /r/. The labiality of /r/ appears to lead to the production of a rounded vowel or to result in a PVP form. The fragility of Max's vowel representations may play a role, since the mid front vowel /e/ is uncommon in his speech at 1;11 (only the templatic form [gek] for *gate* and *shake* is realized with the vowel [e]). The target word *truck* has velar specification in the coda, and this appears to be the salient feature which influences his word production for several months, until the labial influence of /r/ takes over at 2;4. In the case of *grass*, Max hesitates between the velar and the labial at the beginning (2;0) but later chooses the labial. Note that /r/ is produced in a phonetically target-like form for several months but is gradually replaced by the glide [w]. That Max's production patterns relate to his analysis of /r/ as labial is confirmed by his production patterns of the near minimal pair *glasses*. It is produced either as velar- or coronal-initial (during the "no velar" period) but never as labial-initial. Thus, we observe that Max's later cluster reduction patterns are already determined at the early stages of word production, although the labial-left effect becomes more pronounced over time.

In sum, the findings show that when given the chance, labials surface at the left side of the word at the later stages of development: (1) Max preserves the labial element of /Cw/ clusters in English and French; and (2) Max preserves the sonorant element of /Cr/ clusters in English but not in French and German, a pattern which relates to the place specification of /r/ as labial.

DISCUSSION

This study focused on the speech production patterns of a single child, Max, with the aim of contrasting Universal and Language-Specific (input-based) accounts of phonological acquisition. During a period in which whole-word templates predominated, we saw the emergence of CV forms and the decline of velar forms. Later, we saw the establishment of PoA restrictions such as Labial-Left and No Initial Velars. If we consider Max's speech in terms of Fikkert and Levelt's (2008) stages of PoA development, there was evidence for a long period (1;10–2;5/2;6) in which PoA was not segmentalized within the word—consonants and vowels shared the same PoA feature, or consonants shared the same PoA feature—and a later period (2;6 onwards) in which PoA restrictions emerged. It seems no coincidence that place-determined cluster reduction and positional velar fronting occur together in Max's system, as both are processes that lead to output patterns with PoA restrictions. We now explore the importance of markedness or input-based frequency in accounting for the linguistic patterns in Max's speech.

Early Stage (1;9 to 2;6): (C)V Forms, the Decline of Velars, and the Rise of Labials

Max displayed a U-shaped pattern of development in terms of the shape of his word forms and the production of velars. (C)V forms became more frequent rather than less frequent over time, and output forms containing initial velars declined in frequency until they almost disappeared. We also observed a tendency for output forms containing initial labials to become more frequent during the early period (see examples in (11)).

In order to determine whether frequency may explain these patterns, we examine the frequency of lexical targets consisting of CV forms, initial labials, and initial velars selected by Max during this period. We also examine the frequency of Max's realizations of these forms. The findings on CV forms are straightforward. Lexical words consisting of CV forms were not frequent in the data, representing on average 9% of lexical types during the period 1;10 through 2;6. On a monthly basis, their frequency ranged from 4% (6 out of 146 types at 2;3) to 18% (13 out of 74 types at 1;11). Our percentages are slightly greater than the 6% reported by Stoel-Gammon (1998) on the basis of a phonological analysis of 598 words in the MacArthur Communicative Development Inventories (MCDI) (Fenson et al., 1993). Differences may be due to the fact that Max was acquiring a form of English which does not contain postvocalic /r/. Thus, words like *car* and *door* were coded as CVs. Regardless, the average percentage of 9% for CV forms is considerably less than the percentage of lexical types that Max realized as CV during this period: 44% of lexical forms were realized as CV at 1;10, and this frequency rose to 86% at 2;2 (see Figure 8.1).

Figure 8.3 presents the percentage of lexical targets containing initial labials and initial velars in Max's lexicon, and the percentage of output forms consisting of initial labials and initial velars in Max's speech. Words containing initial labials represented on average 34% of lexical types, with percentages fluctuating from 25% (4 out of 16 types at 1;10) to 40% (93 out of 235 types at 2;4) on a monthly basis. This value is similar to the percentage reported by Stoel-Gammon (1998) based on a phonological analysis of the MCDI: 33% of words begin with a labial phoneme (/p, b, m, w, f, v/). Max produced 25% of words with initial labials at 1;10, but by 1;11 over 40% of his output types consisted of initial labials, and this increased to 50% at the end of the period. Thus, Max's preference for initial labials became stronger towards the end of this period. Turning to velars, words containing initial velars represented on average 11% of the total number of lexical types, with percentages fluctuating from 9% (17 out of 190 types at 2;2) to 19% (3 out of 16 types at 1;10) on a monthly basis. This value is similar to the 12% reported by Stoel-Gammon (1998) for initial velars based on an analysis of the MCDI. Max's realization of word-initial velars declined during this period. He realized 25% of his lexical types with initial velars at 1;10 (4 out of 16 types), 14% at 2;0 (14

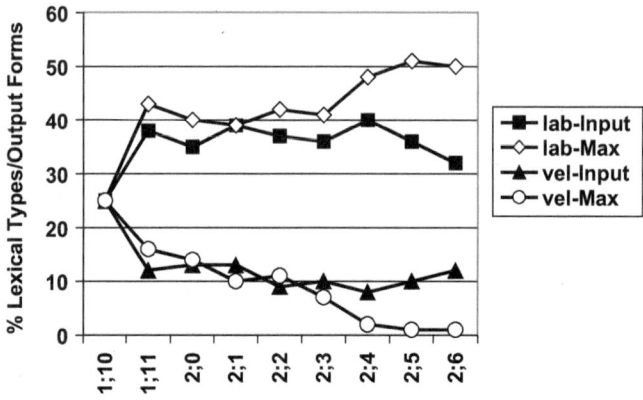

Figure 8.3 Percentage of lexical (input) types produced with initial labials and initial velars (lab-Input and vel-Input) and percentage of output forms produced with initial labials and initial velars (lab-Max and vel-Max) during the period 1;10 and 2;6.

out of 102 types), and 1% at 2;6 (4 out of 311 types). Thus, the changes observed in Max's productions of CV forms, initial labials, and initial velars were not accompanied by similar changes in the frequency of these word types in his lexicon.

The clearest explanation of these patterns is "the emergence of the unmarked". The (C)V form is the unmarked word form, and velars are the most marked segments in terms of PoA. Words containing initial labials are reported to be frequent in the first words of children across a variety of languages (Davis et al., 2002; Locke, 1983), suggesting that initial labials are also unmarked. While many children start off with unmarked structures at the beginning (CV forms, no velars, word-initial labials), other children may first produce marked (often faithful) forms and produce unmarked (unfaithful) forms later on (Fikkert & Levelt, 2008; Vihman & Croft, 2007). Max did not necessarily produce faithful forms at the beginning. Rather, his patterns were consistent with a limited number of whole-word templates (final sibilant, velar template), similar to those described in the research by Vihman and colleagues. We cannot determine to what extent these templates are influenced by pre-linguistic motor patterns or inductive learning of the ambient Thai language, because these data are unavailable; however, it is tempting to speculate that these patterns may be residual articulatory schemas from his earlier period of language exposure. What is clear, however, is that these templates are transient. They are dispensed with quickly in favor of unmarked forms, the appearance of which is unrelated to frequency effects in the input.

Later Stage: Labial-Left and No Initial Velars

Max's later phonological development was marked by a fixed order of PoA development, similar to that described by Fikkert and Levelt (2008) for normally developing (Dutch) children. Following a lengthy period in which words were characterized by a single consonantal PoA, Max's first variegated forms were PVT, consistent with a preference for initial labials. The next variegated forms included TVK and PVK, in which velars were realized in final position and avoided in initial position. Max's preference for initial labials and avoidance of initial velars became entrenched in his phonology, giving it the quality of a disordered system. At first, the labial-left effect was achieved via a variety of processes such as metathesis, consonant harmony, and cluster reduction. Later on, it was maintained largely via the process of (place-determined) cluster reduction. This pattern was observed in Max's French and English words, but it was particularly pronounced in his English words due to the labial representation of /r/.

In terms of Max's velar production, we observed that Max passed through several stages in the acquisition of velars: a stage in which initial and final velars were present, albeit in restricted templatic forms; a stage in which velars (almost) disappeared; and a later stage in which velars reappeared in final position and only minimally in initial position. Their appearance in initial position was conditioned by the presence of dorsal vowels. This final stage lasted until the end of his third year or later. Given that initial velars were present at one point in time and not at another, a speech-motor basis to this positional velar fronting process, as has recently been proposed (Inkelas & Rose, 2008; McAllister Byun, 2012), seems unlikely, although a speech-motor account may explain certain aspects of his pattern, such as the association of velar consonants with dorsal vowels.

Fikkert and Levelt (2008) hypothesize that PoA restrictions such as Labial-Left and No Initial Velars are grammaticized constraints which emerge once the child makes a frequency analysis of the lexicon. They observe that PVT forms are the most frequent, followed by K-final patterns. Stoel-Gammon's (1998) analysis of the English MCDI also revealed high proportions of words containing labials in initial position and coronals in final position, implicating the role of frequency in explaining developmental trends. Thus, Max's PoA restrictions and their manifestation in the form of phonological processes may stem from PoA distribution effects in the adult input. Nevertheless, several aspects of Max's data cannot be explained by frequency alone. At the end of the first period, Max produced more word-initial labial forms and fewer word-initial velar forms compared to input forms with these patterns

(see earlier discussion and Figure 8.3). Later on, Max's labial-left preference was more pronounced in English than in his other languages due
to the phonetic/phonological feature differences between his languages,
supporting the importance of language-specific grammatical factors.[9]
In addition, his preference for final velars was not reflected in similar
effects in his own lexical intake. Target words containing initial velars
were slightly more frequent than words containing final velars in Max's
diary entries (2;9: Initial = 78 target words, Final = 54 target words; 3;0:
Initial = 70, Final = 55; 3;6: Initial = 46, Final = 36), yet Max realized
initial velars less accurately than final velars. In sum, while it cannot
be excluded that children may grammaticalize certain PoA constraints
on the basis of frequency patterns across their lexicons, the way these
constraints manifest in individual children appears to reflect an intricate
balance between both grammar and frequency.

Incomplete Phonological Representation

Fikkert and Levelt's (2008) account of the acquisition of PoA assumes
that children's underlying representations are initially incomplete.
Max's phonetic forms are consistent with many of Fikkert and Levelt's
(2008) observations, suggesting that his early representation of place
was also incomplete. On the basis of his phonetic patterns, we hypothesize that individual segmentation of PoA for consonants and vowels occurs only at the end of the early period, at 2;6. This is when we
observe the realization of variegated PVT patterns and when certain
"one word, one feature" patterns resolve into differentiated forms (e.g.,
the [wo] form for *train* changes to [wen]). A certain global or holistic stage of phonological representation has frequently been associated
with the first-word period of language acquisition. We speculate that
this period may be particularly prolonged in the case of Max due to his
early language input, which was reduced and variable. Indeed, most
children have already acquired a great deal of phonological information
prior to the production of their first words, whereas this "run-up period"
was reduced in the case of Max. The phonological constraints active in
his system might have arisen out of a certain need for salient structure,
which, once established, remained entrenched within his system at several levels (e.g., whole word and word edges).

Conclusion

This study reported detailed findings on the phonological development
of Max, an internationally adopted trilingual child, from the onset of his
word production. His phonological development was characterized by

the emergence of unmarked patterns as well as language-specific ones reflecting grammatical differences.

Max's acquisition of words proceeded at a faster rate than his acquisition of phonemes, suggesting a disassociation between phonological and lexical development, the trademark of a phonological disorder. We do not dwell on the disordered aspect of his speech, since his individual history makes it difficult to compare his results to phonological normative data. Importantly, all of his phonological patterns have been documented in normally developing children across several different languages. We believe that the current findings confirm the role of emergent markedness constraints in phonological acquisition, most likely occurring in interaction with frequency.

NOTES

1 In fact, Max's exposure to French came at 2;0 years when he started spending time with a Maman-de-Jour.
2 Consonant-vowel associations were present in individual words (e.g., *milk* [nɪ], *bear* [dɛ]), but they did not manifest in all words.
3 In categorizing front, rounded and dorsal, and low vowels, the following decisions were made: [i, ɪ, e, ɛ] are front vowels; [u, ʊ, ɔ, ɒ, o] are rounded and dorsal vowels; [æ, a, ʌ, aɪ, aʊ] are low vowels. The vowels [æ] and [ʌ] patterned with the low vowel [a] in Max's phonology; therefore, they were grouped with the low vowels.
4 In this instance, we refer to diary entries to provide an example of the frequency of early velar forms.
5 Diary entries indicate that velar fronting is also present in Max's other languages (German: *Klavier* [davɪɐ], *Katze* [dajɛ] vs. *Flugzeug* [dudɔɪk]; French: *caillou* [taɪjou], *cuillère* [tijɛɐ] vs. *Titanic* [titanik]).
6 /Sw/ sequences were also reduced to the labial element in German (e.g., *schwimmen* /ʃvɪmən/ [wɪmɛn]), but we do not include them here since this reduction pattern may relate to a ban on initial fricatives.
7 Max does not produce fricatives in syllable-initial position. Initial /f/ is replaced by [w] (e.g., *fork* [wɔʔ]). Thus, it cannot be determined which segment, C_1 or C_2, is retained in Max's output forms.
8 Max has a positional velar fronting process, so /kl/ and /gl/ clusters are sometimes realized as coronals (e.g., *cleaning* [dinɪn]). Max also produces some target /tr/ and /dr/ words with initial velars, a process that appears to be related to the presence of a velar-like segment (e.g., postvocalic /l/) or dorsal vowel (e.g., *drill* [guː] 3;1.24, *trolley* [gɒ.i] 3;6.01) in the word. We simplify the analysis by excluding these additional details.

9   It may be possible that frequency nevertheless influenced these results: words starting with labials may be more frequent in English than in French and German. We cannot make a comparable analysis of the frequency of word types beginning with labials in Max's German and French as we did in English, since the diary did not include this information. A phonological analysis of words in the French MCDI indicates comparable (or even higher) percentages of words with initial labials in French compared to English (45% of the nouns of 2;0-year-olds and 42% of the nouns of 2;6-year-olds contain initial labials according to Gayraud and Kern, 2007, vs. 32% for MCDI words ($n = 498$) acquired by children 1;8 to 2;6 according to Stoel-Gammon, 1998), suggesting that, at least in the case of French, initial labials are highly frequent in lexical targets as well.

REFERENCES

Barlow, J. (2001). The structure of /s/-sequences: Evidence from a disordered system. *Journal of Child Language, 28*, 291–324.

Davis, B., MacNeilage, P., & Matyear, C. (2002). Acquisition of serial complexity in speech production: A comparison of phonetic and phonological approaches to first word production. *Phonetica, 59*, 75–107.

Fenson, L., Dale, P., Reznick, J., Thal, D., Bates, E., Hartung, J., Pethick, S., & Reilly, J. (1993). *MacArthur Communicative Development Inventories (CDI)*. San Diego: Singular Publishing.

Ferguson, C., & Farwell, C. (1975). Words and sounds in early language acquisition. *Language, 51*, 419–439.

Fikkert, P., & Levelt, C. (2008). How does place fall into place? The lexicon and emergent constraints in the developing phonological grammar. In P. Avery, B. E. Dresher, & K. Rice (Eds.), *Contrast in phonology: Perception and acquisition* (pp. 219–256). Berlin: Mouton.

Gayraud, F. & Kern, S. (2007). Caractéristiques phonologiques des noms en fonction de l'âge d'acquisition. *Enfance, 59*, 324–338.

Glennen, S. (2007). Predicting language outcomes for internationally adopted children. *Journal of Speech, Language, and Hearing Research, 50*, 529–548.

Gnanadesikan, A. (2004). Markedness and faithfulness constraints in child phonology. In R. Kager, J. Pater, & W. Zonneveld (Eds.), *Constraints in phonological acquisition* (pp. 73–108). Cambridge: Cambridge University Press. Available (1995) on Rutgers Optimality Archive.

Goad, H., & Rose, Y. (2004). Input elaboration, head faithfulness and evidence for representation in the acquisition of left-edge clusters in West-Germanic. In R. Kager, J. Pater, & W. Zonneveld (Eds.), *Constraints in phonological acquisition* (pp. 109–157). Cambridge: Cambridge University Press.

Goldstein, M., King, A., & West, M. (2003). Social interaction shapes babbling: Testing parallels between birdsong and speech. *Proceedings of the Natural Academy of Sciences, 100,* 8030–8035.

Inkelas, S., & Rose, Y. (2008). Positional neutralization: A case study from child language. *Language, 83,* 707–736.

Keren-Portnoy, T., Majorano, M., & Vihman, M. (2009). From phonetics to phonology: The emergence of first words in Italian. *Journal of Child Language, 36,* 235–265.

Levelt, C. (1994). *On the acquisition of place.* Doctoral dissertation. Holland Institute of Generative Linguistics, Leiden University.

Locke, J. (1983). *Phonological acquisition and change.* New York: Academic Press.

Macken, M. (1979). Developmental reorganization of phonology. *Lingua, 49,* 11–49.

MacNeilage, P., & Davis, B. (2000). Origin of the internal structure of word forms. *Science, 288,* 527–531.

Marshall, C., & Chiat, S. (2003). A foot domain account of prosodically conditioned substitutions. *Clinical Linguistics and Phonetics, 17,* 645–657.

McAllister Byun, T. (2012). Positional velar fronting: An updated articulatory account. *Journal of Child Language, 39,* 1043–1076.

Menn, L. (1983). Development of articulatory, phonetic, and phonological capabilities. In B. Butterworth (Ed.), *Language production, Volume 2* (pp. 3–49). London: Academic Press.

Pater, J., & Barlow, J. (2003). Constraint conflict in cluster reduction. *Journal of Child Language, 30,* 487–526.

Pollock, K., & Price, J. (2005). Phonological skills of children adopted from China: Implications for assessment. *Seminars in Speech and Language, 26,* 54–63.

Pollock, K.E., Price, J.R., & Fulmer, K.C. (2003). Speech-language acquisition in children adopted from China: A longitudinal investigation of two children. *Journal of Multilingual Communication Disorders, 1,* 184–193.

Rose, Y. (2000). *Headedness and prosodic licensing in the L1 acquisition of phonology.* Unpublished doctoral dissertation. McGill University, Montreal, Canada.

Rose, Y., & Brittain, J. (2011). Grammar matters: Evidence from phonological and morphological development in Northern East Cree. In M. Pirvulescu et al. (Ed.), *Selected proceedings of the 4th Conference on Generative Approaches to Language Acquisition North America (GALANA 2010)* (pp. 198–208). Somerville, MA: Cascadilla Proceedings Project.

Stoel-Gammon, C. (1996). On the acquisition of velars in English. In B. Bernhardt, J. Gilbert, & D. Ingram (Eds.), *Proceedings of the UBC International Conference on Phonological Acquisition* (pp. 201–214). Somerville, MA: Cascadilla.

Stoel-Gammon, C. (1998). Sounds and words in early language acquisition: The relationship between lexical and phonological development. In R. Paul (Ed.), *Exploring the speech-language connection* (pp. 25–52). Baltimore: Brookes.

Stoel-Gammon, C., & Dunn, K. (1985). *Normal and disordered phonology in children.* Austin, TX: Pro-Ed.

Velleman, S. (1996). Metathesis highlights feature-by-position constraints. In B. Bernhardt, J. Gilbert, & D. Ingram (Eds.), *Proceedings of the UBC International Conference on Phonological Acquisition* (pp. 173–186). Somerville, MA: Cascadilla.

Velleman, S., & Vihman, M. (2002). Whole-word phonology and templates. *Language, Speech, & Hearing Services in Schools, 33*, 9–23.

Vihman, M. (2002). Getting started without a system: From phonetics to phonology in bilingual development. *International Journal of Bilingualism, 6*, 239–254.

Vihman, M. (2010). *Templates in adult and child language.* Paper presented at the Workshop on Templates, Old World Conference in Phonology 7, Nice, France.

Vihman, M., & Croft, W. (2007). Phonological development: Toward a "radical" templatic phonology. *Linguistics, 45*, 683–725.

Vihman, M., & Velleman, S. (2000). The construction of a first phonology. *Phonetica, 57*, 255–266.

Waterson, N. (1971). Child phonology: A prosodic view. *Journal of Linguistics, 7*, 179–211.

Zamuner, T. (2003). *Input-based phonological acquisition.* New York: Routledge.

Zamuner, T., Gerken, L.-A., & Hammond, M. (2005). The acquisition of phonology based on input: A closer look at the relation of cross-linguistic and child language data. *Lingua, 115*, 1403–1426.

9

THE PRODUCTION OF /.sC/ ONSETS IN A MARKEDNESS RELATIONSHIP

Investigating the Ontogeny Phylogeny Model with Longitudinal Data

Robert S. Carlisle and Juan Antonio Cutillas Espinosa

BACKGROUND

Markedness

Markedness relationships among onsets have been examined using two different approaches. In the first approach, investigators such as Greenberg (1978) examined large samples of cross-linguistic data and found implicational patterns. For example, if a language has a biliteral onset consisting of an obstruent (O) followed by a nasal (N), then it also has one consisting of an O followed by a liquid (L), meaning that the OL onset is less marked than the ON onset. As another example, if a language has triliteral onsets, it will also have biliteral onsets, demonstrating that the biliteral onsets are less marked than the triliteral ones. Relying on evidence such as this, Eckman (1977) proposed that less marked structures would be easier for L2 learners to acquire than more marked structures, a claim that has been investigated fairly extensively for more than three decades.

In the second approach to establishing the markedness relationships among onsets, Clements (1990) examined initial demisyllables that adhered to the Core Syllabification Principle (CSP; i.e. those with consistent rising sonority), assigned different values to the segments in the demisyllable based on their sonority, and calculated dispersion values: the greater the dispersion value, the greater the markedness.[1] Clements's approach creates a ranking of onsets that closely approximates the implicational relationships found by Greenberg, reinforcing the idea that markedness relationships among onsets are based on both sonority profiles and their length. (1) displays some of the some of the documented markedness relationships among onsets that have inspired research in second language acquisition (SLA):

(1)   OL < ON < OO < CCC

As displayed in (1) OL onsets are less marked than ON onsets, which in turn are less marked than OO onsets because the latter violate the CSP (Clements, 1990). In addition, all biliteral onsets are less marked than triliteral onsets.

If markedness plays a role in L2 acquisition, as asserted by Eckman (1977, 1991) and Major (2001), then L2 learners should modify less marked onsets significantly less frequently than they modify more marked onsets, and more marked onsets should not reach the criterion of acquisition before less marked onsets do. An impressive amount of research (including the results of the current study) supports both general predictions.

The Ontogeny Phylogeny Model

The Ontogeny Phylogeny Model (OPM; Major, 2001) describes the process of SLA and accounts for the various stages of interlanguage development by appealing to interacting influences from the L1, the L2, and universal grammar, which Major refers to as U. The OPM is composed of four corollaries which deal with the chronology of acquisition, the influence of style on production, the similarity of structures between the L1 and L2, and the influence of markedness. Of these, only the first and fourth are relevant to the current study.

The Chronological Corollary of the OPM

This corollary of the OPM states that "IL [interlanguage] develops chronologically in the following manner: (a) L2 increases, (b) L1 decreases, and (c) U increases and then decreases" (Major, 2001, p. 85). Parts (a) and (b) of the corollary involve the interaction between L1 and L2 in SLA. At the beginning of the acquisition process, the influence of the L1 is very strong, meaning that transfer is most common at the beginning stages, a phenomenon that has been well documented in SLA research. As noted by Major (2001), entire volumes in the 1980s and 1990s were devoted to the topic (Gass & Selinker, 1983, 1992; Kellerman & Sharwood Smith, 1986; Odlin, 1989). The research revealed that L2 learners transfer not only segments from the L1 into the L2 but also phonological rules. For example, as will be discussed more fully in a later section, both Spanish and Portuguese have syllable structure conditions that disallow /.sC(C)/ onsets, and speakers of these languages transfer a rule which inserts a prothetic vowel before the extrasyllabic /s/. As the process of SLA continues, the influence of the L1 diminishes, and the evidence of transfer wanes.

In contrast to the influence of the L1, the influence of the L2 is not readily evident at the beginning of the SLA process simply because the L2 learners have not had sufficient time to acquire its structures or rules. As the L2 learners continue to acquire more of the L2, the structure of the interlanguage will approach native-like norms though it will probably never reach them, especially in phonology. For example, when speakers of a language with relatively short voice onset times (VOTs) as in Spanish attempt to learn a language with substantially longer VOTs, they will lengthen their VOTs, but most never quite reach native-like norms (Yavaş, 1996).

Part (c) of the Chronological Corollary states that U increases and then decreases over time, which is evident in the intermediate stages of acquisition. In the beginning stages of SLA, L1 transfer is so dominant that U is not manifest. Conversely, in the later stages of acquisition, the influence of U diminishes because the L2 learner has come to acquire more native-like pronunciations. Much more will be stated about the influence of U on the L2 production of intermediate learners in the following section.

The Markedness Corollary of the OPM

"In marked phenomena, IL [interlanguage] develops chronologically in the following manner: (a) L2 increases slowly, (b) L1 decreases and then decreases slowly, and (c) U increases rapidly and then decreases slowly. Thus, except for the earliest stages, the role of U is much greater than L1, compared to less-marked phenomena" (Major, 2001, p. 85). For the current study the important part of the corollary is part (c). Markedness relationships are part of U, and U manifests itself once the suppressing influence of L1 transfer has diminished. The influence of U will continue until the later stages of SLA when more native-like structures replace those affected by U. Several consequences of the of Markedness Corollary are that in the intermediate stages of language acquisition, L2 learners will correctly produce less marked structures more frequently than they will produce more marked structures, and that less marked structures will reach a criterion level of acquisition before more marked onsets, findings that are well documented in research involving onsets.

Markedness by Length of Onset

Phonologists universally recognize that the markedness of onsets increases with length (Clements, 1990; Greenberg, 1978; Morelli, 2003), and research in SLA has consistently shown that shorter onsets are less frequently modified and reach a criterion level of acquisition before longer onsets do. Anderson (1987) examined the frequency with which 20 speakers each of Amoy Chinese, Mandarin Chinese, and Egyptian Arabic modified English onsets, finding that both groups of participants made significantly more modifications of onsets as their length increased. Arabic speakers did not modify simple onsets at all, but they modified over 7% of the biliteral onsets. In turn, the Chinese speakers modified only 0.8% of simple onsets but 10.4% of the biliteral onsets.

Eckman (1991) examined the production of three triliteral onsets and their biliteral sub-sequences by 11 participants who were native speakers of Japanese, Cantonese, and Korean, none of which allow complex onsets. Instead of using a test of statistical significance to determine whether the participants modified more marked onsets more frequently than less marked onsets, Eckman used a criterion level of 80% correct production to determine whether the participants had acquired the structure under investigation. For example, if a participant produced any of the target onsets (/.spr/ and its two sub-sequences /.sp/ and /.pr/) correctly 80% of the time, it was regarded as acquired. The hypothesis was that more marked onsets would not reach the criterion level before less marked onsets, a hypothesis that could have been falsified if the triliteral onset had reached the criterion level while neither of the biliteral subsequences had. Eckman examined three triliteral onsets across 11 participants and four tasks and found one falsification; in one case, a triliteral onset was present at the criterion level, but both biliteral subsequences were absent. Given only one falsification in approximately 130 cases, this study provided evidence that less marked onsets are acquired before more marked onsets.

A few longitudinal studies have examined the effect of markedness on the production of onsets differing in length (Carlisle, 1997, 1998, 2002). The series of studies examined the production of two pairs of /.sC/ and /.sCC/ onsets: /.sk/ and /.skr/, and /.sp/ and /.spr/, the first member of each pair being less marked than the second. All participants were native Spanish speakers and were defined as intermediate at Time 1 according to their overall rate of correct production, between 21% and 79%. At Time 1 the data was analyzed in two ways. First, the frequency of prothesis was compared across the biliteral and triliteral pairs. Second, acquisition was examined by investigating whether the less marked member of a pair would reach the criterion level of 80% correct production before the more marked member of the pair would.

Results at Time 1 revealed that the 11 participants modified the triliteral onset of both pairs significantly more frequently than they modified the biliteral onset. In addition, Participants 3 and 6 produced /.sk/ but not /.skr/ at the criterion level, and Participants 2, 3, 6, and 10 produced /.sp/ at the criterion level but not /.spr/. These results agreed with those of previous studies in that more marked structures were correctly produced significantly less frequently than were less marked structures, and more marked structures did not reach a criterion level of acquisition before less marked structures did.

Time 2 data from the remaining 10 participants was gathered 10 months after Time 1. At Time 2, even though nearly all participants correctly produced the less marked onsets more frequently than they produced the more marked onsets, the increase in correct production was not significant. At Time 2, Participant 6 produced all four onsets at the criterion level, and Participant 2 produced /.sp/ at the criterion level but not /.spr/. In contrast, Participants 3 and 10, who had produced onsets at the criterion level at Time 1, actually displayed decreased frequencies of correct production at Time 2, decreases that were so large that the onsets were no longer at the criterion level.

Time 3 data from the four remaining participants was gathered nearly 3.5 years after Time 2. One participant was producing all four onsets with complete accuracy; two had increased frequency of correct production, but none of the onsets had reached the criterion level; and the fourth participant had a lower frequency of correct production even though the data gathering was years apart. Finally, the last three participants were still producing the less marked onsets with a greater frequency of correct production than they were the more marked onsets.

These findings clearly indicate two points. First, at all three times of data gathering, the participants as a group produced less marked onsets with greater frequency of correct production than more marked onsets, revealing the very strong influence that markedness has on production. Second, L2 learners do not uniformly improve. In fact, frequencies of correct production can reach a criterion level at one time and then fall below it the next.

Finally, in a longitudinal case study, Abrahamsson (1999) tracked the production of /.sC(C)/ onsets in Swedish by a native Spanish speaker. Over a 10-month period, the participant modified .77 of the triliteral onsets and .59 of the biliteral onsets, a statistically significant difference.

Markedness by Sonority Sequencing

Another set of studies held length constant, examining just biliteral onsets that were in a markedness relationship according to their sonority profile. Carlisle (1988) examined the frequency of prothesis before OL and ON onsets. Even though both onsets abide by the CSP of continuously rising sonority through the nucleus (Clements, 1990), OL onsets are still less marked because they have a lower dispersion value, (0.56), than do ON onsets (1.17) according to the Feature Dispersion Principle (Clements, 1990). To test the possible influence of this markedness relationship, Carlisle examined the frequency of prothesis before the onsets /.sl/, /.sm/, and /.sn/, the hypothesis being that prothesis would occur less frequently before the OL onset than the ON onsets. The mean proportions of prothesis before the three onsets were .29 for /.sl/, .38 for /.sm/, and .33 for /.sn/, a significant difference among the three means. Pairwise comparisons revealed that the mean frequency of prothesis before /.sl/ was significantly less than before /.sm/ or /.sn/, as hypothesized. In addition, /.sm/ was also more frequently modified than was /.sn/, although the two onsets are not in any known implicational relationship. However, a possible explanation may be found in Clements's Sequential Markedness Principle (1990, p. 313), stated below:

(2) For any two segments A and B and any given context X Y, if A is simpler than B, then XAY is simpler than XBY.

Given that anterior coronals are less marked than are labials, the sequence /.sn/ is less marked than /.sm/ and should therefore be modified less frequently.

In a later study, Carlisle (1991b) examined the production of /.sl/ and /.st/ onsets by 11 native Spanish-speaking adults; the two onsets differ in that /.sl/ conforms to the CSP and /.st/ does not, making the former less marked than the latter. The frequency of prothesis was .36 before /.st/ and .25 before /.sl/, a significant difference. So again the less marked onset was modified less frequently than was the more marked onset.

Another study finding that complex onsets with a lower dispersion value are modified less frequently than those with a higher one was conducted by Eckman and Iverson (1993). They investigated the production of four onsets ranked in terms of their dispersion value and the Sequential Markedness Principle. The least marked onset was a voiceless stop + liquid with a dispersion value of 0.56, and the most marked was a voiceless stop + glide with a dispersion value of 1.17. The two intermediate onsets were voiced stop + liquid and voiceless fricative +

liquid. Eckman and Iverson gathered data for their study by interviewing 11 participants, three speakers of Cantonese and four speakers each of Japanese and Korean.

To test their predicted markedness ranking, the researchers measured their participants' production against a criterion of 80% correct production, hypothesizing that more marked onsets would reach the criterion level only if the corresponding less marked onsets also reached the criterion level. The study contained 55 potential tests of the hypothesis, but 5 of the tests could not be conducted because some participants did not produce the minimum number of tokens for one of the target onsets. Of the 50 remaining tests, 46 supported the general hypothesis that a more marked onset would not reach the criterion threshold unless a corresponding less marked onset had also reached the criterion level.

Criterion Level of Acquisition

If the OPM is accurate, less marked structures should reach a criterion level of acquisition before more marked structures, and three studies already reviewed above—Eckman (1991), Carlisle (1998), and Eckman and Iverson (1993)—have provided evidence for this position. The current study will also examine acquisition using the criterion level of 80% correct production.

THE STUDY

Purpose

As discussed by Major (2001, p. 92), the claims of the OPM are difficult to support because they can be validly investigated only with the use of longitudinal studies or the use of clearly defined groups of participants with different levels of proficiency. Consequently, the major purpose of the current study is to fill a void in SLA research by explicitly testing the OPM using both longitudinal data and data from groups with different levels of ability, beginning learners and advanced, as determined by how frequently they correctly produce onsets in a markedness relationship while reading a list of sentences containing the target onsets.[2]

Hypotheses

The following six hypotheses were tested based on the markedness relationships among the three target onsets. /.st/ is the most marked of three; in turn, /.sn/ is more marked than /.sl/ (Clements, 1990).

1. Participants will correctly produce onsets more frequently at Time 2 than at Time 1.

2. Participants will correctly produce /.sl/ significantly more frequently than they will produce /.sn/ and /.st/.
3. Participants will correctly produce /.sn/ significantly more frequently than they will produce /.st/.
4. Beginning English learners will correctly produce the three onsets with the same frequency.
5. Advanced English learners will correctly produce the three onsets with the same frequency.
6. Participants will not acquire more marked onsets before less marked onsets as determined by a criterion level of 80% correct production.

The hypotheses are in non-null format because the findings of previous research provide evidence for particular expectations. Specifically, the second and third hypotheses have been written in non-null format under the assumption that most, or even all, of the participants will be in the intermediate stages of SLA; that is, their overall correct production of the onsets will still be between 21% and 79%. This is a fairly safe assumption given that the data for Time 2 was gathered only one year after that for Time 1. In addition, the fourth and fifth hypotheses are written in non-null format because the OPM asserts that language universals do not exert much influence on the interlanguage of beginning and advanced learners, here defined as those who respectively produce less than 21% of the onsets or at least 80% of the onsets correctly.

Methodology

Participants

All the participants in the study were native Spanish speakers. Only native Spanish speakers participated because the syllable structure conditions of Spanish prohibit word-initial onsets of the form /sC(C)-/ (Harris, 1983). Spanish speakers treat the initial /s/ or /ʃ/ of complex onsets as an extrasyllabic consonant. Studies investigating the acquisition of these complex onsets in English (Carlisle, 1988, 1991a, 1991b, 1997, 1998, 2006, 2010; Rauber, 2006), Swedish (Abrahamsson, 1999), German (Tropf, 1987), and Italian (Schmid, 1997) have found that native Spanish speakers modify the onsets almost exclusively by prothesis. Spanish speakers then resyllabify the extrasyllabic consonant with the prothetic vowel (Clements & Keyser, 1983).

All the participants were enrolled in intermediate English as a second language courses at Bakersfield College at Time 1. The students were placed in the intermediate classes based on their scores on the

Secondary Level English Proficiency Test, which consists only of listening and reading comprehension sections; students were never placed according to their proficiency in pronunciation.

Because the students were not placed because of their pronunciation, at Time 1 the participants' overall frequency of correct production of the onsets had to fall within a certain range. All of the participants had to produce at least 21% of the onsets correctly but no more than 79%. This range of production to identify intermediate learners can be defended because previous research has used 80% correct production of any particular structure as the criterion level for acquisition (Andersen, 1978; Cancino, Rosansky, & Schumann, 1975; Carlisle, 1997; Eckman, 1991; Eckman & Iverson, 1993).[3]

At Time 1, 34 potential participants were taped, but 17 were eliminated because their frequency of correct production was below 21% or above 79%, meaning that they were classified as beginning and advanced learners respectively. Their data is used in the current study to test hypotheses 4 and 5.[4]

Data Gathering Instruments

The data gathering instrument used at both Time 1 and Time 2 consisted of 375 randomly ordered sentences, 125 each for /.sl/, /.sn/, and /.st/. The environments before the three onsets were strictly controlled; 25 environments each appeared exactly five times before each onset. Each sheet contained 25 sentences for the participants to read. At Time 2, participants read the sentences in different orders than they had at Time 1.

Procedure

The 12 participants at Time 2 were individually taped exactly one year after they were originally taped and in the same language laboratory at Bakersfield College. Participants were taped with a Sony TC-D5PROII recorder with Sony ECM-530 microphone.

Transcription and Reliability

The two researchers independently transcribed the tapes of the 12 participants, specifically noting the quality of the preceding environment, the presence of a prothetic vowel, and the quality of the onset. Interrater reliability coefficients ranged from .87 to .97, with the average being .92. Another faculty member with training in phonetics and experience in transcribing independently resolved the differences between the first two transcribers. Participants in the study either skipped a sentence or misread the word containing the target onset 118 times. These items were removed from the statistical analysis.

Analysis

A two-way ANOVA with repeated measures was calculated with onset and time as the independent variables. This analysis enabled the researchers to determine whether the markedness relationships among the three onsets were still influencing the frequency of correct production at Time 2. The analysis also enabled the researchers to determine whether the participants were producing a significantly greater percentage of the onsets correctly at Time 2 than at Time 1. We also examined acquisition against a criterion level of 80% correct production.

Results and Discussion

Results from the ANOVA

The main effect for time. The main effect for time was not significant; at Time 1, the participants produced 52.7% of all onsets correctly, and at Time 2, they produced 56.7% of them correctly, a difference of only 4% in the year between data gathering. However, even though the overall increase in correct production was only 4%, individual participants differed greatly in their performance from Time 1 to Time 2, as displayed in Figures 9.1 and 9.2. Between Time 1 and Time 2, nine participants experienced gains; Participant 15 displayed little or no difference; and Participants 7 and 16 displayed dramatic decreases in correct production over time, 33.7% and 16.9% respectively.

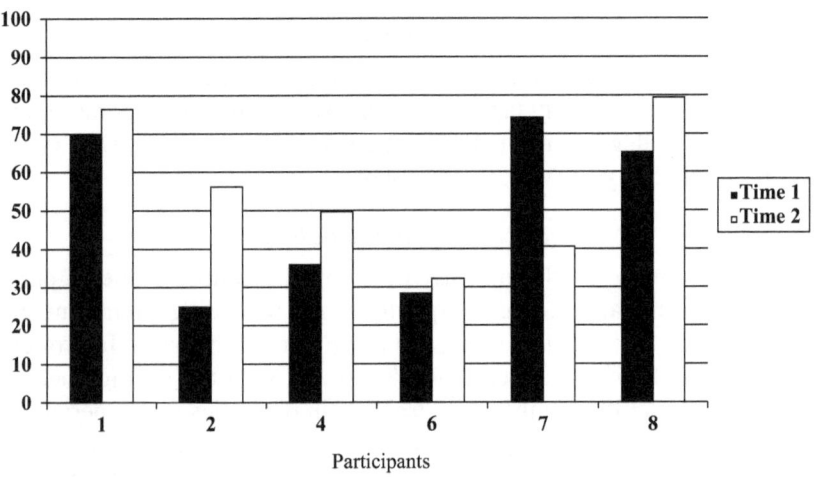

Figure 9.1 Percentage of overall correct production at Time 1 and Time 2: Participants 1, 2, 4, 6, 7, and 8.

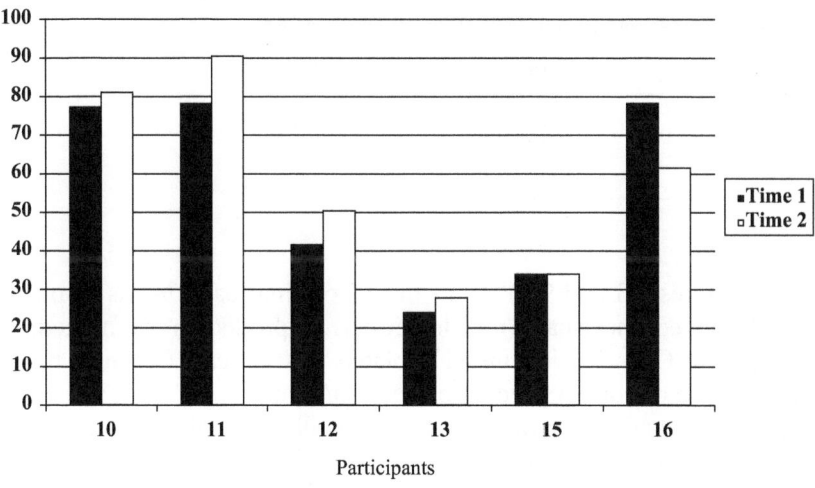

Figure 9.2 Percentage of overall correct production at Time 1 and Time 2: Participants 10, 11, 12, 13, 15, and 16.

The importance of these findings is that 10 of the 12 participants were still in the intermediate stages of SLA, with only Participants 10 and 11 having passed the threshold of 80% correct production. Consequently, given that the participants were still intermediate learners, the OPM predicts that a significant difference among the means of correct production for the onsets will still hold.

The main effect for onset. Table 9.1 displays the frequency of correct production for the three onsets at Time 1 and Time 2. As revealed in the table, the frequency of correct production is in the expected order according to the markedness relationships. At Time 2, participants produced 62.9% of the /.sl/ onsets correctly, 58.1% of the /.sn/ onsets correctly, and 49.2% of the /.st/ onsets correctly. These mean differences produced a significant result for onset: $F(2,22) = 13.070$, $p < .0005$. These results are in accordance with those found at Time 1 (Carlisle, 2006). At both times, markedness had a significant influence on the correct production of the onsets. The influence of markedness did not diminish over the time of the study, which supports the OPM given that the participants were still in the intermediate stages of SLA, when the influence of markedness is most pronounced.

The consistency in the pattern of individual production reaffirms the statistical finding that less marked onsets are correctly produced significantly more frequently than are more marked onsets. At Time 1

Table 9.1 The percentage of correct production at Time 1 and Time 2

	Time 1	Time 2
.sl	61.3	62.9
.sn	54.0	58.1
.st	42.7	49.2

(see Figures 9.3 and 9.4), 16 of the 17 original participants displayed the expected linear pattern of lower correct production as markedness increased. Only Participant 11 violated this pattern, having a higher percentage of correct production for /.sn/ than for /.sl/. At Time 2 (see Figures 9.5 and 9.6), 8 of 12 participants adhered to the expected linear pattern of lower frequencies of correct production with the increase of markedness; four participants—1, 11, 12, and 16—did not.

The interaction effect. A significant interaction effect obtained between the main variables of onset and time: $F(2, 22) = 21.881, p = .0005$, indicating that the pattern of correct production was different from Time 1 to Time 2. Table 9.1 indicates that even though Time 2 means are higher than those for Time 1, the differences in correct production were not uniform across the three onsets: 1.6% for /.sl/, 4.1% for /.sn/, and 6.5% for /.st/. This pattern of improvement is related to the markedness

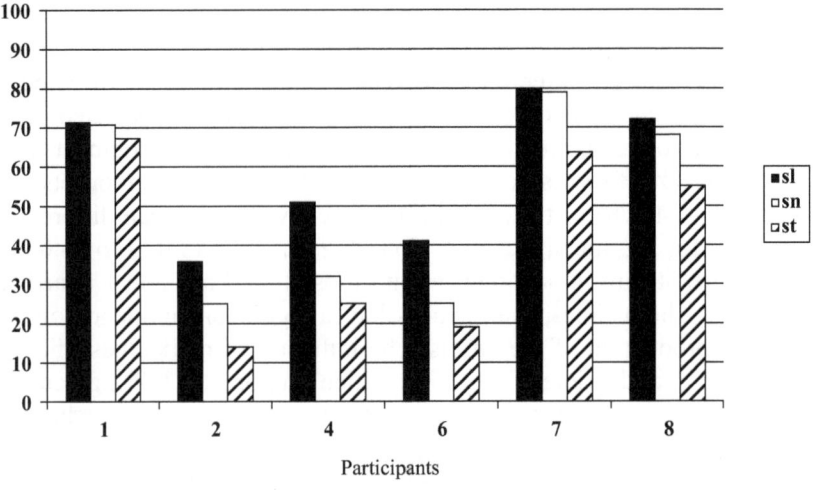

Figure 9.3 Percentage of /.sl/, /.sn/, and /.st/ correctly produced at Time 1: Participants 1, 2, 4, 6, 7, and 8.

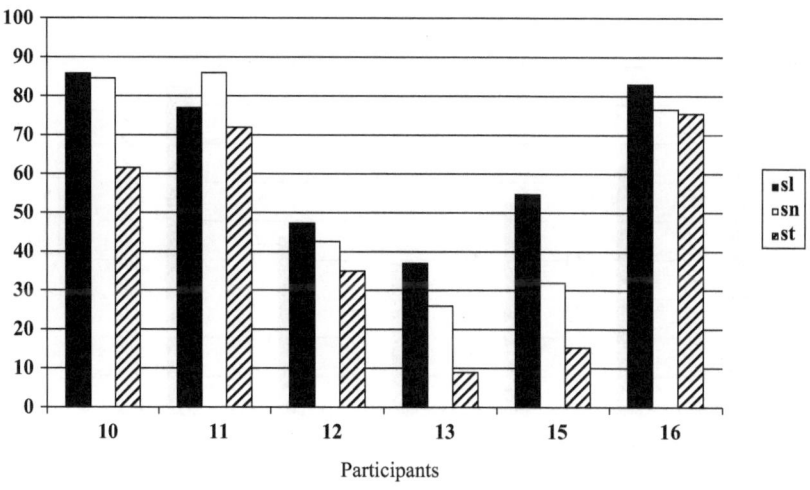

Figure 9.4 Percentage of /.sl/, /.sn/, and /.st/ correctly produced at Time 1: Participants 10, 11, 12, 13, 15, and 16.

relationships: the more marked the onset, the greater the increase in correct production. If this trend were to continue over time, the means for the correct production of the onsets would converge, a finding that would be in accordance with the OPM, which postulates that the influence of markedness is weak in the early stages in L2 acquisition, increases in the intermediates stages, and declines in the later stages.

Criterion Level of Acquisition

The researchers also examined the means of individual participants against an acquisition level of 80% correct production. At Time 1 (see Figures 9.3 and 9.4), Participants 7 and 16 produced /.sl/ at the criterion level but neither of the more marked onsets. Participant 10 produced both /.sl/ and /.sn/ at the criterion level but not /.st/. However, at Time 1 Participant 11 violated the expectation in that /.sn/ reached the criterion level before /.sl/.

At Time 2 (see Figures 9.5 and 9.6) Participant 8 produced /.sl/ at the criterion level, Participant 10 produced both /.sl/ and /.sn/ at the criterion level, and Participant 11 produced all three onsets at the criterion level. All of these findings conform to the expectation that more marked onsets will not reach a criterion level before less marked onsets. However, an onset's reaching of the criterion level at Time 1 does not guarantee that it will remain at the criterion level at Time 2. Both

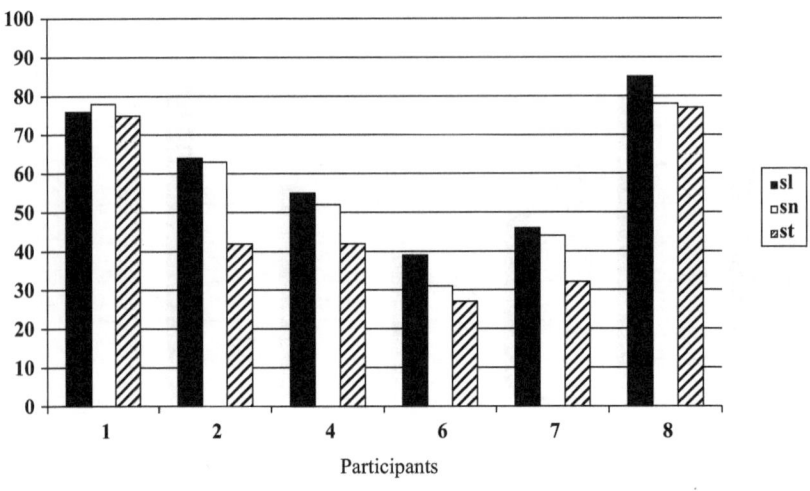

Figure 9.5 Percentage of /.sl/, /.sn/, and /.st/ correctly produced at Time 2: Participants 1, 2, 4, 6, 7, and 8.

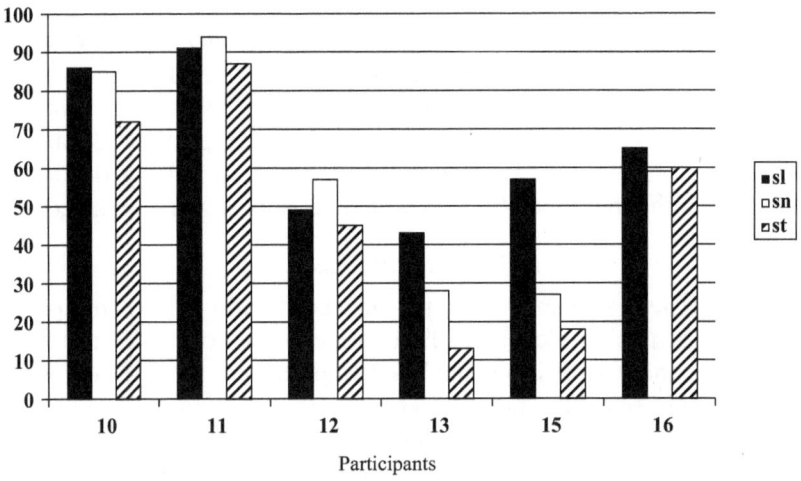

Figure 9.6 Percentage of /.sl/, /.sn/, and /.st/ correctly produced at Time 2: Participants 10, 11, 12, 13, 15, and 16.

Participants 7 and 16 produced /.sl/ at the criterion level at Time 1 but not at Time 2. In fact, both participants displayed a uniform decrease in the correct production of the onsets. The finding that frequencies of correct production can reach a criterion level at one time and then fall below it the next has been documented in a previous study (Carlisle, 1998).

Time 1 and Time 2 data allowed for 87 tests of the hypothesis that more marked onsets would not reach the criterion level of 80% correct production before less marked onsets.[5] Ten tests (11.5%) supported the hypothesis; 76 tests (87.4%) were consistent with the hypothesis in that they neither supported nor falsified it; and only 1 test (1.1%) failed to support the hypothesis. These findings are in accordance with previous findings that more marked onsets do not normally reach the criterion level before less marked onsets (Eckman, 1991; Eckman & Iverson, 1993; Carlisle, 1998).

Beginning and Advanced Learners

The OPM claims that the effect of markedness is clearly evident during the intermediate stages of SLA, a claim which the results of Time 1 and Time 2 clearly supported. As discussed above, the means of correct production of the three onsets were significantly different, and the pattern of correct production was in the expected direction, with less marked onsets being correctly produced more frequently than more marked onsets: /.sl/ > /.sn/ > /.st/.

The OPM also claims that the influence of markedness is weak in the beginning stages of SLA, the interlanguage instead being characterized by transference from the L1. The current study also supports this claim. As displayed in Figure 9.7, at Time 1 six participants correctly produced less than 20% of the onsets correctly: 15.2% for /.sl/, 17.9% for /.sn/, and 16.2% for /.st/. Given the small number of participants, we did not attempt to show statistical differences among the means, but the differences are quite small, only 2.7% between the highest and the lowest means. In addition, the means of correct production did not vary in the expected direction if markedness was an influence; the least marked onset, /.sl/, had the lowest frequency of correct production. As predicted by the OPM, transference was the most powerful factor in structuring the interlanguage in the beginning stages. The native Spanish-speaking participants transferred the rule of prothesis from their L1, applying it to modify well over 80% of the target onsets in English.

According to the OPM, the influence of markedness should not be evident in the latter stages of SLA, a claim that is also supported in the current study. As displayed in Figure 9.8, three participants at Time 1 correctly produced 80% or more the target onsets; also included in Figure 9.8 is Participant 11, who at Time 2 produced all three onsets at the criterion level. The means of correct production for the three onsets

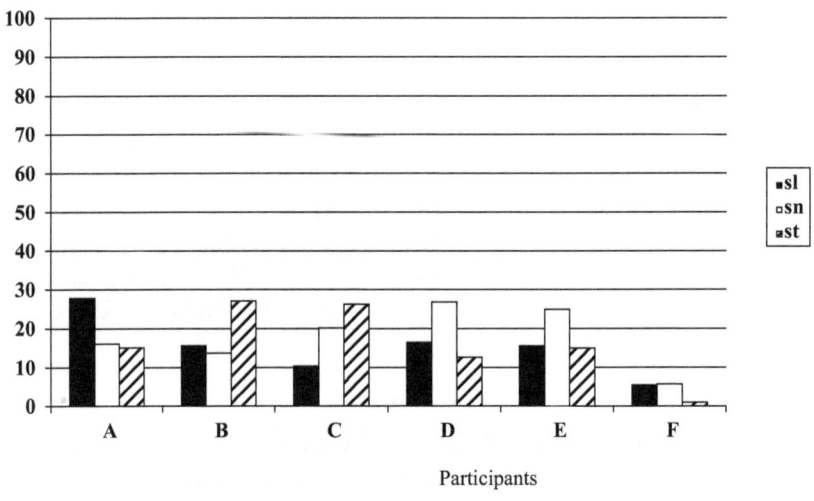

Figure 9.7 Percentage of /.sl/, /.sn/, and /.st/ correctly produced at Time 1 by advanced learners: Participants A, B, C, D, E, and F.

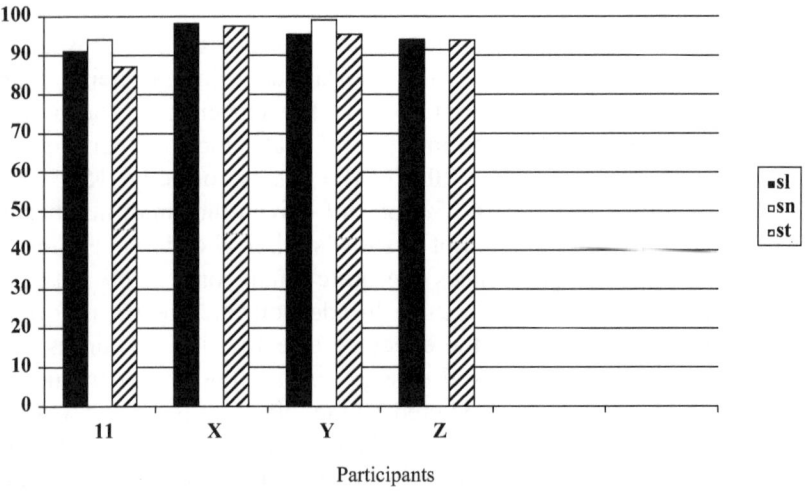

Figure 9.8 Percentage of /.sl/, /.sn/, and /.st/ correctly produced at Time 1 by beginning learners: Participants 11, X, Y, and Z.

were 94.7% for /.sl/, 94.4% for /sn/, and 93.5% for /.st/. Again, we did not perform a statistical analysis on this data because the number of participants was too small. However, the highest and lowest means are only 1.2% apart, suggesting that, as predicted by the OPM, markedness is not a significant influence on the structure of the interlanguage in the advanced stages of SLA.

THE INTERACTION OF LANGUAGE UNIVERSALS AND LANGUAGE SPECIFIC RULES

The current volume is devoted to the influences of language universals and language specific factors on SLA. We take the position that the influences of language universals are crucial in accounting for the acquisitional patterns found in interlanguage, patterns that are completely in accordance with established markedness relationships and the predictions that derive from them. These patterns are particularly evident in the interlanguage of intermediate learners as postulated in the OPM, and advocates of language specific influences would be hard pressed to explain the presence of the documented patterns without referring to language universals, especially given the fact that some onsets that violate sonority sequencing such as /.st/ occur more frequently in the language than those that adhere to sonority sequencing (Vitevitch & Luce, 2004). In the following discussion, we reassert the obviously strong impact that language universals have on the structuring of the interlanguage while acknowledging that in some cases the transfer of language specific rules may actually attenuate the expected influence of language universals. We will concentrate on studies that have compared the production of OL, ON, and OO onsets in English by native speakers of Spanish and Portuguese.

At least four studies examining native Spanish speakers learning English support the predictions based on markedness relationships that less marked onsets will be modified less frequently than will more marked onsets. Carlisle (1991b) examined the production of OL and OO onsets, finding that the participants produced a significantly greater percentage of OL onsets correctly than they did OO onsets. Carlisle (1992) found that participants also produced a significantly greater percentage of OL onsets correctly than ON onsets. In addition, Carlisle (2006) found that at Time 1 of a longitudinal study participants produced a significantly greater percentage of OL onsets correctly than either ON or OO onsets and that they produced a greater percentage of ON onsets correctly than OO onsets, a finding that was duplicated at Time 2 in the current study because nearly all of the participants were still intermediate learners. Finally, Rauber (2006) found that participants modified OO onsets significantly more frequently than they modified onsets that abided by the CSP.

Three studies of Portuguese speakers learning English (Major, 1996; Rauber, 2006; Rebello & Baptista, 2006) produced findings that contradict the finding that L2 learners modify OO onsets significantly more frequently than they do onsets that abide by the CSP. Using a VARBRUL analysis, Major found that OL onsets, specifically realized as FL, promoted errors most frequently, and OO onsets, specifically realized as /s/ followed by a voiceless stop, promoted errors least frequently. In the second study, Rebello and Baptista compared the production of biliteral onsets abiding by the CSP—OL and ON—against those that did not—OO—and found that the six participants modified 63% of the less marked onsets as opposed to 54% of the more marked onsets, a significant difference. Finally, in the third study, Rauber (2006) found that 10 participants modified 27.6% of the OL and ON onsets and 30.9% of the OO onsets. Unlike the first two studies, the frequency of modification was in the correct direction, but it did not reach significance.

The researchers of all three studies argue that the seemingly aberrant findings may be attributed to the positive transfer of two interacting rules, prothesis and voicing assimilation. Major (1996, p. 88) points out that in the underlying representation, Brazilian Portuguese does not have any word-initial onsets of the form /.sC/; instead, the underlying form is /s.C/, where /s/ is an extrasyllabic consonant that must resyllabify at some point in the derivation (Clements & Keyser, 1983). Portuguese has a rule of prothesis triggered by the extrasyllabic consonant that inserts /i/ before the /s/, to which the latter sound resyllabifies, resulting in structures such as /is.C/.

In addition, Portuguese also has a rule that voices voiceless obstruents, such as /s/, when they are in syllable-final position and followed by a voiced consonant either within the same word or across a word boundary. Consequently, underlying structures such as /s.l/ will be pronounced as [zl], but underlying /s.k/ will never be pronounced as *[zk]. Furthermore, in running speech the prothetic vowel is frequently devoiced and subsequently deleted, but only when /s/ has not been voiced, so a word beginning with /sC$_1$/ (where C$_1$ represents a voiceless stop) variably goes through the following derivation:

(3) /s.C$_1$/ underlying representation (/s/ is extrasyllabic)
[s.C$_1$] voicing assimilation (does not apply)
[is.C$_1$] prothesis and resyllabification with the extrasyllabic consonant
[sC$_1$] devoicing of the prothetic vowel and subsequent deletion

The derivation above reveals that even though Portuguese does not allow /.sC$_1$/ onsets in the underlying representation, they may occur on the surface because of the devoicing of the prothetic vowel and its subsequent deletion. Note that the derivation in (3) applies only to onsets that violate the CSP, with the result that more marked onsets appear to be modified less frequently than expected.

The derivation of OL and ON onsets can have quite a different outcome, as displayed in (4), where C_2 represents any voiced consonant.

(4) /s.C_2/ underlying representation (/s/ is extrasyllabic)
[z.C_2] voicing assimilation
[iz.C_2] prothesis and resyllabification with the extrasyllabic consonant
[iz.C_2] devoicing of the prothetic vowel and deletion (do not apply)

Because of two language specific rules in Portuguese, the apparently aberrant finding that onsets violating sonority sequencing are modified less frequently than those that do not becomes explicable. In Portuguese the prothetic vowel would never be deleted before clusters such as /s.l/ and /s.N/ because the extrasyllabic consonant voices before the sonorant, consequently bleeding the environment for the application of the devoicing rule and the subsequent deletion of the vowel. In contrast, the extrasyllabic /s/ of [s.C_1] would never be voiced. Thus, the prothetic vowel would undergo devoicing and subsequent deletion, resulting in a marked surface form that is not found in the underlying representation.

The frequency of the modification of less marked clusters such as OL and ON is unusually high because the voicing of the syllabic /s/ induces a higher frequency of prothesis. Rebello and Baptista (2006) found that their participants voiced 58% of the occurrences of /s/ in /s/ + sonorant clusters, and prothesis occurred before 79% of those. In contrast, prothesis occurred before only 39% of the clusters whose first member was not voiced. Also, Rauber (2006) found that 55.6% of the initial segments in /sN/ onsets were voiced and that prothesis occurred before 56.4% of them. In contrast, prothesis occurred before only 11.7% of the /sN/ onsets whose first member was not voiced. She also found that 59.3% of the initial segments in /sL/ onsets were voiced and that epenthesis occurred before 53.4% of them, whereas prothesis occurred before only 12% of the initial segments that were not voiced.

The different results obtained with studies involving Spanish and Portuguese learners of English clearly indicate that while language universals play an important role in structuring the interlanguage of intermediate learners, their influence may be attenuated by the transference of L1 rules. These results do not falsify the predictions of the OPM;

they reveal that transference still has an influence on L2 acquisition though it is not as strong in the intermediate stages as in the beginning stages.

SUMMARY

The major purpose of the current study was to explicitly test the OPM by using both longitudinal data and data from groups with different levels of ability. The results from the longitudinal study revealed that the influence of markedness remained as strong at Time 2 as at Time 1. At both times less marked onsets were modified significantly less frequently than were the more marked onsets. These findings should not be surprising given that Time 1 and Time 2 were only one year apart, and nearly all the participants were still intermediate learners, which also explains why time was not a significant factor even though the overall mean of correct production was 4% higher at Time 2 than at Time 1. In spite of the non-significance of time, 8 of the 12 participants had the expected order of correct production, and the finding that the increase in correct production was greater for more marked onsets supports Major's (2001) claims that the influence of markedness declines in later stages of acquisition.

The analysis of the beginning and advanced groups revealed that both groups produced the three onsets correctly with nearly the same frequency, which supports the claim of the OPM that language universals do not strongly influence the interlanguage of beginning and advanced learners.

Though the results from the current study strongly support the OPM, all the participants spoke the same native language, Spanish. Research on the same onsets that has used native Portuguese speakers as participants has found that more marked onsets may actually have a higher percentage of correct production due to the transference of L1 rules that may attenuate the influence on markedness.

NOTES

1 An initial demisyllable consists of the onset and the nucleus. Because all of the initial demisyllables have a nucleus, its value is held constant so that the dispersion values reveal the markedness relationships among onsets. For a much more complete discussion of Clements's approach, see Carlisle (2010).

2 It is very difficult to determine the frequency of correct production of truly beginning students using a reading instrument because they do not know enough of the L2 to read very well. It is also difficult to elicit more

natural examples of language because their vocabularies tend to be small and may not contain many of the target structures under investigation.

3 For more detailed background information on the participants, see Carlisle (2006).

4 Not all of the data could be used, especially for the 'advanced' learners, because the frequency of correct production was 100% for all three onsets. It is possible to examine the hypothesis that universals no longer influence advanced learners' interlanguage only if there is still variation among the means of correct production for the target onsets.

5 The number of tests was determined in the following manner. The use of three onsets permitted three tests for each subject: /.sl/ to /.sn/, /.sl/ to /.st/, and /.sn/ to /.st/. Time 1 had 17 participants, resulting in 51 tests, and Time 2 had 12 participants, resulting in another 36 tests.

REFERENCES

Abrahamsson, N. (1999). Vowel epenthesis of /sC(C)/ onsets in Spanish/ Swedish interphonology: A longitudinal study. *Language Learning, 49,* 473–508.

Andersen, R. (1978). An implicational model for second language research. *Language Learning, 28,* 221–281.

Anderson, J. (1987). The markedness differential hypothesis and syllable structure difficulty. In G. Ioup & S. Weinberger (Eds.), *Interlanguage phonology: The acquisition of a second language sound system* (pp. 279–291). Cambridge, MA: Newbury House.

Cancino, H., Rosansky, E., & Schumann, J. (1975). The acquisition of the English auxiliary by native Spanish speakers. *TESOL Quarterly, 4,* 421–430.

Carlisle, R. (1988). The effect of markedness on epenthesis in Spanish/English interlanguage phonology. *Issues and Developments in English and Applied Linguistics, 3,* 15–23.

Carlisle, R. (1991a). The influence of environment on vowel epenthesis in Spanish/English interphonology. *Applied Linguistics, 12,* 76–95.

Carlisle, R. (1991b). The influence of syllable structure universals on the variability of interlanguage phonology. In A. Volpe (Ed.), *The seventeenth LACUS forum 1990* (pp. 135–145). Lake Bluff, IL: Linguistic Association of Canada and the United States.

Carlisle, R. (1992). Environment and markedness as interacting constraints on vowel epenthesis. In J. Leather & A. James (Eds.), *New Sounds 92* (pp. 64–75). Amsterdam: University of Amsterdam Press.

Carlisle, R. (1997). The modification of onsets in a markedness relationship: Testing the interlanguage structural conformity hypothesis. *Language Learning, 47,* 327–361.

Carlisle, R. (1998). The acquisition of onsets in a markedness relationship: A longitudinal study. *Studies in Second Language Acquisition, 20,* 245–260.

Carlisle, R. (2002). The acquisition of two and three member onsets: Time III of a longitudinal study. In A. James & J. Leather (Eds.), *New Sounds 2000* (pp. 42–47). Klagenfurt, Austria: University of Klagenfurt Press.

Carlisle, R. (2006). The sonority cycle and the acquisition of complex onsets. In B. Baptista & A. Watkins (Eds.), *English with a Latin beat: Studies in Portuguese/Spanish-English interphonology* (pp. 105–137). Amsterdam: John Benjamins.

Carlisle, R. S. (2010). Word-final sonority as an environmental constraint on prothesis. In A. Rauber, M. Watkins, R. Silveira, & R. Koerich (Eds.), *The acquisition of second language speech: Studies in honor of Professor Barbara O. Baptista* (pp. 243–266). Santa Catarina, Brazil: Universidade Federal de Santa Catarina.

Clements, G. (1990). The role of the sonority cycle in core syllabification. In J. Kingston & M. Beckman (Eds.), *Papers in laboratory phonology I: Between the grammar and physics of speech* (pp. 283–333). Cambridge: Cambridge University Press.

Clements, G., & Keyser, S. (1983). *CV phonology: A generative theory of the syllable.* Cambridge, MA: MIT Press.

Eckman, F. (1977). Markedness and the contrastive analysis hypothesis. *Language Learning, 27,* 315–330.

Eckman, F. (1991). The structural conformity hypothesis and the acquisition of consonant clusters in the interlanguage of ESL learners. *Studies in Second Language Acquisition, 13,* 23–41.

Eckman, F., & Iverson, G. (1993). Sonority and markedness among onset clusters in the interlanguage of ESL learners. *Second Language Research, 9,* 234–252.

Gass, S. M., & Selinker, L. (Eds.). (1983). *Language transfer in language learning.* Rowley, MA: Newbury House.

Gass, S. M., & Selinker, L. (Eds.). (1992). *Language transfer in language learning.* Amsterdam: John Benjamins.

Greenberg, J. (1978). Some generalizations concerning initial and final consonant clusters. In J. Greenberg, C. Ferguson, & E. Moravcsik (Eds.), *Universals of human language (Vol. 2)* (pp. 243–279). Stanford, CA: Stanford University Press.

Harris, J. (1983). *Syllable structure and stress in Spanish: A non-linear analysis.* Cambridge, MA: MIT Press.

Kellerman, E., & Sharwood Smith, M. (Eds.). (1986). *Cross-linguistic influence in second language acquisition.* New York: Pergamon.

Major, R. (1996). Markedness in second language acquisition of consonant clusters. In Dennis R. Preston and Robert Bayley (Eds.), *Variation and second language acquisition* (pp. 75–96). Amsterdam: John Benjamins.

Major, R. (2001). *Foreign accent: The ontogeny and phylogeny of second language phonology*. Mahwah, NJ: Lawrence Erlbaum.

Morelli, F. (2003). The relative harmony of /s+stop/ onsets: Obstruent clusters and the sonority sequencing principle. In C. Fery & R. van de Vijver (Eds.), *The syllable in Optimality Theory* (pp. 356–371). Cambridge: Cambridge University Press.

Odlin, T. (1989). *Language transfer: Cross-linguistic influence in language learning.* Cambridge: Cambridge University Press.

Rauber, A. (2006). Production of English initial /s/-clusters by speakers of Brazilian Portuguese and Argentine Spanish. In B. Baptista & A. Watkins (Eds.), *English with a Latin beat: Studies in Portuguese/Spanish-English interphonology* (pp. 155–167). Amsterdam: John Benjamins.

Rebello, J., & Baptista, B. (2006). The influence of voicing on the production of initial /s/-clusters by Brazilian learners. In B. Baptista & A. Watkins (Eds.), *English with a Latin beat: Studies in Portuguese/Spanish-English interphonology* (pp. 139–154). Amsterdam: John Benjamins.

Schmid, S. (1997). Phonological processes in Spanish-Italian interlanguages. In J. Leather & A. James (Eds.), *New Sounds 97* (pp. 286–293). Klagenfurt, Austria: University of Klagenfurt.

Tropf, H. (1987). Sonority as a variability factor in second language phonology. In A. James & J. Leather (Eds.), *Sound patterns in second language acquisition* (pp. 173–191). Providence, RI: Foris.

Vitevitch, M., & Luce, P. (2004). A Web-based interface to calculate phonotactic probability for words and nonwords in English. *Behavior Research Methods, Instruments & Computers, 36*, 481–487.

Yavaş, M. (1996). Differences in voice onset time in early and later Spanish English bilinguals. In A. Roca & J. B. Jensen (Eds.), *Spanish in contact: Issues in bilingualism* (pp. 131–141). Somerville, MA: Cascadilla.

10

THE ROLE OF INPUT FREQUENCY, UNIVERSALS, AND L1 TRANSFER IN THE ACQUISITION OF ENGLISH L2 ONSETS BY NATIVE SPEAKERS OF CANTONESE, MANDARIN CHINESE, AND VIETNAMESE

Jette G. Hansen Edwards

This chapter focuses on universal and language-specific patterns in the acquisition of English second language (L2) onsets by native speakers of three Asian languages: Mandarin Chinese, Cantonese, and Vietnamese. In specific, the purpose of this chapter is to examine whether the acquisition orders found for the English onsets /sl sn st/ for native speakers of these three languages as well as the modifications found in the production of the onsets can be best explained by input frequency of the onsets, universal constraints, or L1 transfer. In terms of the first, the chapter examines whether the frequency of a particular form in the input affects acquisition orders. The chapter also examines whether linguistic universals, which are innate and devoid of influence from the input, provide a better explanation for the acquisition orders found in the data. As the L2 research to date that has examined input frequency versus markedness has not examined the role of L1 transfer, although it has been found to have a prominent role in the acquisition of L2 phonology, the current study will examine the role of the participants' native language in comparison with the role of input frequency and markedness in the acquisition and production of these onsets.

BACKGROUND TO THE STUDY

The primary objective of this chapter is to examine whether language-universal constraints, input frequency, or L1 transfer provides a better explanation for the acquisition sequences found for English onsets produced by native speakers of Cantonese, Mandarin Chinese, and Vietnamese. The roles of L1 transfer and markedness in the L2 acquisition of all domains of phonology have been supported by a significant number of studies (cf. Eckman, 2008; Major, 2008), with a consensus among researchers that both of these factors, particularly L1 transfer in the early stages and markedness in later stages of acquisition, are major constraints on the development of an L2 sound system. In contrast, very little is known about the role of input frequency in L2 phonological acquisition although it has been found to play a significant role in acquisition orders for child L1 phonology (cf. Zamuner, Gerken, & Hammond, 2004, 2005; Zamuner, Morin-Lessard, & Bouchat-Laird, this volume) as well as being an important constraint in the acquisition of other domains of second language acquisition (cf. Ellis & Ferreira-Junior, 2009). In specific, in the area of child L1 acquisition, research on input frequency typically examines the role of the Universal Grammar Hypothesis (UGH) versus the Language-Specific Grammar Hypothesis on the acquisition sequences of L1 sounds. As Zamuner, Gerken, and Hammond (2005) note:

> In the domain of phonology, the UGH predicts that children should initially produce those sound patterns that are unmarked or frequent across languages before those patterns that are marked or infrequent. The SLGH predicts that children should initially produce the most frequently occurring sound patterns in their ambient language before producing the less frequent ones. . . .
>
> (p. 1406)

Research (cf. Zamuner, Gerken, Hammond, 2004, 2005; Zamuner, Morin-Lessard, & Bouchat-Laird, this volume) has provided substantive evidence that the input frequency of sound structures can override universal constraints in the acquisition of L1 sound structures. It is therefore important to investigate the role of input frequency in the acquisition of L2 sound structures.

To date, only a few studies have examined the effect of input frequency on L2 phonological acquisition, in particular in contrast to universal constraints such as markedness. L2 researchers who examine input frequency:

. . . hold that language users are sensitive to the frequency of lexical items in linguistic input and that language acquisition involves the learning of phonological, morphological, semantic, and other regularities from input. With respect to L2 phonology, the logic here is that certain aspects of speech (e.g., speech sounds, stress patterns, intonation contours) are easier to learn when they occur within and across a variety of recurrent familiar lexical items. The more frequently L2 learners experience a given phonological pattern in the input, especially across a range of lexical items, the more accurately they will perceive and produce this pattern.

(Trofimovich, Collins, Cardoso, White, & Horst, 2012, pp. 176–177)

The findings on the role of input frequency in L2 phonological acquisition are limited for a number of reasons: First, there have been only a few studies on the effect of input frequency on L2 phonological acquisition to date; second, the findings from these studies have been mixed. A study by Flege, Takagi, and Mann (1996) which did not specifically focus on input frequency nevertheless found that frequency may have an impact as the L2 learners in their study had a higher accuracy in identifying sounds in more frequently used words than in less frequently used words. In research on the acquisition of voiceless versus voiced obstruent codas, Broselow and Xu (2004) found that frequency of the L2 structure itself did not have an impact on acquisition but that the L2 structures that were 'perceived' to be more frequent by the learners were produced with more accuracy. This study implies that learners themselves are active agents in perceiving which structures are more frequent, and possibly more important for acquisition, and that this perception can override actual input frequency rankings. Finally, a study by Cardoso (2008) that examined the effects of input frequency versus markedness on the acquisition of /sl sn st/ onsets found that markedness, which would predict an /sl/ > /sn/ > /st/ accuracy order, provided a better explanation for his findings. Therefore, it appears that the findings for the effect of input frequency on L2 phonology are not as clear-cut as for child L1 phonology, which may not be surprising given that more factors, extraneous and internal, impact L2 than L1 acquisition.

PREVIOUS RESEARCH ON /SC/ ONSETS

As the focus of the current study is the acquisition of /sC/ onsets, the findings from previous studies that have focused on those onsets will be reviewed briefly. There has been a great deal of research on the acquisition of /sC/ onsets and in particular the acquisition orders of onsets such as /sl sn st/. One reason for interest in these onsets is that they can be studied in a markedness relationship based on sonority. The sonority sequencing principle (SSP) (Selkirk, 1984) states that optimal, and thus less marked, onsets are those that increase in sonority from the margin into the nucleus (usually a vowel) of the syllable. Both /l/ and /n/ are considered to be sonorous while /t/ is not; in addition, /l/ is considered to be more sonorous than /n/. Therefore, on a sonority scale, the onset preference would be for /sl/ > /sn/ > /st/, with the /st/ onset violating the SSP as stops are less sonorous than fricatives and therefore there is a decrease rather than an increase in sonority for this onset. Researchers have been interested in examining to what extent sonority plays a role in acquisition orders for these onsets, as the SSP would predict the following acquisition order based on sonority rankings: /sl/ > /sn/ > /st/.

The majority of the L2 research on these onsets has focused on learners of L2 English whose L1 is Spanish or Brazilian Portuguese as neither Spanish nor Portuguese permits /sC(C)/ sequences though they do have some complex onsets. Additionally, both these languages have the initial sequence *esC(C)* (Abrahamsson, 1999), which provides researchers with a good opportunity to examine not only the effect of markedness on the acquisition of these structures in terms of length (e.g., /sC/ is shorter and thus less marked than /sCC/ and would be hypothesized to be acquired earlier) but also the effect of the linguistic environment in promoting vowel epenthesis, which is likely to occur as a transfer from the L1. In particular, for Brazilian Portuguese L1 speakers of English, it could be predicted that epenthesis would be more likely to occur in /st/ over /sl sn/ clusters as it occurs only in a voiceless obstruent cluster, and in Portuguese, /sl sn/ are voiced clusters (Rebello & Baptista, 2006).

A series of studies on Spanish L1 speakers' production of English L2 /sC/ and /sCC/ onsets by Carlisle (1988, 1991, 1992, 1997, 2006; see also Carlisle & Cutillas Espinosa, this volume) found that the /sC/ onsets had higher accuracy ratings than the longer, and more marked, /sCC/ onsets, and that epenthesis occurred significantly more often after a consonant (before the onset) than after a vowel (and before the onset). Carlisle also found that the more sonorous, and thus less marked, /sl/ was more accurate than /st/ and that the more sonorous /sl/ was produced more accurately than either /sn/ or /sm/. Markedness in terms of sonority thus provided the best explanation for the patterns found in Carlisle's studies. Abrahamsson (1999) examined the production of /sC(C)/ onsets by L1 speakers of Spanish who were learning Swedish as an L2. Like English, Swedish also allows /sC(C)/ onsets. Abrahamsson found the following sequence of modification, and therefore level of accuracy (from least modified, and thus most accurate, to most modified): /s/ plus nasal > /s/ plus stop > /s/ plus /l/. In other words, /sl/ was modified the most, followed by /s/ plus stop sequences, while /sn/ and /sm/ were modified the least. This accuracy hierarchy could only partially be explained by sonority. Rebello and Baptista (2006) examined the acquisition of English /sC(C)/ clusters by native speakers of Brazilian Portuguese and found that error rates were higher for /sn/ > /sl/ > /st/ onsets, resulting in the accuracy hierarchy, from most to least, of /st/ > /sl/ > /sn/, which provides only partial support for the SSP but could be explained by markedness in terms of voicing, as /st/ as a voiceless cluster could be argued to be less marked than either the heterogeneously voiced /sl/ or /sn/ cluster. Rauber (2006) examined the production of these English onsets by L1 speakers of both Argentine Spanish and Brazilian Portuguese. Rauber found that both groups modified the /st/ onset more often than either the /sl/ or /sn/ onset although this was significant only for the Argentine Spanish speakers. Both groups also had more modification for the /sn/ over the /sl/ cluster, although this was not significant for either group.

A series of studies by Cardoso and colleagues (Cardoso, 2008; Cardoso, John, & French, 2008; Cardoso & Liakin, 2009) focusing on production and perception of these clusters, also with Brazilian Portuguese L1 learners of English L2, examined the role of input frequency versus sonority in the production of these onsets. In both production studies (Cardoso, 2008; Cardoso & Liakin, 2009), the researchers found that accuracy orders followed a sonority pattern of /sl/ > /sn/ > /st/, rather than input frequency, which would have predicted an accuracy order of /st/ > /sn/ > /sl/. This is similar to the majority of the findings from the previous studies discussed above. Interestingly, however, in the perception study (Cardoso, John, & French, 2008), the researchers found that input frequency best explained the accuracy orders, as the most accurately identified onset was /st/, followed by /sn/, with /sl/ the least accurately identified onset. This finding provides evidence that the constraints governing perception and production may differ and that even though participants may be able to correctly perceive /st/ onsets, sonority constraints may override frequency effects when it comes to production. Finally, Enochson (2014) focused on the acquisition of the English L2 onsets /sl sn st/ by L1 Japanese, Cantonese, and Mandarin Chinese speakers and also found that sonority did not explain her participants' accuracy orders of /st/ > /sn/ > /sl/, which did not vary across the three L1 groups. Enochson's findings indicate that the L1 of the participants may be an important factor and, to some extent, that language-specific constraints such as L1 transfer may override language-universal constraints such as sonority. This deserves more investigation.

In summary, the majority of the L2 studies to date have found that sonority provides the best explanation for the acquisition orders in their studies, typically /sl/ > /sn/ > /st/. However, these findings may be relevant only to the domain of production as Cardoso, John, and French (2008) found that input frequency, and not sonority, may be a more powerful constraint on learners' abilities to perceive the three onsets. Finally, the findings on /sC/ onsets in L2 research also come from a relatively homogeneous population of learners as the L1 of the participants has been either Brazilian Portuguese or Spanish, and the L2 typically English and in one case Swedish. Conflicting findings come from Enochson (2014), which examines the acquisition of English L2 onsets by speakers of three different Asian languages: Japanese, Cantonese, and Mandarin Chinese. Enochson's findings demonstrate the need to examine the acquisition of these onsets by learners from various L1s as the role of sonority in the acquisition of these onsets may not be a universal constraint but may be governed by the L1 to some extent. This needs further exploration.

THE CURRENT STUDY

The study examines the acquisition of English /sl sn st/ onsets by native speakers of Mandarin Chinese, Vietnamese, and Cantonese, as well as the role of input frequency, markedness, and L1 transfer in the acquisition of these onsets. Similar to previous research (cf. Cardoso, 2008), this study adopts the following markedness hierarchy, from least to most marked, based on sonority as nasals are less sonorous than liquids and stops are less sonorous than either liquids or nasals: /sl/ > /sn/ > /st/. In terms of input frequency, a number of previous investigations, including Cardoso's (2008) analysis of teacher talk, an L2 textbook analysis, and a corpus analysis, have found that /st/ onsets occur more frequently than either /sl/ or /sn/ onsets and that /sl/ onsets are more frequent than /sn/ onsets, with the following frequency hierarchy found, from most to least frequent: /st/ > /sl/ > /sn/. As this ordering was consistent across the teacher talk analysis, an L2 textbook analysis, and an analysis of both a spoken (ALERT Corpus) and a written corpus (the Brown Corpus) (see Cardoso, 2008), the current study will adopt this input frequency hierarchy.

As this study also examines the role of the L1 in onset acquisition, it is important to examine the onset structures in the three languages in the current study. An overview of the phonotactic constraints for English, as well as Vietnamese, Cantonese, and Mandarin Chinese onsets, is given in Table 10.1. As Table 10.1 indicates, all three speaker

Table 10.1 A comparison of English, Vietnamese, Mandarin Chinese, and Cantonese onset structure

Structure	English	Vietnamese**	Mandarin Chinese	Cantonese
Singleton onsets	Stops: /p t k b d g/ Fricatives: /s z f v ʃ ʒ θ ð h/ Affricates: /tʃ dʒ/ Nasals: /m n ŋ*/ Approximants: / ɹ l j w/	Stops: /b̥ t̪ t̪ʰ d̪ t̪ c k/ Fricatives: /f v ş ʃ ʒ x ɣ h/ Nasals: /m ɱ ɲ ŋ/ Approximants: /l j w/ Trill: /r/	Stops: /p pʰ t tʰ k kʰ/ Fricatives: /f s ɕ ş x/ Affricates: /ts tsʰ tɕ tɕʰ tʂ tʂʰ/ Nasals: /m n ŋ/ Approximants: /l ɹ w j/	Stops: /p t k kw pʰ tʰ kʰ kwʰ/ Fricatives: /f s h/ Affricates: /ts tsʰ/ Nasals: /m n ŋ/ Approximants: /l j w/
Complex onsets	CC, CCC	Not allowed	Not allowed	Not allowed

*Only in medial position. **Saigon dialect, the language of the participants of the study.

Sources: Cheng (1973), Nguyen (1970), Roach (2009), Santry (1997).

L1 languages are similar to each other and to English in that they allow a single consonant in the onset position. These singleton onset consonants include the voiceless alveolar fricative /s/, the voiceless stop /t/, the liquid /l/, and the nasal /n/. In short, all three L1s in the study allow the constituents of the onsets in the study, /sl sn st/, in singleton form. Unlike English, however, none of the L1s allows complex onsets, and therefore, on the basis of L1 transfer, all speakers from all three L1 groups would be similar in the predicted effect of L1 transfer, in that all three onsets would be equally difficult for all three speaker groups.

To summarize, markedness would predict that participants in the study would acquire the onsets in question in the following order: /sl/ > /sn/ > /st/, while input frequency based on the order found in Cardoso (2008) would predict the acquisition order as /st/ > /sl/ > /sn/. As none of the three languages in the study allows complex onsets, L1 transfer would predict that speakers of all three languages would find the three onset clusters to be equally difficult.

Three different speech samples comprise the data. As the three data sets are drawn from a larger research study, there is a disparity in the number of participants and therefore the number of tokens across the three L1s. However, since the frequency of /sl sn st/ onsets in speech is not very high, and the language samples within each L1 group are homogeneous in terms of both accuracy rates and modifications, all the available data were employed for this study in order to increase the robustness of the findings. The first data sample is taken from 33 native speakers of Cantonese who were all first year English majors at a tertiary institution in Hong Kong. All the participants were required to take the Hong Kong Advanced Level Examination for university admission and based on these scores were considered to have an advanced proficiency level in English speaking skills. They were also all living in a context where English is one of three official languages and the language of their university study. The second data sample is taken from three native speakers of Mandarin Chinese, all of whom were postgraduate students at a large tertiary institution in the US. The participants were required to take a Test of Spoken English upon admission to their postgraduate program; based on this test, the participants were rated as being high intermediate speakers of English. The third data sample is taken from two native speakers of Vietnamese residing in the US at the time of the study. These two L2 speakers of English had a low intermediate proficiency in English based on a proficiency test given at the community college where they were studying at the time of the research.

Although the three data sets differ in both the number of speakers and the spoken English proficiency level of the participants, there are a number of commonalities in the data sets that are beneficial for a comparative study such as this. First, all three data sets are exclusively based on naturalistic, spoken conversational data drawn from one-on-one interviews between the participants and the researcher; this is different from the previous research, which has primarily relied on word lists or sentence reading tasks. The conversational data of the current study allow for the analysis of naturalistic production of the onsets in question, which may yield greater insights into the acquisition of these onsets than more structured and controlled speech tasks. Second, the participants are all speakers of Asian languages. These languages both differ and have similarities in terms of their phonemic/phonetic inventories as well as phonotactic constraints, which will allow the examination of both the role of universals and L1 transfer in the acquisition of the onsets in question.

All data were based on one-on-one interviews between the researcher and each participant. The interviews between the researcher and the Mandarin Chinese and Cantonese speaking participants lasted approximately 30 minutes per participant, while the interviews between the researcher and the Vietnamese participants lasted approximately 1.5 hours each. The interviews did not attempt to specifically elicit /sC/ forms; rather, the focus was on the participants' English language use, motivation to study English, opportunities to study English, favorite books, favorite movies, travel, and hobbies. Therefore, the frequency of use of each of the /sC/ onsets was not controlled for; rather, their frequency was as naturalistic as possible. The caveat of employing a conversational task rather than a word list and/or reading passage is that the participants may use only a small range of words with which they are familiar, which may create an inaccurate picture of their ability to produce a given type of sound structure. To minimize this occurrence, the researcher focused the interviews on a broad range of topics (see above) in order to promote the use of a wide range of vocabulary.

The interview data were transcribed first by the researcher and then by a research assistant trained in English phonetic transcription in order to increase the accuracy of the phonemic and phonetic transcriptions. Inter-rater reliability was calculated with an agreement percentage of 93.10%. Where there was disagreement between the two raters, another research assistant transcribed the tokens/words. If there was disagreement among all three raters, the word in question was eliminated from the data set. All in all, 145 tokens from the Mandarin Chinese data set, 511 tokens from the Cantonese L1 data set, and 280 tokens from the Vietnamese data set were analyzed, for a total of 936 tokens.

FINDINGS

Table 10.2 outlines the production of each onset type by speaker L1 group and by type of production: accurate, deletion (of either the entire onset or one member of the onset), epenthesis, or modification of one or more of the members of the onset. As Table 10.2 indicates, aside from Cantonese speakers' production of /sl/ and /sn/ onsets, the onsets are overall produced with a high accuracy of over 80% and, for some onsets, 100%. Interestingly, however, none of the participants in the three speaker groups produced all of the onsets with 100% accuracy.

The accuracy hierarchy for each speaker group is as follows:

Cantonese L1:	/st/ (100%) > /sn/ (53%) > /sl/ (43%)
Mandarin Chinese L1:	/st/ (89%) > /sl/ (86%) > /sn/ (82%)
Vietnamese L1:	/sl/, /sn/ (100%) > /st/ (84%)

As these hierarchies indicate, the three speaker groups varied in their hierarchies, although for both the Mandarin Chinese speakers and the Cantonese speakers, /st/ was the most accurate onset of the three, indicating that input frequency may be a stronger constraint than markedness (and L1 transfer) in the acquisition of these onset structures by this group of learners. In contrast, for the Vietnamese speakers in the study, the less marked structures /sl/ and /sn/ were both produced with 100% accuracy, while the more marked structure /st/ was produced with a slightly lower accuracy. For the Vietnamese speakers, then, markedness may have more impact on acquisition than input frequency; it is possible

Table 10.2 Onset production by speaker groups

Onset	Cantonese L1				Mandarin Chinese L1				Vietnamese L1			
	Accurate	Deleted	Epen-thesized	Modified	Accurate	Deleted	Epen-thesized	Modified	Accurate	Deleted	Epen-thesized	Modified
/st/	417 100%	0	0	0	58 89%	3 5% →/t/	4 6% →/sə.t/	0	145 84%	27 16% →/s/	0	0
/sn/	25 53%	0	0	23 47% →/sl/	31 82%	7 18% →/n/	0	0	49 100%	0	0	0
/sl/	20 43%	0	0	26 57% →/sn/	36 86%	0	6 14% →/sə.l/	0	59 100%	0	0	0
Total	462 90%	0 0%	0 0%	49 10%	125 86%	10 7%	10 7%	0 0%	253 90%	27 10%	0 0%	0 0%

that the role of input frequency versus markedness is related to the language proficiency of the learner. Just as L1 transfer is hypothesized to be a more powerful constraint in the early stages of L2 acquisition, it may be that input frequency becomes a more powerful constraint on L2 acquisition in later stages, with markedness possibly a more dominant factor in the middle stages of acquisition. This supports Major's (2001) Ontogeny Phylogeny Model, which predicts that L1 transfer is initially the most powerful constraint on L2 phonological acquisition; across time, however, L1 transfer effects decrease, and universal constraints, such as sonority, become more powerful constraints on acquisition. In their research on the acquisition of /sl sn st/ onsets, Carlisle and Cutillas Espinosa (this volume) also found that markedness, and the OPM, provided the best explanation for the acquisition orders of /sl/ > /sn/ > /st/ for their Spanish L1, English L2 participants, and particularly for the intermediate learners in their study as these learners appeared to be affected more by markedness than L1 transfer effects, in contrast to beginning learners, who were affected more by L1 transfer. Carlisle and Cutillas Espinosa state that their findings confirm the OPM; the current study also partially confirms the OPM, with the extension that it may be that input frequency effects become dominant in later stages of acquisition as the influence of universal constraints lessens.

Another interesting finding is that the modifications employed by the participants differed by L1 and were consistent within each L1 group. As Table 10.2 illustrates, the most difficult onsets for Cantonese speakers were /sl/ and /sn/, and for both of these clusters, there was feature change, with /sl/ changed to /sn/ and /sn/ to /sl/. There were no cases of deletion or epenthesis in this data set, even though it comprised 511 tokens. For the Mandarin Chinese speakers, deletion was employed for both /sn/ (to /n/) and /st/ (to /t/) onsets, and epenthesis for /sl/ and /st/ (there was slightly more epenthesis than deletion for /st/ onsets for this speaker group). Finally, the only onset Vietnamese speakers had difficulty with was the /st/ onset, which they deleted to /s/. As these patterns were different for each speaker group, and since they were remarkably consistent for all members of each L1 group, these group patterns will be discussed in turn below.

As noted previously, the Cantonese L1 speakers of English do not appear to have difficulty with complex onsets, in particular the /sC/ onset. Nor do they have difficulty with sonorants as they can produce both an /sl/ and an /sn/ onset. In other words, if we disregard the actual modifications of /l/ to /n/ and vice versa, the Cantonese speakers do not have any difference in their production of an /s/ plus sonorant versus an /s/ plus obstruent onset. Therefore, neither input frequency nor markedness seems to have an effect on their onset production. What explains the /n/-/l/ variation then? In fact, /n/-/l/ variation is a phenomenon that has been found to occur in Cantonese for native speakers of Cantonese (cf. Bauer & Benedict, 1997; Matthews & Yip, 1994) as well as in the English of native speakers of Cantonese (cf. Hung, 2000). In specific, /n/-/l/ variation in onsets has been found to be common among young (e.g., young adult) Cantonese speakers (cf. Bauer & Benedict, 1997), such as the participants in this study. Interestingly, /n/-/l/ variation in Cantonese is not solely based on articulation difficulties; Bauer and Benedict (1997) have also found that Cantonese speakers also have difficulty perceiving a difference in the two sounds in Cantonese. Therefore, transfer of L1 variation patterns appears to impact English L2 /n/-/l/ production (and mostly likely perception, which was not tested in this study). Research on the English of Cantonese speakers (cf. Hung, 2000; Leung, 2011) has also found /n/-/l/ variation to occur in English L2 onsets; therefore, it appears to be a common phenomenon for some (though not all) speakers of Cantonese. In sum, for the Cantonese data set, the accuracy order of /st/ > /sl/ > /sn/ may on the surface appear to be based on input frequency. However, a closer examination of the data, and the L1 of the speakers, offers a more plausible explanation, that the learners are transferring /n/-/l/ variation patterns from their native Cantonese into English. L1 transfer is thus the best explanation for the modifications found in this data set and, by default, for the low accuracy for /sl/ and /sn/ onsets for L1 speakers of Cantonese. Overall, the Cantonese L1 speakers of English can produce all three onset structures with a high level of accuracy but may vary between /n/ and /l/ in /sl/ and /sn/ onsets, leading to a lower accuracy rating for these onsets, due to L1 transfer of Cantonese variation patterns.

Interestingly, though they had the lowest proficiency of the three groups of speakers, the Vietnamese participants had the most accurate onset production overall. The best explanation for the findings from this data set is that the participants found the less sonorous, and thus less marked, /sl sn/ onsets easier than the /st/ onset, which violates the SSP. The only onset they had difficulty with was /st/, which they consistently modified to /s/, though only 16% of the time. The question arises as to why the participants modified /st/ to /s/ rather than /t/. This choice cannot be explained by the SSP, which would predict retention of the least sonorous consonant, in this case /t/ rather than /s/, in order to make an optimal syllable due to a greater rise in sonority between the onset consonant and the nucleus of the syllable (cf. Hefter, 2012). Although retention of /s/ rather than /t/ is not predicted by the SSP, it is not a rare occurrence and has been attested in a number of studies of child L1 acquisition of /sC/ onsets. Hefter (2012), for example, in research on L1 English children acquiring /sl sn st/ onsets, found that children typically reduced all three onsets to /s/ in the early stages of acquisition. Hefter explains her findings by noting that the perceptual salience of the /s/ versus the /t/ may explain its retention rather than the stop; as she states, ". . . it may be possible that perceptual salience . . . played a role in eliciting the preservation of /s/, which vis-à-vis /t/, is acoustically more salient . . ." (p. 57). This is an interesting observation in light of the findings of the perceptual study on /sC/ onsets by Cardoso, John, and French (2008), which also indicates that perception of these onsets is not related to sonority but rather to input frequency. The role of both these factors—perceptual salience and input frequency—is relatively unexplored for L2 learners' acquisition of these onsets, but the findings of both Hefter (2012) and Cardoso, John, and French (2008) indicate that these factors are important areas for future research.

Research by Yavaş and colleagues (Yavaş, 2013; Yavaş & Marecka, 2013) on child L1 acquisition of these onsets has also found that L1 child learners of Dutch, English, Hebrew, Croatian, and Polish may modify /st/ onsets to /s/, though reduction to /t/ is preferred. This indicates that when children are developing their L1 sound system, reduction of /st/ to /t/ is not categorical; for some children, and possibly in some contexts, reduction to /s/ also occurs. Another study, by Jongstra (2003), on child L1 acquisition of Dutch, found variation both among children and within one child's data in terms of strategies for cluster reduction—including which consonant was reduced within each cluster. For /s/ + stop onset clusters, Jongstra found that while the preference was for stop retention, for all three /s/ + stop clusters /st sk sp/, some children retained the /s/ rather than the stop. In particular, Jongstra found that the /st/ cluster was realized as both /s/ and /t/. Because of the variable nature of the child language data, it is difficult to offer a cohesive theory to explain cluster reduction; sonority appears to be a preference, though it is not categorical. In sum, children learning their L1 may not necessarily adhere to SSP principles when dealing with difficult clusters; other factors, such as salience, may affect how clusters are reduced. It is possible that, similar to the child L1 learners in Hefter's study, the Vietnamese participants in the current study found /s/ to be more salient than /t/, and this impacted their production of the /st/ cluster. It is also possible that the Vietnamese participants in the study behaved more similarly to child L1 learners due to their lower L2 proficiency overall and were evidencing developmental modification patterns in reducing /st/ to /s/, similar to child L1 learners. While the data from the Vietnamese learners in the current study do not show variation in cluster reduction, this could be due to the fact that the data set is limited to two participants. Perhaps more data—and the analysis of more factors—would shed more light on why these participants reduced the /st/ cluster to /s/.

For the Mandarin Chinese speakers in the current study, the most accurately produced onset was /st/, followed by /sl/ and then /sn/. This suggests that input frequency may provide the best explanation for this data set. Another possible explanation for the data is the Syllable Contact Law, which Enochson (2014) posits as an explanation for the /st/ > /sn/ > /sl/ accuracy order she found for her participants. The Syllable Contact Law posits that the greater the sonority drop between the /s/ and the next consonant, the greater the harmonic relationship (Murray & Vennemann, 1983). As Enochson notes, while both /sn/ and /sl/ produce a sonority rise, /st/ results in a sonority drop, which thus creates a more harmonic cluster. While both input frequency and the Syllable Contact Law, as well as a combination of factors, could explain the findings from the Mandarin Chinese data set in the current study, it is possible that since both part of Enochson's data and this data set stem from L1 speakers of Mandarin Chinese, the L1 of the participants was a factor as well.

For the Mandarin Chinese speakers in the current study, although all three onsets had a high accuracy rating, all three were modified; in fact, the Mandarin Chinese speakers had the most variation in production modifications. The onset /st/ was both modified to /t/, which can be explained by the SSP, and epenthesized to /sə.t/; the next most accurate onset, /sl/, was epenthesized to /sə.l/; and the least accurate (though still highly accurate) /sn/ deleted to /n/. Interestingly, Enochson (2014) also found that the Asian L1 learners of English in her study—speakers of Cantonese, Mandarin Chinese, and Japanese—employed epenthesis to modify all three consonant clusters. The Mandarin Chinese learners in her study also had an intermediate proficiency level. It is possible that epenthesis is a more advanced strategy for dealing with these onsets for the Mandarin Chinese speakers, as both consonants are produced in the epenthesized form, though as singleton onsets. Deletion, on the other hand, could be a modification strategy that is employed in the initial stages of the acquisition of each onset structure, which may gradually increase as the onset begins to be acquired, at which point epenthesis may become a more dominant strategy. In other words, for the Mandarin Chinese participants in this study, the acquisition order appears to be:

Initial stage: deletion > middle stage: epenthesis > final stage: accurate production

How do the results of the current study compare with the results of previous studies of /sC/ onsets, and in particular with those of Cardoso (2008), which also examined input frequency? Table 10.3 provides a

Table 10.3 Onset production hierarchies across studies

Speaker group	Proficiency level	L1/L2	Accuracy hierarchy (most to least)	Possible explanation
Current study	Advanced	Cantonese L1 English L2	/st/ > /sn/ > /sl/	L1 transfer
Current study	High intermediate	Mandarin Chinese L1 English L2	/st/ > /sl/ > /sn/	Input frequency
Current study	Low Intermediate	Vietnamese L1 English L2	/sl/, /sn/ > /st/	Sonority (markedness)
Abrahamsson (1999)	Beginner	Spanish L1 Swedish L2	/sn/ > /st/ > /sl/	Partly sonority (markedness)
Cardoso (2008)	Low intermediate & advanced	Brazilian Portuguese L1 English L2	/sl/ > /sn/ > /st/	Sonority (markedness)
Cardoso, John, & French (2008)	No English, intermediate, advanced	Brazilian Portuguese L1 English L2	Perception: /st/ > /sl/ > /sn/	Input frequency
Cardoso & Liakin (2009)	Low intermediate & advanced	Brazilian Portuguese L1 English L2	/sl/ > /sn/ > /st/	Sonority (markedness)
Carlisle (1988)	Not given	Spanish L1 English L2	/sl/ > /sn/	Sonority (markedness)
Carlisle (1991)	Not given	Spanish L1 English L2	/sl/ > /st/	Sonority (markedness)
Carlisle (1992)	Not given	Spanish L1 English L2	/sl/ > /sm/, /sn/	Sonority (markedness)
Carlisle (1997)	Intermediate	Spanish L1 English L2	/sl/ > /sn/, /sm/	Sonority (markedness)
Carlisle (2006)	Intermediate	Spanish L1 English L2	/sl/ > /sn/ > /st/	Sonority (markedness)
Carlisle & Cutillas Espinosa (this volume)	Intermediate	Spanish L1 English L2	/sl/ > /sn/ > /st/	Sonority (markedness)
Enochson (2014)	Intermediate	Mandarin Chinese L1 Japanese L1 Cantonese L1 English L2	/st/ > /sn/ > /sl/	Syllable Contact Law
Hefter (2012)	2;3 years old to 3;10 (acquisition across time)	Child L1 learners of English	/sl/ > /sn/ > /st/	Sonority (markedness)
Major (1996)	Beginner	Brazilian Portuguese L1 English L2	/st > /sl/	Input frequency

Speaker group	Proficiency level	L1/L2	Accuracy hierarchy (most to least)	Possible explanation
Rauber (2006)	Not known	Brazilian Portuguese L1 Spanish L1 English L2	/sl/ > /sn/ > /st/	Sonority (markedness)
Rebello & Baptista (2006)	Intermediate	Brazilian Portuguese L1 English L2	/st/ > /sl/ > /sn/	Markedness (by voicing, not sonority) Input frequency
Yavaş & Marecka (2013)	Child L1	Polish L1	/s/ + nasal > /s/ + stop > /sw/ > /sx/	Continuancy

Source: Table based partly on Cardoso (2008).

synthesis of these findings for the three speaker groups from the current study and from previous research on /sC/ onsets.

As Table 10.3 indicates, sonority provides the best explanation for the findings for the majority, though not all, of the previous studies of /sC/. Cardoso (2008), which was the only previous study on /sC/ onsets to examine the role of input frequency, also found that sonority provided the best explanation for his findings and that input frequency was not a significant factor. It therefore appears that either markedness overrides frequency effects for L2 phonology, or, as mentioned previously, the effects of L1 transfer, markedness, and input frequency are dependent on the proficiency level of the participants, with the caveat that some L1 effects, such as those for /n/-/l/ variation for Cantonese speakers, are dominant in the L2 if they are also dominant in the L1.

For the three data sets in the current study, markedness provides the best explanation only for the Vietnamese data set, with L1 transfer the best explanation for the Cantonese data, and input frequency providing the best explanation for the Mandarin Chinese data. One major difference between the current study and the previous research is that the current study employed only naturalistic data; the other studies employed word lists or sentence reading tasks in order to obtain sufficient tokens of each onset type as these onsets may not occur frequently in natural conversation. Therefore, one of the differences between the findings of the current study and those of previous studies could be the type of data collected. Another difference is the language type: The majority of the previous studies focused on either Brazilian Portuguese or Spanish, as these two L1s have complex onsets but do not allow /s(C)/ onsets. Speakers of both L1s are also hypothesized to employ epenthesis in order to manage these onsets, as both these L1s have an /esC/ structure in the L1. However, the current study focused on three Asian languages that did not allow complex onsets and are overall fairly dissimilar to the two Romance languages in terms of their phonotactic constraints. Overall, the picture that Table 10.3 presents is that markedness, and not input frequency or L1 transfer, has the greatest effect on the acquisition of /sC/ onset structures.

CONCLUSION

This study investigated the role of input frequency, markedness, and L1 transfer in the acquisition of the English /sl sn st/ onsets by native speakers of Cantonese, Mandarin Chinese, and Vietnamese. The study found that all three constraints played a role in both the accuracy orders and production modifications employed by the speakers of the study, in that L1 transfer had a dominant role for Cantonese speakers, input frequency for the Mandarin Chinese speakers, and markedness for the Vietnamese speakers. Only the findings for the Vietnamese speakers, that sonority plays a more significant role than the other factors in the acquisition of /sl sn st/ onset sequences, corroborate previous research on the role of input frequency and markedness in the acquisition of these onsets, as well as previous research on /sC/ onsets in general. A major difference between this study and previous research is the L1 background of the participants, which may affect the results of the study and explain differences among studies. Another difference is the nature of the data collected as this study relied on conversational data rather than more controlled word lists and reading passages. Finally, the proficiency level of the learners may impact which factors—sonority, input frequency, or L1 transfer—affect the acquisition and modification of /sl sn st/ onsets. These findings demonstrate that further research is required in order to fully understand the role of input frequency, sonority, and L1 transfer in L2 phonological acquisition.

REFERENCES

Abrahamsson, N. (1999). Vowel epenthesis of /sC(C)/ onsets in Spanish/Swedish interphonology: A longitudinal case study. *Language Learning 49*, 473–508.

Bauer, R. S., & Benedict, P. K. (1997). *Modern Cantonese phonology*. New York: Mouton de Gruyter.

Broselow, E., & Xu, Z. (2004). Differential difficulty in the acquisition of second language phonology. *International Journal of English Studies 4*(2), 135–163.

Cardoso, W. (2008). The development of sC onset clusters in interlanguage: Markedness vs. frequency effects. In R. Slabakova et al. (Eds.), *Proceedings of the 9th Generative Approaches to Second Language Acquisition Conference (GASLA) 2007*, pp. 15–29. Somerville, MA: Cascadilla Proceedings Project.

Cardoso, W., John, P., & French, L. (2008). The variable perception of /s/ + coronal onset clusters in Brazilian Portuguese English. In M. A. Watkins, A. S. Rauber, & B. O. Baptista (Eds.), *Recent research in second language phonetics/phonology: Perception and production*, pp. 203–231. Newcastle upon Tyne, UK: Cambridge Scholars Publishing.

Cardoso, W., & Liakin, D. (2009). When input frequency patterns fail to drive learning: The acquisition of sC onset clusters. In M. A. Watkins, A. S. Rauber, & B. O. Baptista (Eds.), *Recent research in second language phonetics/phonology: Perception and production*, pp. 174–202. Newcastle upon Tyne, UK: Cambridge Scholars Publishing.

Carlisle, R. S. (1988). The effect of markedness on epenthesis in Spanish/English interlanguage phonology. *Issues and Developments in English and Applied Linguistics 3*, 15–23.

Carlisle, R. S. (1991). The influence of environment on vowel epenthesis in Spanish/English interphonology. *Applied Linguistics 12*(1), 76–95.

Carlisle, R. S. (1992). Environment and markedness as interacting constraints on vowel epenthesis. In J. Leather & A. James (Eds.), *New sounds '92*, pp. 64–75. Amsterdam: University of Amsterdam Press.

Carlisle, R. S. (1997). The modification of onsets in a markedness relationship: Testing the interlanguage structural conformity hypothesis. *Language Learning 47*(2), 327–361.

Carlisle, R. S. (2006). The sonority cycle and the acquisition of complex onsets. In B. Baptista and M. Watkins (Eds.), *English with a Latin beat: Studies in Portuguese/Spanish English interphonology*, pp. 105–138. Amsterdam: John Benjamins.

Carlisle, R. S., & Cutillas Espinosa, J. A. (This volume). The production of /sC/ onsets in a markedness relationship: Investigating the Ontogeny Phylogeny Model with longitudinal data.

Cheng, C.-C. (1973). *A synchronic phonology of Mandarin Chinese.* The Hague: Mouton.

Eckman, F. R. (2008). Typological markedness and second language phonology. In J. G. Hansen Edwards and M. L. Zampini (Eds.), *Phonology and second language acquisition*, pp. 95–115. Amsterdam: John Benjamins.

Ellis, N. C., & Ferreira-Junior, F. (2009). Construction learning as a function of frequency, frequency distribution, and function. *Modern Language Journal 93*(3), 370–385.

Enochson, K. (2014). The effect of continuance on the L2 production of onset clusters. In U. Minai, A. Tremblay, C. Coughlin, C.-Y. Chu, and B. Lopez Prego (Eds.), *Selected proceedings of the 5th Conference on Generative Approaches to Language Acquisition—North America,* pp. 1–9. Somerville, MA: Cascadilla Press.

Flege, F. E., Takagi, N., and Mann, V. (1996). Lexical familiarity and English-language experience affect Japanese adults' perception of /r/ and /l/. *Journal of the Acoustical Society of America, 97,* 3125–3134.

Hefter, H. (2012). *The acquisition of /s/ + consonant onset clusters: A longitudinal study.* MPhil thesis, Concordia University, Montreal, Québec, Canada.

Hung, T. T. N. (2000). Toward a phonology of Hong Kong English. *World Englishes 19*(3), 337–356.

Jongstra, W. (2003). Variable and stable clusters: Variation in the realization of consonant clusters. *Canadian Journal of Linguistics 48*(3–4), 265–288.

Leung, M. M. (2011). *Phonological variation of consonant by Hong Kong Cantonese speakers of English: A sociolinguistic perspective.* Unpublished doctoral dissertation, The Chinese University of Hong Kong.

Major, R. C. (1996). Markedness in second language acquisition of consonant clusters. In R. Bayley and D. R. Preston (Eds.), *Variation and second language acquisition,* pp. 75–96. Amsterdam: John Benjamins.

Major, R. C. (2001). *Foreign accent: The ontogeny and phylogeny of second language phonology.* Mahwah, NJ: Lawrence Erlbaum.

Major, R. C. (2008). Transfer in second language phonology: A review. In J. G. Hansen Edwards and M. L. Zampini (Eds.), *Phonology and second language acquisition,* pp. 63–94. Amsterdam: John Benjamins.

Matthews, S., & Yip, V. (1994). *Cantonese: A comprehensive grammar.* London: Routledge.

Murray, R., & Vennemann, T. (1983). Sound change and syllable structure in Germanic phonology. *Language 59,* 514–528.

Nguyen, D. L. (1970). *Vietnamese pronunciation.* Kolawalu: University of Hawaii Press.

Rauber, A. S. (2006). Production of English initial /s/ clusters by speakers of Brazilian Portuguese and Argentine Spanish. In B. Baptista and M. Watkins (Eds.), *English with a Latin beat: Studies in Portuguese/Spanish English interphonology,* pp. 155–167. Amsterdam: John Benjamins.

Rebello, J. T., & Baptista, B. O. (2006). The influence of voicing on the production of initial /s/-clusters by Brazilian learners. In B. Baptista and M. Watkins (Eds.), *English with a Latin beat: Studies in Portuguese/Spanish English interphonology,* pp. 139–167. Amsterdam: John Benjamins.

Roach, P. (2009). *English phonetics and phonology: A practical course.* 4th Edition. Cambridge: Cambridge University Press.

Santry, P. A. (1997). *The way South Vietnamese pronounce English.* Frankfurt am Main: Hector.

Selkirk, E. (1984). On the major class features and syllable theory. In M. Aronoff and R. Oerhle (Eds.), *Language sound structure*, pp. 107–136. Cambridge, MA: MIT Press.

Trofimovich, P., Collins, L., Cardoso, W., White, J., & Horst, M. (2012). A frequency-based approach to L2 phonological learning: Teacher input and student output in an intensive ESL context. *TESOL Quarterly 46*(1), 176–187.

Yavaş, M. (2013). What explains the reductions in /s/-clusters: Sonority or [continuant]? *Clinical Linguistics & Phonetics 27*(6), 151–161.

Yavaş, M., & Marecka, M. (2013). Acquisition of Polish #sC clusters in typically-developing children and children with phonological disorders. *International Journal of Speech-Language Pathology 16*(2), 132–141.

Zamuner, T. S., Gerken, L., & Hammond, M. (2004). Phonotactic probabilities in young children's speech production. *Journal of Child Language 31*, 515–536.

Zamuner, T. S., Gerken, L., & Hammond, M. (2005). The acquisition of phonology based on input: A closer look at the relation of cross-linguistic and child language data. *Lingua 115*, 1403–1426.

Zamuner, T. S., Morin-Lessard, E., & Bouchat-Laird, N. (This volume). Phonological patterns in the lexical development of French.

11

STOP VOT PRODUCTIONS BY YOUNG BILINGUAL SPANISH-ENGLISH CHILDREN AND THEIR MONOLINGUAL PEERS

Amanda L. Procter, Ferenc Bunta, and Rachel Aghara

Bilingual children acquiring the phonological systems of their target languages are sometimes faced with conflicting acoustic cues regarding phonemic contrasts in those languages. One such example of conflicting cross-language cues exists in the production of voiced and voiceless stops in English and Spanish. Specifically, an English voiced stop consonant in initial, stressed, singleton onset position (such as /d/ in the word *do*) may share physical properties with its Spanish voiceless counterpart (as /t/ in the word *taza* "cup"). Thus, Spanish voiceless stops and English voiced stops in initial position may be acoustically similar regarding their voice onset times (cf. Lisker & Abramson, 1964). The present study addresses this issue by focusing on the production of stop voice onset time in bilingual children acquiring Spanish and English and their monolingual peers in each language.

Voice onset time (VOT) has been identified as the primary cue to differentiating voiced and voiceless initial, singleton stops in stressed position across various languages (Lisker & Abramson, 1964). VOT is defined as the time interval between the stop release (burst) and the onset of vocal fold vibration (voicing) of the sound that follows the stop. Languages vary in how they differentiate voiced and voiceless stops. Some languages (such as English or German) differentiate initial, stressed, singleton voiced and voiceless stops by assigning short VOT to voiced stops and long VOT to voiceless stops. Other languages (such as Spanish, French, or Italian) have voiced stops with a voicing lead, and voiceless stops have short VOTs. In English, the initial, stressed, singleton voiceless stops (/p t k/) generally have long VOT values, while their voiced counterparts (/b d g/) show relatively shorter VOT values. However, Spanish voiceless stops (/p t k/) generally have short VOT durations, while the voiced stops (/b d g/) show prevoiced values (Lisker & Abramson, 1964). This overlap in VOT values between English voiced and Spanish voiceless stops poses a unique problem for Spanish- and English-speaking bilinguals.

Investigating the production of VOT and lead voicing in the target languages of bilingual children can provide valuable insights into bilingual phonological acquisition, especially because these acoustic cues are not consistent across the target languages. Examining such phenomena may reveal information regarding how conflicting cross-linguistic cues are resolved by bilingual children. Although there has been a fair amount of research conducted on the topic of VOT acquisition in bilingual children and adults (Flege & Eefting, 1987; Fowler, Sramko, Ostry, Rowland, & Hallé, 2008; Kehoe, Lleó, & Rakow, 2004), research is still on-going as to how bilingual children resolve conflicting patterns between two languages. By looking at VOT productions of preschool-age Spanish- and English-speaking bilingual children and their monolingual peers in each language, this study will provide insights into how bilingual children acquire voiced and voiceless stop consonants in languages that present them with conflicting cues that need to be resolved during phonological acquisition.

ACQUISITION OF VOT BY MONOLINGUAL CHILDREN

Kewley-Port and Preston (1974) examined the VOT of /t/ and /d/ of three monolingual English-speaking children. The three children were recorded at separate intervals from the time they were approximately six months old to four and a half years of age. At six months of age, the infants' vocalizations of /t/ and /d/ ranged from prevoicing to short-lag to long-lag values with no clear categorical differentiation. However, after only a few months, the children began to produce both alveolar stops in the short-lag category only. By four and a half years, the children were producing both /d/ and /t/ stops; however, only /d/ showed adult-like values, with some errors, and the distribution of /t/ had not stabilized despite the categories of /d/ and /t/ becoming more differentiated over time.

In another study investigating the acquisition of voiced and voiceless stop differentiation in English, Macken and Barton (1980a) identified three stages of VOT contrast acquisition of initial stops in four mono-lingual English-speaking children. In stage I, the children produced all stops in the short-lag range with no difference in VOT values between voiced and voiceless stops. In stage II, children produced the voiced and voiceless stops with a significant contrast, but both values fell in the short-lag range. In stage III, the children produced adult-like voiced and voiceless stops. The authors also noted gradual transitions between the stages over two to four months with a more abrupt change from stage II to III. By approximately 1;9, three of the four participants had rela-tively adult-like VOT values, and the fourth child had acquired the con-trast by 2;6.19. Although Macken and Barton's (1980a) study differs in some respects from Kewley-Port and Preston's (1974) work, both stud-ies indicate that monolingual English-speaking children master short-lag stops (/b d g/) first and then differentiate voiced and voiceless stop VOTs in the short-lag range before producing longer VOTs.

Macken and Barton (1980b) also examined the voiced and voiceless stop contrast acquisition of monolingual Spanish-speaking children. The researchers showed that monolingual Spanish-speaking children acquired short-lag values (/p t k/, in Spanish) first. This finding was comparable to monolingual English-speaking children's patterns in that short-lag VOT stops occurred earliest in production. However, the monolingual Spanish-speaking children did not acquire adult-like contrasts by four years of age for their Spanish voiced (/b d g/) stops. Instead, some of the children used spirantization of their voiced con-sonants to create a voicing contrast. It must be noted that in Spanish, voiced stops may be spirantized (/b/ → [β], /d/ → [ð], and /g/ → [ɣ]) in certain phonetic environments but typically not in word-initial position, with significant dialectal variation (see Lleó & Rakow, 2005). Further-more, Macken and Barton (1980b) also found examples of spirantiza-tion among adults who spoke Mexican Spanish, even word-initially.

ACQUISITION OF VOT BY BILINGUALS

Kehoe, Lleó, and Rakow (2004) examined German and Spanish stop voicing contrasts in four bilingual children between the ages of two and three years and compared the results to three monolingual German-speaking children. Similarly to English, German /b d g/ have short-lag stop VOTs, while /p t k/ have long-lag ones. According to the study, the monolingual German children acquired a target-like voicing contrast, similar to English monolinguals, by around two years of age. However, only two of the bilingual German-Spanish children acquired the voic-ing contrast in German. Furthermore, none of the bilingual children showed target-like voicing contrast in Spanish. Thus, similarly to the findings presented by Macken and Barton (1980b) for monolingual Spanish-speaking children, Kehoe et al. (2004) found that bilingual Spanish-German children also have difficulty with Spanish prevoiced stops. Kehoe et al. offered three explanations: (1) bilingual children may experience a delay in acquiring the German and Spanish voicing distinction due to learning two languages, (2) there were examples of the transfer of rules of one language to another in that one child showed prevoicing in German stops and another child showed long-lag values for Spanish voiceless stops, and (3) there may not be cross-language influence in acquiring target-like voicing contrast distinctions, as shown by one child.

Flege and Eefting (1987) studied stop VOT values in seven groups of participants and found evidence of intermediate VOT values in the productions of the bilingual participants. The three bilingual groups were (1) children who were early sequential bilinguals with Spanish as the L1 and English as the L2, (2) adults who learned English as their L2 in early childhood, and (3) adults who were simultaneous Spanish-English bilinguals. The monolingual control groups included adult and child groups in each language. The researchers found that both groups of sequential bilingual learners used intermediate values for English /p t k/ that were shorter than the observed values for monolingual English speakers. The simultaneous bilingual adult group did not produce monolingual-like values of English voiceless stops either, but their values were significantly closer to English monolingual values than the sequential bilinguals' VOT values, suggesting that age of acquisition has a significant effect on voiced and voiceless stop productions in Spanish- and English-speaking bilinguals.

Fowler, Sramko, Ostry, Rowland, and Hallé (2008) also found instances of bilingual speakers using intermediate instead of monolingual-like VOT values. The authors examined French-English bilinguals' VOT values of /p t k/ and compared them to the values of their monolingual English and monolingual French peers. French VOT values of /p t k/ fall in the short-lag durations (similar to Spanish), overlapping with their English voiced counterparts. The authors found that monolingual French speakers produced the shortest VOT values, well within the short-lag category. Regarding the performance of the bilingual participants, sequential bilinguals whose L1 was French displayed VOT values closest to monolingual French values. Simultaneous bilinguals and sequential bilinguals whose L1 was English produced intermediate VOT values. Last, monolingual English speakers showed the longest VOT values, clearly within the long-lag duration category. These results show that as the bilingual participants' language dominance shifted from French to English, so did the VOT values. Specifically, as dominance shifted from French to English, VOT values became longer as a result of more English influence.

The results found by Fowler et al. (2008) differ from what has been found by other researchers. Flege (1991) compared sequential late Spanish-English bilingual adults to sequential early bilingual adults on the VOT duration of /t/. The results showed that late bilingual learners produced intermediate VOT values for /t/. In contrast, early bilingual adults produced values that were similar to those produced by monolingual English speakers. In the Fowler et al. (2008) study, early bilinguals did not achieve monolingual-like values but instead created intermediate values that did not exactly match monolinguals' VOT values. However, supporting Flege's (1991) findings, Antoniou, Best, Tyler, and Kroos (2010) provide evidence of adult early sequential bilingual speakers who produced monolingual-like values in Australian English and Greek. Just as in Spanish, Greek voiced and voiceless VOT values are in the short-lag range, with prevoicing on the voiced stop consonants. It appears that bilingual speakers can obtain values that match their monolingual peers in both languages, but only if there is early enough acquisition and adequate usage of both languages.

RESEARCH QUESTIONS AND HYPOTHESES

Two questions are addressed in the current study. First, do bilingual Spanish-English children acquire voicing contrasts similarly to their monolingual peers? Studies on how bilingual children acquire their stop VOT values indicate that when compared to their monolingual peers, bilingual children's VOT values may differ from those of their monolingual peers (e.g., Fabiano-Smith & Bunta, 2012; Harada, 2007; Kehoe et al., 2004). We hypothesize that the stop VOT values of the bilingual children would be different from those of their monolingual peers.

Second, is there evidence of cross-language interaction in the production of VOT in bilingual children's productions? The studies by Flege and Eefting (1987) and Fowler et al. (2008) found intermediate VOT values of voiceless /p t k/ stop consonants for both sequential and simultaneous bilinguals. However, studies also found that while some of the VOT values of bilinguals may not match the VOT values of their monolingual peers, bilinguals do differentiate the two languages based on VOT values (Harada, 2007; MacLeod & Stoel-Gammon, 2009). We predict that there will be a difference between the Spanish and English VOT values for voiced and voiceless stops in bilingual children's productions, irrespective of whether or not those values are monolingual-like.

METHOD

Participants

Fourteen three- to seven-year-old children participated in the present study. Participants were divided into three groups: five monolingual English (ME; mean age = 5;0; range 3;11–6;9), four monolingual Spanish (MS; mean age = 3;10; range 3;6–4;6), and five bilingual Spanish-English (BSE; mean age = 5;5; range 3;9–6;11) speakers. The method of data collection was consistent with the Bunta, DiLuca, and Branum-Martin (2011) study because we used a sub-set of the same data, but different analyses were performed. Recruitment for participants occurred in the Houston, Texas, USA metropolitan area. Participants were given a language background questionnaire, a pure tone hearing screening, and the Preschool Language Scales—Fourth Edition (PLS-4) (Zimmerman, Steiner, & Pond 2002a, 2002b) to ensure typically developing language.

Information on socio-economic status, parental education, language development history, and the language environment (including language use and proficiency) of the child was gathered via a language background questionnaire given to the parents of the participants. For bilingual children, information was collected on the use of and exposure to both languages. All participants passed a pure tone hearing screening at 500, 1000, 2000, and 4000 Hz at 25 dB.

Children were assessed for age-appropriate typical language development in expressive language with the PLS-4. Monolingual participants had to complete the expressive language assessment at an age-appropriate level in order to participate in the study. Bilingual participants had to pass the expressive language assessment of the PLS-4 only in their stronger language. Parent reports also showed no concerns regarding the children's speech, language, and cognitive abilities.

Division of participants into their language groups was completed based on percentage of exposure to each language according to parental reports. Participants who spoke English were placed in the ME group if less than 20% exposure to Spanish was reported and they had no functional knowledge of or ability in another language. The same criterion was required of MS participants, for less than 20% exposure to English. Participants in the BSE group had to have more than 20% exposure to both languages in their environment. All of the bilingual participants were also able to communicate in both languages.

Materials and Procedure

Elicitation of a comprehensive list of words with target phonemes was achieved through a picture naming task. There were a total of 280 stop VOTs measured (170 in English and 110 in Spanish), and at least two different target items were presented to each child per stop consonant to elicit more than one form. Audio samples were recorded digitally at 44 kHz and 16 bits onto a laptop computer equipped with a Sennheiser EW300 G2 wireless lavalier microphone system and an Echo Indigo IO external sound card. The microphone was positioned approximately eight inches from the participants' mouths to ensure consistency.

Black-and-white line drawings were used for both English and Spanish elicitation. The drawings were age-appropriate for young children and were not culturally biased. A total of 60 line drawings for Spanish and 90 line drawings for English were shown to children via a laptop computer screen. The vocabulary was determined to be common, effective, and appropriate to the age range being tested (Bunta et al., 2011). First, each child was asked to independently name each picture presented to them. If the picture was not named independently by the child, delayed imitation was used to elicit the target word.

Monolingual children were asked to provide their language sample during the course of one session lasting approximately 45 minutes. Bilingual children required two separate sessions, lasting 90 minutes in total, in which only one language was used per session. A different investigator collected the data in each language from the participants in separate language sessions to minimize code-switching and code mixing. The experimenters were proficient in the languages they tested and were also aware of how to interact appropriately with children from culturally and linguistically diverse backgrounds. Parental consent and the child's verbal assent were obtained before sampling, and the study was approved by the Institutional Review Board of the University of Houston.

VOT Measurements

The VOTs of /p t k/ and /b d g/ were measured on the selection of samples that had the targeted phonemes in the initial, singleton position of words elicited during the picture naming task, targeting each phoneme at least twice, with 170 English and 110 Spanish tokens. VOT duration was measured by finding the time between the beginning of the burst and the onset of voicing for the following vowel using a time waveform and a spectrogram; the latter had the following parameters: 350 Hz bandwidth, 0.8 pre-emphasis factor, and frequency range from 0–5000 Hz with Wavesurfer (Sjölander & Beskow, 2010).

The first author performed all of the VOT measurements. The second author measured 40% of the data for inter-rater agreement. Inter-rater agreement exceeded 98.2% with an error window of 10 milliseconds, which is an acceptable level of disagreement, according to Peterson and Lehiste (1960).

RESULTS

Two sets of comparative analyses were conducted: (1) contrasts between the VOT values of monolingual versus bilingual participants and (2) comparisons of the Spanish and English VOT values of the bilingual participants. Due to the exploratory nature of the study, the alpha level was set at 0.05 despite the fact that the number of comparisons does increase the risk of encountering experimentwise Type I error. In order to alleviate the problem, we are also reporting the effect sizes to allow us and the reader to interpret the findings in the context of our pilot study. We are also including the standard errors of measurement in our figures (see Figures 11.1, 11.2, and 11.3) to assist the readers in judging our findings.

Monolingual versus Bilingual Participants

According to the first hypothesis, the VOT values of the bilingual children were expected to differ from the VOT values of the monolingual children for the same stop consonants. Independent-samples t-tests were conducted to compare monolingual English and bilingual English VOT values for voiced (/b d g/) and voiceless (/p t k/) stop consonants. The results provide partial support for the first hypothesis. Significant differences were found only in English when comparing the VOT values for the bilingual participants and their monolingual peers. Specifically, monolingual English-speaking children produced longer VOTs (mean = 0.014 sec) for their voiced bilabial stops (/b/) than their bilingual peers speaking English (mean = 0.009 sec; t (28) = 2.16 at p = 0.020 with a large effect size of d = 0.82). Monolingual English-speaking children also had longer VOT values (mean = 0.060 sec) for their voiceless bilabial stops (/p/) than their bilingual peers speaking English (mean = 0.040 sec; t (28) = 2.08 at p = 0.023 with an effect size d = 0.78). A significant difference in the VOT values of /g/ was also found between the monolingual English-speaking children (mean = 0.018 sec) and the bilingual children speaking English (mean = 0.035 sec; t (28) = −2.85 at p = 0.005 with a large effect size of d = −1.34). However, this difference in the VOT of /g/ between monolingual English-speaking and bilingual children's English productions was in a direction contrary to our

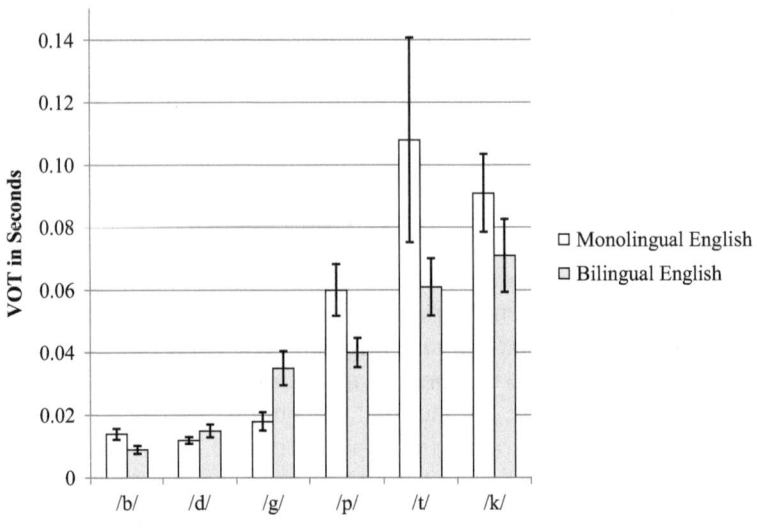

Figure 11.1 Monolingual English and bilingual English VOT values with standard error bars.

expectation. This unique pattern is further discussed in the next section. No significant differences were found between the monolingual English-speaking and the bilingual participants regarding the VOT values of the English /d/, /t/, and /k/ stops. Figure 11.1 illustrates the mean differences between the VOT values of the monolingual English-speaking children and their bilingual peers who spoke English.

In comparisons of the VOT values of the Spanish stops of the monolingual Spanish-speaking children and their bilingual peers speaking Spanish, no statistically significant differences were found (see Figure 11.2).

Overall, the results only partially supported the first hypothesis. There was a distinct language-based pattern indicating that the VOT values of the bilingual children do differ for half of the stops in English; however, there were no significant differences between the VOT values for the Spanish stops of the bilingual children and their monolingual Spanish-speaking peers.

English versus Spanish Productions of Bilingual Participants

According to the second hypothesis, we expected to find differences between the Spanish and English VOT values for voiced and voiceless stops in the bilingual children's productions. The second hypothesis was partially supported by the data. Analyses were conducted comparing

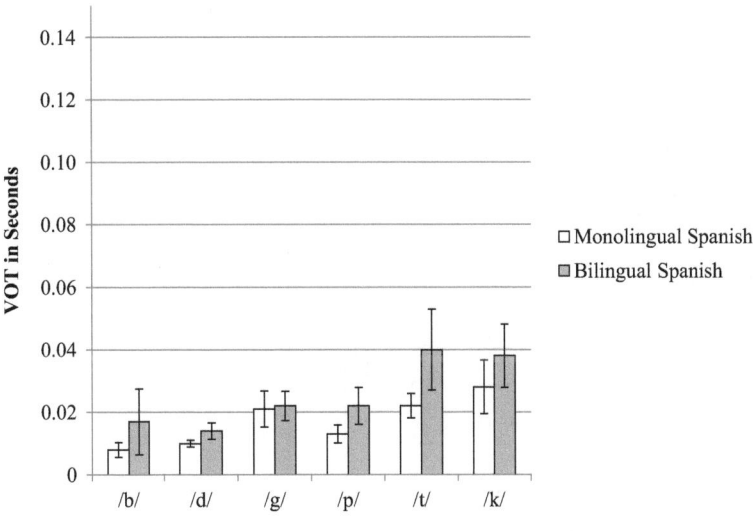

Figure 11.2 Monolingual Spanish and bilingual Spanish VOT values with standard error bars.

the English to the Spanish VOTs for the analogous stop consonants produced by the bilingual children. For example, the VOT values of the English and Spanish /p/ were compared in the bilingual children's productions. Of the six contrasts, three were statistically significant. When we compared the English and Spanish VOTs for /g/ in each language, the English VOT values (mean = 0.035 sec) were significantly longer than their Spanish counterparts (mean = 0.022 sec; t (17) = 1.81 at p = 0.044 with a large effect size of d = 0.88). The VOT for the English /p/ (mean = 0.040 sec) also exceeded the VOT for its Spanish analog (mean = 0.022 sec; t (27) = 2.48 at p = 0.009 with a large effect size of d = 0.95). There was also a significant difference regarding the VOT for the English /k/ (mean = 0.071 sec) and its Spanish counterpart (mean = 0.038 sec; t (22) = 1.92 at p = 0.033 with a large effect size of d = 0.82). The language-based VOT contrasts were not statistically significantly different for /b/, /d/, and /t/. Figure 11.3 illustrates the differences in VOT values for the six stop consonants in English and Spanish, as realized by the bilingual children.

Overall, it appears that the bilingual children did display signs of differentiating their VOT values in their target languages, but those differences appear to be selective, an issue that will be further explored in the Discussion section.

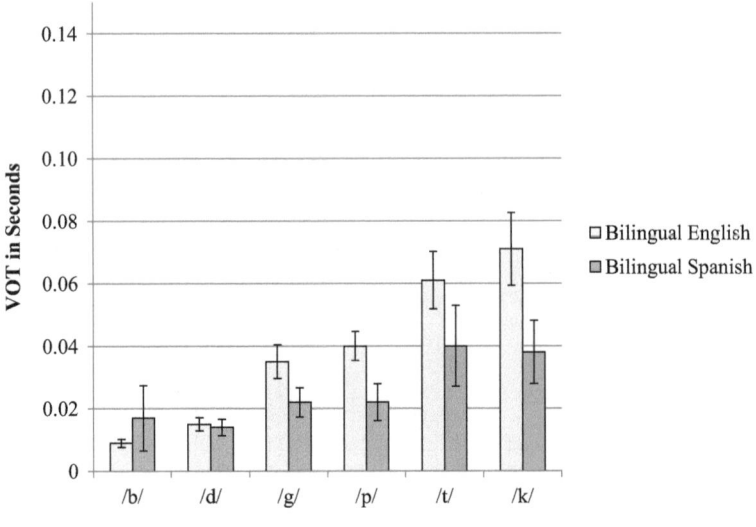

Figure 11.3 English versus Spanish VOT values of the bilingual participants with standard error bars.

DISCUSSION

Our findings indicate that there were select differences in VOT between bilingual and monolingual English speakers in the production of /b/, /p/, and /g/. The VOT of /b/ fell in the short-lag range, but the VOT productions of monolingual English-speaking children were significantly longer than those produced by the children in the bilingual group. The monolingual productions of /p/ were also significantly longer than bilingual English productions, with both averages fitting into the long-lag range. In a study focusing on the VOT productions of /p/ and /k/ in the speech of younger participants, Fabiano-Smith and Bunta (2012) found similar results for the English productions of /p/, such that monolingual English productions of /p/ were significantly longer than bilingual English productions of /p/. A large effect size for /k/ was also found in the Fabiano-Smith and Bunta (2012) study but not in the present study, despite the fact that the group means were different in this study as well.

The significant difference between the monolingual and bilingual English productions of the bilabial (/p/ and /b/) stop VOT values may be an example of cross-language interaction. While the bilingual productions were within the correct range of English productions, they were still significantly shorter than the English monolingual productions, likely due to the influence of the shorter Spanish VOTs.

Unlike the results found for the bilabial stop productions, the bilingual children's English mean VOT values of /g/ (0.035 sec) were significantly longer than their monolingual English peers' values for the same phoneme (0.017 sec), a finding contrary to our expectations. Interestingly, the bilingual English productions were above the short-lag range expected for both English and Spanish productions of /g/. One possible explanation for this unique pattern of /g/ VOT production by the bilingual group was to keep the Spanish and English /g/ phonemes separate in their two phonological systems. In order to maintain differentiation between the Spanish and English /g/ phonemes, bilingual children "overshot" the VOT for the /g/ in English, keeping it distinct from its Spanish counterpart by making the former excessively long. This may be an example of phonetic category dissimilation described by Flege (1995), whereby some bilinguals deflect certain phoneme categories away from existing ones to maintain differentiation. Flege, Schirru, and MacKay (2003) found evidence of phonetic category dissimilation in their study of vowel productions in adult bilingual English-Italian speakers. Interestingly, Flege et al. (2003) observed dissimilation phenomena only with early bilinguals who used their L2 more frequently than their L1. The difference, however, between the Flege et al. (2003) study and the current one is that the former assessed only adults, while the current study evaluated the productions of young children.

Although there were differences between the VOT productions of the stop consonants in the English samples of the bilinguals and their monolingual English-speaking peers, there were no such differences between the bilingual children's Spanish samples and those of their monolingual Spanish-speaking peers. As observed by Fowler et al. (2008), language dominance and use influences VOT length. The bilingual participants sampled for the present study all learned Spanish from birth, and while some were bilingual as first language learners, the home language was mostly Spanish. Because of the predominant use of Spanish at home, the participants' Spanish productions more closely resembled monolingual values than their English productions. The finding that Spanish productions of young bilinguals better approximate their monolingual peers' values was also found by other studies on bilingual phonological development (e.g., Bunta, Fabiano, Ingram, & Goldstein, 2009; Bunta & Ingram, 2007).

In the present study, analyses were also conducted on the differences between the English and Spanish VOT productions of the bilingual participants. The English VOT productions of all stop consonants were longer than the Spanish productions in the bilingual participants' samples. However, only the contrasts for /g/, /p/, and /k/ reached statistical significance. The VOT values for the /p t k/ of the bilingual partici-pants' English samples were within the long-lag stop category, but the Spanish VOT values of the voiceless stops were closer to the long-lag stop category as well. Although the differences in values between the Spanish productions of the monolingual and bilingual speakers were not statistically significant, the values were still longer than would be expected based on the study by Lisker and Abramson (1964). These findings provide further support for bilingual children who are exposed to their languages early having autonomous phonological systems that also interact (cf. Fabiano-Smith & Goldstein, 2010).

In terms of universal versus language-specific effects on bilingual child phonological acquisition, our study appears to support the existence of both. In their paper, Bunta, Davidovich, and Ingram (2006) argued that language-specific manifestations of certain phonological phenomena relied—at least to some extent—on building blocks that were universal in nature (such as phonological features). Considering our present data, it seems that a universal phonological feature (i.e., voicing) that manifests itself differentially in Spanish and English drives the unique production patterns attested in both monolingual and bilingual children. Resolving the cross-linguistic conflict promotes unique productions in bilingual children that resemble those of their monolingual peers in some respects but also differ in specific ways. It appears that bilingual children gener-ally maintain phonemic voicing differentiation and keep their target lan-guage patterns separate. However, it is also evident that the productions of bilingual children display selective and language-specific differences from their monolingual peers that are at least partially due to the input and acquiring two languages at the same time.

The present study provides valuable insights into bilingual pho-nological development in preschool-age children through the lens of VOT productions to mark voicing differences within and across languages. Nonetheless, our study does have limitations that should be noted. One of the limitations is that our study was a retrospective one based on an existing data set originally designed for a different purpose (cf. Bunta et al., 2011). Although we had a sufficient number of tokens whose VOT values were analyzed (280 items in total), future studies should include pre-selected test items specifically designed with VOT analyses in mind and with multiple repetitions of each item. Also, the monolingual Spanish-speaking participants were younger than the members of the other two groups, but despite the age discrep-ancy, the younger monolingual Spanish group displayed more mono-lingual Spanish adult-like VOTs than their bilingual peers speaking Spanish did (cf. Lisker & Abramson, 1964).

Yavaş (2002, 2009) points out that stop VOT values are affected not only by voicing and place of articulation but also by the following vowel, to some extent. In our study, we did not control for the vowel following the stop consonant because the original list of lexical items did not specifically target stop consonants, so some caution needs to be exercised in interpreting our results.

Finally, a larger number of participants would have allowed for more robust findings and may have increased our ability to generalize to the larger population, but such low numbers of participants are not at all unusual in similar studies. Despite the limitations of the present study, the results contribute to our knowledge of how bilingual Spanish- and English-speaking children and their monolingual peers produce stops in initial position. Further research should expand on the current findings by collecting longitudinal data from a larger number of bilingual and monolingual children to observe the patterns of VOT acquisition.

Research on bilingual phonological acquisition still has many unanswered questions. With more research on bilingual acquisition, more concrete patterns of phonological development will begin to emerge. New results in the field will have significant ramifications not only for basic research but also for clinical work in communication sciences and disorders, as well as education. Deciphering phonological interaction in bilingual children will aid in distinguishing a language *difference* from a language *disorder*, preventing the over- and under-diagnosis of communication disorders in bilingual children. Educators will also benefit from a better understanding of phonological development in bilingual children, because the patterns attested in bilingual children differ in specific ways from those of their monolingual peers, and, sometimes, acquisition of certain structures is even aided by being bilingual, if those structures are transferable. Future studies on the acquisition of the stop voicing contrast may use a longitudinal approach, include more participants, and add language combinations other than Spanish and English to gain a more precise and complete understanding of bilingual phonological acquisition.

REFERENCES

Antoniou, M., Best, C. T., Tyler, M. D., & Kroos, C. (2010). Language context elicits native-like stop voicing in early bilinguals' productions in both L1 and L2. *Journal of Phonetics,* 38, 640–653. doi:10.1016/j.wocn.2010.09.005

Bunta, F., Davidovich, I., & Ingram, D. (2006). The relationship between the phonological complexity of a bilingual child's words and those of the target languages. *International Journal of Bilingualism, 10*(1), 71–88.

Bunta, F., DiLuca, C., & Branum-Martin, L. (2011). The acquisition of voice-less post-alveolar fricatives and affricates by bilingual children and their monolingual peers. *The Phonetician, 103/104*, 36–56.

Bunta, F., Fabiano, L., Ingram, D., & Goldstein, B. (2009). Phonological whole-word measures in three-year-old bilingual children and their monolingual peers. *Clinical Linguistics and Phonetics, 23*(2), 156–175.

Bunta, F., & Ingram, D. (2007). The acquisition of speech rhythm by bilingual Spanish- and English-speaking four-and five-year-old children. *Journal of Speech, Language, and Hearing Research, 50*(4), 999–1014.

Fabiano-Smith, L., & Bunta, F. (2012). Voice onset time of voiceless bilabial and velar stops in three-year-old bilingual children and their age-matched monolingual peers. *Clinical Linguistics and Phonetics, 26*(2), 148–163. doi:10.3109/02699206.2011.595526.

Fabiano-Smith, L., & Goldstein, B. A. (2010). Early-, middle-, and late-developing sounds in monolingual and bilingual children: An exploratory investigation. *American Journal of Speech-Language Pathology, 19*, 66–77. doi:10.1044/1058-0360(2009/08-0036)

Flege, J. E. (1991). Age of learning affects the authenticity of voice-onset time (VOT) in stop consonants produced in a second language. *Journal of Acoustic Society of America, 89*, 395–411.

Flege, J. E. (1995). Second-language speech learning: Theory, findings, and problems. In W. Strange (Ed.), *Speech perception and linguistic experience: Issues in cross-language research* (pp. 233–372). Timonium, MD: York.

Flege, J. E., & Eefting, W. (1987). The production and perception English stops by Spanish speakers in English. *Journal of Phonetics, 15*, 67–83.

Flege, J. E., Schirru, C., & MacKay, I. (2003). Interaction between the native and second language phonetic subsystems. *Speech Communication, 40*, 467–491. doi:10.1016/S0167-6393(02)00128-0

Fowler, C. A., Sramko, V., Ostry, D. J., Rowland, S. A., & Hallé, P. (2008). Cross language phonetic influences on the speech of French-English bilinguals. *Journal of Phonetics, 36*, 649–663. doi:10.1016/j.wocn.2008.04.001

Harada, T. (2007). The production of voice onset time (VOT) by English-speaking children in a Japanese immersion program. *International Review of Applied Linguistics in Language Teaching, 45*(4), 353–378. doi:10.1515/IRAL.2007.015

Kehoe, M. M., Lleó, C., & Rakow, M. (2004). Voice onset time in bilingual German-Spanish children. *Bilingualism: Language and Cognition, 7*(1), 71–88. doi:10.1017/S1366728904001282

Kewley-Port, D., & Preston, M. S. (1974). Early apical stop production: A voice onset time analysis. *Journal of Phonetics, 2*, 195–210.

Lisker, L., & Abramson, A. (1964). A cross-language study of voicing in initial stops: Acoustical measurements. *Word, 20*, 384–422.

Lleó, C., & Rakow, M. (2005). Markedness effects in the acquisition of voiced stop spirantization by Spanish-German bilinguals. In J. Cohen, K. McAlister, K. Rolstad, & J. MacSwan (Eds.), *The Proceedings of the 4th International Symposium on Bilingualism* (pp. 1353–1371). Somerville, MA: Cascadilla.

Macken, M., & Barton, D. (1980a). The acquisition of the voicing contrast in English: A study of voice onset time in word-initial stop consonants. *Journal of Child Language, 7*, 41–47.

Macken, M., & Barton, D. (1980b). The acquisition of the voicing contrast in Spanish: A phonetic and phonological study of word-initial stop consonants. *Journal of Child Language, 7*, 433–478.

MacLeod, A. A. N., & Stoel-Gammon, C. (2009). The use of voice onset time by early bilinguals to distinguish homorganic stops in Canadian English and Canadian French. *Applied Psycholinguistics, 30*(1), 53–77. doi:10.1017/S0142716408090036

Peterson, G. E., & Lehiste, I. (1960). Duration of syllable nuclei in English. *Journal of the Acoustical Society of America, 32*, 693–703.

Sjölander, K., & Beskow, J. (2010). WaveSurfer (Version 1.8.8p2) [Computer software]. Retrieved December 7, 2010, at http.sourceforge.net/projects/wavesurfer/.

Yavaş, M. (2002). VOT patterns in bilingual phonological development. In F. Windsor, L. Kelly, & N. Hewlett (Eds.), *Themes in clinical linguistics* (pp. 341–349). Mahwah, NJ: Lawrence Erlbaum.

Yavaş, M. (2009). Factors influencing the VOT of English long lag stops in interlanguage phonology. In M. Watkins, A. Reuber, & B. Baptista (Eds.), *Recent research in second language phonetics/phonology: Perception and production* (pp. 244–255). Newcastle upon Tyne: Cambridge Scholars Publishing.

Zimmerman, I.L., Steiner, V.G., & Pond, R.E. (2002a). *Preschool Language Scales-4.* San Antonio, TX: Pearson.

Zimmerman, I.L., Steiner, V.G., & Pond, R.E. (2002b). *Preschool Language Scales-4 (Spanish Edition).* San Antonio, TX: Pearson.

12

PRODUCTION OF VOICELESS STOPS IN EARLY SEQUENTIAL SPANISH-ENGLISH BILINGUALS

Mehmet Yavaş and Emily Byers

Bilinguals, conventionally defined as speakers who regularly use more than one language (Grosjean, 1982), must balance the task of managing two lexicons and two grammars for use in separate domains. The extent to which bilinguals possess two phonologies, however, and how these phonological systems interact with one another, is a discussion that is still very much alive. Contemporary research in bilingualism is divided along four basic hypotheses concerning the relationship between a speaker's first and second language: (a) the L1 may display a unidirectional influence on the L2; (b) the L2 may be able to operate independently of the L1 (in the case of second-language dominance); (c) the L1 and L2 may reciprocally affect one another, resulting in a bidirectional relationship; or (d) there may be no clear relationship between the L1 and L2 in bilingual speech production.

Antoniou et al. (2011) explore the commonly held belief that the L1 phonetic system has a heavy unidirectional influence on L2 production, resulting in a noticeable foreign accent for the L2 speaker. When languages are not acquired simultaneously, the L2 must be acquired through the filter of the L1, a process termed "interference" (Flege, 1981, 1987, 1991; Flege & Eefting, 1987). Here, depending on the amount of experience the speaker has with the L2, we may see L1-like productions or compromise values. While acquiring the second language earlier in life is thought to minimize the effects of interference on L2 phonetic production, studies have shown that certain phonetic effects persist even in those who acquired their L2 very early in life. Fowler et al. (2008) discovered that sequential bilinguals displayed longer-lag VOT times than simultaneous bilinguals, indicating that even the earliest consecutive bilinguals displayed effects of processing the L2 through the L1's "filter."

It is suggested that an individual bilingual's pattern of L1/L2 acquisition contributes to the presence (and direction) of interlanguage interference. One area of phonetic influence that has been repeatedly tested, due to the relative ease of obtaining stable values, is voice onset timing (VOT)—defined as the time that elapses following a complete closure of the articulators between a release burst and the onset of vocal cord vibration (Lisker & Abramson, 1964). Both English and Spanish contain voiceless stops in their phonological inventories; however, the phonetic realizations of these sounds differ systematically between the two languages. English stops can be characterized as "long-lag" stops, averaging 60–120 milliseconds in duration, whereas the voiceless stops of Spanish are known as "short-lag," spanning roughly 0–30 milliseconds in duration. Flege and Eefting (1987) found that Spanish-English bilinguals who came to the United States as infants and very young children continued to display shorter VOT values for /p, t, k/ than English-only speakers. Others have established the existence of separate phonetic categories for the L1 and L2 but maintain that the L1 continues to "interfere" in phonetic processes such as achieving native-like VOT values (Flege, 1992, 1995; Sancier & Fowler, 1997; Bialystok & Miller, 1998).

While claims have been made that L1 interference in L2 production is inevitable due to its chronological precedence, others have suggested that the predominant interference of the L1 seen in so many studies is actually the result of L1 dominance affecting L2 phonetic output. It stands to reason, then, that L2 dominant bilinguals, those who are truly immersed in their L2 and experience limited to no use of their first language, may experience L2 interference in the L1 instead. Flege, MacKay, and Piske (2002) redefined interlanguage interference as a situation where dominance, not order of acquisition, is the crucial factor in determining which language interferes with the other. Thus, we find in several studies that early bilinguals who became dominant in L2 were able to develop speech patterns that closely resembled those of native speakers of the L2 (Flege & MacKay, 2004; Guion, Flege, & Loftin, 2000; Piske et al., 2002). From this perspective, the explanation that the L2 is processed through the L1 filter can be viewed as the result of L1 dominance (i.e., the dominant language exerts influence over the non-dominant one).

It is important to acknowledge that bilinguals' productions may vary when the language environment changes. Sancier and Fowler (1997), for example, noted this in the VOT productions of a Portuguese-English bilingual. In what is called the "gestural drift," their subject's L1 Portuguese voiceless stops (typically short-lag) drifted by 5–6 milliseconds toward the longer VOT values when in an English-speaking environment in the United States. Her VOT values, however, shifted back (shorter) in both languages when she returned to Portuguese-speaking Brazil. These findings support the "language mode" framework of Grosjean (2001), which posits a continuum whereby bilinguals move along from "unilingual" to "bilingual" in language activation depending on the linguistic environment.

The notion of a bidirectional influence was refuted by the study of Antoniou et al. (2011), who found an asymmetrical influence in English-dominant Greek-English bilinguals where the VOTs of L1 Greek continued to influence voiceless stop production in English, though when English became the base language for the code-switching sentence, the same effect was not present. These findings contrast greatly with Flege et al. (2002) and Piske et al. (2002), who suggested that bilinguals who become dominant in their L2 may be able to suppress L1 interference when pronouncing L2 sentences, as was found in the case of L2 dominant Italian-English bilinguals.

It is not necessary when measuring interlanguage influence in bilingual speech production to determine that either the L1 or the L2 is entirely responsible for a bilingual's perceived foreign accent in one of her languages. It is quite possible that the languages are involved in a reciprocal relationship whereby they affect one another. Flege's Speech Learning Model (1995) postulates that a bilingual's language-specific phonetic categories are stored within a common phonological space and that these categories may influence each other through a variety of merging and dissimilation processes. According to this model, the phonetic categories of even a speaker's first language may be altered if similar sounds are acquired in a new language; hence, the acquisition of another language exhibits a bidirectional influence on a speaker's phonetic inventory. An example of this bidirectional influence involves cases where two sounds may be "deflected" away from one another to preserve contrast between L1 and L2 phones. It is possible, therefore, that even the L1 phonemic inventory of a bilingual may systematically vary from the inventory of a monolingual. To summarize, predictions from the SLM would be that the L1 and L2 pronunciation of bilinguals will not be the same as that of monolinguals of either language.

Flege's Merger Hypothesis (1987) proposed that similar L1 and L2 phones may merge into a single category in the mind of a bilingual, thus preventing the speaker from creating contrastive sounds for her two languages. Flege (1991) terms this procedure "equivalence classification" of sounds. Equating of the L1 and L2 sounds inhibits the establishment of a separate category for the L2 sound. Because of this, Flege proposes that "similar" L2 sounds may be harder to acquire than L2 sounds that are unlike anything found in the L1. Neither equivalence classification nor "deflection" is the only route a speaker may take when forming phonetic categories, however. Flege (1987), examining the duration of voice onset time (VOT) in Spanish-English bilinguals, concluded that bilinguals who used insufficient aspiration either had failed to form separate categories (indicating that L2 categorical formation is still in progress) or had blended the L1/L2 categories through the equivalence classification process.

There continues to be much debate concerning the separation or convergence of phonetic production and perception systems in the minds of bilinguals, however. The fourth possibility to be examined is that the L1 and L2 operate independently of one another in the production of highly competent, or "balanced," bilinguals (Antoniou et al., 2010; Grosjean & Miller, 1994; Magliore & Green, 1999). Olson (2013) affirms that while the phonetic categories of bilinguals may not be identical to those of two monolinguals (Flege & Port, 1981), a bilingual continues to be in possession of two distinct sets of phonetic categories for the L1 and L2; essentially, the L1 and L2 do not influence one another. In order for two languages not to affect one another, the speaker must have some method for restricting access to the language not currently in use. Lord (2008) found that English-Spanish bilinguals were able to suppress aspiration in their Spanish voiceless stop production. There is some evidence, therefore, that acquiring both languages earlier in life would certainly aid the chances of forming separate phonetic categories, as Thornburg and Ryalls (1998) found that bilinguals who acquired English in childhood were able to make a systematic distinction between their voiced and voiceless stops.

Sundara, Polka, and Baum (2006) examined the speech of French and English simultaneous bilingual adults to see if they maintained language-specific differences similar to monolingual speakers of the two languages. The subjects were balanced bilinguals since they had been exposed to both languages simultaneously since birth, had bilingual schooling, and had lived in a bilingual community in Canada. Results of this study showed that the subjects produced language-specific differences for their French and English recordings, and Sundara et al.

concluded that these findings suggest that simultaneous balanced bilinguals can keep their two phonetic systems separate. Although the subjects in this study had the ability to produce language-specific differences, the researchers found that they still differed from monolinguals in their two languages. This implies that the simultaneous bilinguals and the monolingual speakers differ in the ways in which they produce the phonetic elements of their two languages. MacLeod and Stoel-Gammon (2009) report similar findings in the speech of adult simultaneous French-English bilinguals. Their subjects were balanced bilinguals (i.e., did not display language dominance in either of their languages). The researchers compared the consonant productions of simultaneous bilinguals and monolingual speakers of French and English. The results showed that the simultaneous bilinguals produced language-specific differences that were similar to monolingual productions in most cases. These findings suggest that balanced simultaneous bilinguals may maintain two separate phonetic systems that are comparable to those of monolingual speakers of those languages.

Equating simultaneous bilinguals with early sequential bilinguals may be objected to on the grounds that, typically, the first three years are spent in a primarily monolingual environment for the latter group. While it may also be argued that it is possible to equate simultaneous and early sequential bilinguals' L2 acquisition patterns due to the incomplete formation of the L1 during the earliest years of language learning, many people still believe that differences in the acquisition patterns of sequential bilinguals prevent attainment of balanced bilingualism. However, balanced bilingualism is rarely attained by bilingual speakers, even if both of the languages are acquired simultaneously, since the variation of the language input is influenced by the mother's native language (Mack, Bott, & Boronat, 1995; Sebastian-Galles, Echeverria, & Bosch, 2005).

While analyzing bilinguals' productions in the unilingual modes in either group for the two languages is insightful, such situations do not necessarily force the full activation of both languages. Code-switching offers an exciting opportunity to test the four hypotheses outlined above, as this process requires bilinguals to activate both languages simultaneously. It is expected that speakers would manifest values in code-switched utterances that differ from their productions in monolingual modes. Speakers of more than one language are often tasked with deciding which language to use and how much of the other language is appropriate to most efficiently convey information—a task which is done unconsciously and often without disruption of the temporal structure of the conversation (Grosjean, 2001). The speed and versatility with which bilinguals are able to alternate between languages, often within the course of a single conversation, has been the focus of study for some time (Grosjean, 1982; Sancier & Fowler, 1997; Antoniou et al., 2010).

Code-switching has been operationally defined as a "… within utterance shift from the base language of the established conversational context, to produce a within-sentence target word in their other out-of-context language" (Antoniou et al., 2011, p. 560; cf. Grosjean, 1982, 2008). Indeed, many studies examining the effects of code-switching have adopted this definition and extracted generalizations on the nature of code-switching based on the criteria of single-word language shifts (Flege & Eefting, 1987; Antoniou et al., 2011).[1] Others have provided a definition of code-switching as "the selection by bilinguals or multilinguals of forms of an embedded variety in utterances of a matrix variety during the same conversation" (Myers-Scotton, 1993, p. 3). This definition more closely reflects the linguistic interaction of two bilinguals engaged in casual conversation that drifts between languages seamlessly without any need for conversational repair, as in the following example:

Speaker 1: Tengo que ir al *[computer lab to do my project.]*
Speaker 2: Seriously? Oh hold on, *[mi mama me llama todo el día].*

Productions such as these are common in conversations between bilingual speakers of all ages, professions, and degrees of socio-economic status. Code-switching is not, as many speakers who engage in the practice view it, a sign of "bad Spanish" or "bad English"; rather, it is a complex system of alternating between two (or more) languages within the course of a single conversation in order to pick the most appropriate vocabulary at one's disposal for conveying meaning without causing delay or impairment on the part of the listener.

While much work has been done on the pragmatic, semantic, and syntactic properties of code-switching and the sociolinguistic implications of code-switching in second and third generation bilinguals (Hebblethwaite, 2010), far less is known about the phonological effects of L1-L2 interference on code-switching. Prior studies have investigated L1-L2 phonetic production in the context of code-switching with conflicting results. Toribio et al. (2005) discovered that bilinguals show significantly different VOTs in both code-switched and monolingual Spanish and English sentences, consistent with a pattern of cue use which is present in a given construction's "base language." The implications of the suggestion that bilinguals are alternating between two distinct systems when they code-switch are that these speakers must make phonetic adjustments when they alternate between languages in addition to the more obvious alternations made at the lexical level.

Other studies indicate that the distinction between the L1 and L2 phonetic systems may not be as categorically separate as the previous studies suggest. An alternate view would be that rather than maintaining separate VOT categories for the voiceless stops of both languages, bilinguals may employ a sort of compromise value to be used interchangeably across both languages. Gonzalez-Lopez (2012) found that late English-Spanish bilinguals produced compromise values for /p, t/ but not for /k/. Hazan and Boulakia (1997) further concluded that French-English bilinguals did not always produce monolingual-like VOTs in their self-rated "weaker" language. It is one possibility for the current study that if separate phonetic category formation has failed to occur, then the production of voiceless stops should display nearly identical values in sentences which activate only one language, English-only or Spanish-only. As in the case of Hazan and Boulakia, it is also entirely possible that bilinguals will produce monolingual-like VOTs in only one of the languages activated during code-switching but will fail to achieve monolingual VOTs in their "weaker" language.

There is much evidence from prior studies on code-switching that the L1 continues to affect L2 phonetic production long after the bilingual has achieved fluency in her L2. Flege and Eefting (1987) found that early bilinguals who were either born in the United States or moved there shortly after birth continued to produce short-lag VOTs during code-switching. The situation may be more complex than a simple filtering of the L2 through the phonetic structure of the L1, however, when one considers the effects the ambient language has on the various activation levels that a bilingual may access (Grosjean, 2001; Bullock et al., 2006; Gonzalez-Lopez, 2012). Language activation levels span from "monolingual mode," where only the base language is in use, to a bilingual mode where the L2 is also highly active. Nowhere is the bilingual mode better exemplified than in code-switching, where the speaker/listener dyad engages in a process of switching effortlessly back and forth between languages within the context of a contained utterance, as is seen daily in bilingual cities.

Our focus in this study is to examine the effects of the language mode (monolingual and code-switching sentences) on VOT in early sequential Spanish-English bilinguals. How these speakers adjust their VOT production in sentences that call on them to manipulate both types of voiceless stops in fluent speech is a central focus of our study. As code-switching arguably requires bilinguals to activate both languages simultaneously, it is expected that speakers will manifest VOT values in code-switched tasks that differ from their productions in monolingual modes. In testing the bilinguals in Spanish-English and English-Spanish code-switching sentences, the following research questions were considered:

1. Are there differences between bilinguals' productions and monolingual norms in monolingual sentences?
2. Do bilinguals systematically distinguish between productions in L1 and L2?
3. Does the direction of the code-switch affect the increasing or decreasing of VOT values in the construction? Specifically, do English to Spanish switches create longer VOT values in the Spanish targets, and do Spanish to English switches create shorter VOT values in the English portion when compared with monolingual sentences?
4. Are there within-language differences between VOT values in monolingual versus code-switched sentences?
5. Is one language affected more than the other with respect to VOT?

METHOD

Twenty participants from Miami were recruited to participate in the present study. They were early sequential Spanish-English bilinguals (having acquired English before age 6). Participants mainly consisted of undergraduate students from Florida International University in Miami, Florida. The group consisted of 13 female and 7 male students whose ages ranged from 18 to 30. Within this group, the average age of L2 (English) acquisition was 3;7.

As a group, the average length of residence in the United States was 19.9 years; however, the majority of the participants in this group were born in the United States. They were natives of the following countries: United States (15), Cuba (3), Colombia (1), and Honduras (1). All students who reported being born in the United States were either natives of Miami, Florida, or had moved to Miami from New York City during infancy and did not begin learning English from their parents. In other words, they belong to the very typical local pattern whereby the children are in a Spanish-speaking environment until they begin their education.

Stimulus Materials

The stimulus materials consisted of three different types of sentences: (a) English-only sentences, (b) Spanish-only sentences, and (c) bilingual

(English-Spanish code-switched and Spanish-English code-switched) sentences. The monolingual sentences had 54 target words (9 for each target stop) in 18 sentences. English monolingual sentences contained /p, t, k/ sounds (3 × 9 = 27) (e.g., The **kids** were **taking pictures** at the zoo), as did the Spanish constructions (/p, t, k/ 3 × 9 = 27) (e.g., Mi **tio piense** que estoy en **casa** hoy).

Bilingual sentences were constructed by a balanced bilingual and checked for acceptability by a second bilingual researcher. The sentences were found to be similar with regard to phonotactic characteristics, as well as at the segmental level regarding the phonetic environment of the target sounds. Code-switched sentences were also evaluated for "naturalness" by both bilingual researchers. Whereas several previous studies have relied on singular foreign word insertion into a carrier sentence, the focus of this study was to replicate the type of code-switching constructions found in the everyday conversation of bilinguals. These sentences comprised switches at syntactically felicitous code-switching junctures (e.g., at phrase boundaries). They had 60 target words (30 for each language) for English and Spanish /p, t, k/ in 20 sentences, as illustrated in the following example:

English to Spanish code-switch: "*Today's quiz* era sobre la *política*."
Spanish to English code-switch: "Despues de los *cuatro*, I will *take* my *pills.*"

Procedure

Participants were told that the study involved reading sentences on a computer screen and that their speech would be recorded for later acoustic analysis. They were situated in a quiet room. After signing the consent form, they sat in front of a laptop, and the procedure was explained to them in English. They were instructed to read each individual sentence from a PowerPoint presentation as it appeared on the screen and to self-advance the slides as the experiment was not timed. The first sentences to appear on the screen were English-only. Participants were prompted to read the sentences aloud, and their productions were recorded as MP3s on a Sony digital voice recorder for analysis using PRAAT speech analyzing software.

After the English-only section was completed, participants reached a slide explaining that they should take a 5 minute break. At the conclusion of the break, a slide appeared in Spanish which explained to continue the task in the same manner as before. By changing the language of instruction, we intended to keep participants in monolingual mode and avoid any carryover effects that would accompany an abrupt shift of the base language. Participants then read 10 Spanish-only sentences into the recorder. The purpose of gathering this monolingual data from bilingual participants was to provide a clear picture of each participant's base stop values in each language, to be directly compared with participants' stop production in code-switched sentences, as well as with the values commonly found in the literature for monolingual speakers of English and Spanish.

At the conclusion of the Spanish-only sentences, participants were instructed to take a 20 minute break. During this time an extensive language background questionnaire was administered. At the conclusion of the questionnaire, participants were instructed to leave the room for the remainder of the break. Upon their return, they were placed in front of the computer with no oral instruction from the researchers. The purpose of abstaining from interaction with the participant was to allow each speaker to engage their bilingual language mode as naturally as possible.

In section 2, participants read 10 English-Spanish code-switched sentences. At the conclusion of this portion, a slide appeared in Spanish prompting participants to continue to the next section when they were ready. Participants then read 10 Spanish-English code-switched sentences, thus concluding the experiment.

VOT Measurements

VOT values for /p, t, k/ targets were obtained from the waveform and verified with the corresponding wide-band spectrogram as waveforms are resistant to temporal smearing, whereas the spectrogram is not. In spectrograms, VOT corresponds to the interval between the onset of the energy "burst," representing the release of an articulatory constriction, and the first of the regularly spaced vertical striations representing the vocal cord vibration. Lag time measurements were taken from the burst to the onset of the first formant of the following vowel. In the waveforms, positive VOT (or "lag") exhibited a sharp spike (where the waveform changes from quiescent to transient) in the waveform denoting a release burst, and the onset of voicing was identified as the last extreme negative deviation from 0 in the waveform that preceded the onset of regular voiced pulsation where the waveform becomes periodic (i.e., jagged and "saw-tooth" waveforms). Whenever the spectrogram and the waveform showed double bursts, we considered the first one to measure the VOT.

We examined 2242 tokens. Less than 1% of the productions could not be measured and were discarded. Inter-judge reliability for 10% of the target measurements was over 96% within 8 milliseconds, an error window which is lower than the generally acceptable level of disagreement (Peterson & Lehiste, 1960).

RESULTS AND DISCUSSION

We start with the VOT values produced by the participants in their monolingual utterances of English and Spanish. These are compared with the frequently cited means and ranges reported for the two languages by Lisker and Abramson (1964).

We see from the means in Table 12.1 that the productions of the bilinguals in monolingual sentences are, in general, different from the values given by Lisker and Abramson (1964). Overall, the means for English are lower but within the range nevertheless. The values for Spanish, on the other hand, are very different. For /p/ and /t/ of Spanish, our subjects' productions had much higher VOT means than given by Lisker and Abramson; actually, the means were even beyond the ranges given in parentheses. For /k/, the difference is not so great, and the means is within the range. These numbers do suggest that the participants' Spanish /p/ and /t/ have been affected in a much greater way than their English. Although there is a significant shift in bilinguals' Spanish in the direction of English with the increased VOT values, the two systems are undeniably separated. The values for /p/ are English: 50.18 vs. Spanish: 27.94, $p < .001$; for /t/, English: 65.89 vs. Spanish: 29.69, $p < .001$; and for /k/, English: 65.31 vs. Spanish: 34.39, $p < .001$. While these values are different from the monolingual norms, the VOT values we have from bilinguals' monolingual productions point to a clear distinction of two systems between the two languages.

Table 12.1 English and Spanish VOT Values (in Milliseconds) in Monolingual Utterances

	English		Spanish	
	Lisker and Abramson[a]	Bilinguals	Lisker and Abramson	Bilinguals
/p/	58 (20–120)	50.18	4 (0–15)	27.94
/t/	70 (30–110)	65.89	9 (0–15)	29.69
/k/	80 (30–150)	65.31	29 (15–55)	34.39

[a]At the time of writing this chapter, we had our own VOT measurements from 10 monolingual speakers for each language and thus did not want to compare these statistically with 20 bilinguals. It is worth noting, however, that our means, especially for English, are not very different than those given by Lisker and Abramson.

Table 12.2 Comparison of English /p, t, k/ VOT Values in Monolingual and Code-Switching Utterances

Mean Values	English Only	English → Spanish	Spanish → English
/p/	50.18	59.59	42.95
/t/	65.89	61.93	58.49
/k/	65.31	71.75	60.04

In comparing our subjects' productions in their monolingual and code-switched utterances, we observe different patterns with respect to the two languages. First, we examine the patterns for English mean /p, t, k/ productions (see Table 12.2).

Our subjects' mean VOT values for English /p, t, k/ in monolingual productions differ from the means for those stops as the subjects code-switched from English to Spanish. These are significantly lower for /p/ (50.18 vs. 59.59), $p = .017$, in monolingual productions. The values for /t/ and /k/ are slightly, but non-significantly, different: 65.89 vs. 61.93 for /t/, and 65.31 vs. 71.75 for /k/. When subjects code-switched from Spanish to English, we see the opposite picture: significantly higher VOT values in monolingual productions for /p/ (50.18 vs. 42.95), $p = .037$, and for /t/ (65.89 vs. 58.49), $p = .020$. For /k/, although the means (65.31 vs. 60.04) also indicate some lowering in a Spanish-English switch, there are no significant differences between these and the monolingual utterances.

Figure 12.1, with boxplots, displays the measures of central tendency for the VOT values illustrating the means as well as minimum and maximum values.

When we turn our attention to the values obtained for Spanish /p, t, k/, we have the picture shown in Table 12.3.

Subjects' mean VOT values for Spanish stops in monolingual productions differ significantly from the means for /t/ and /k/ as subjects code-switched from English to Spanish; they were significantly higher in code-switched utterances: for /t/, we have 29.69 vs. 38.77, $p = .001$, and for /k/ 34.39 vs. 42.39, $p = .002$. When we compare subjects' monolingual utterances and the code-switching from Spanish to English, we have significantly higher means for /k/ alone in the latter mode (34.39 vs. 40.72), $p = .020$. The means for /p/ are not affected between the monolingual productions and in any of the directions of the code-switched utterances.

Between the two types of code-switching utterances, the direction of the switch is significant in the following cases: English /p/ and /k/

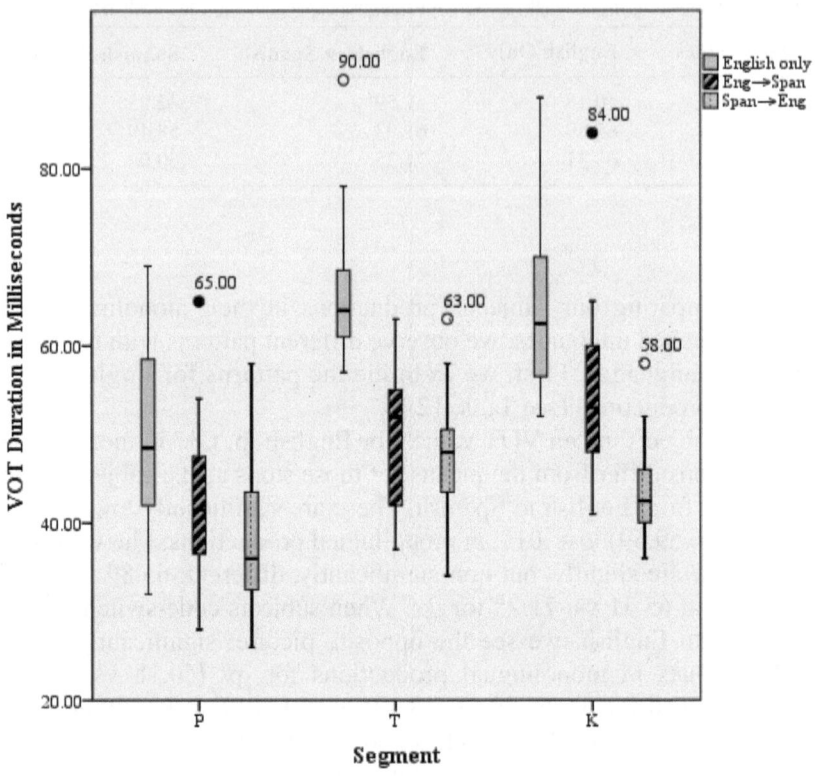

Figure 12.1 Bilinguals' English VOT means in 'English-only', 'English to Spanish switching', and 'Spanish to English switching' utterances.

Table 12.3 Comparison of Spanish /p, t, k/ VOT Values in Monolingual and Code-Switching Utterances

Mean Values	Spanish Only	English → Spanish	Spanish → English
/p/	27.94	29.92	27.44
/t/	29.69	38.77	29.67
/k/	34.39	42.39	40.72

have significantly higher VOT means in English to Spanish switches than in Spanish to English switches: for /p/ there is a decrease from 59.59 to 42.95, $p = .006$, and for /k/ it is 71.75 vs. 60.04, $p = .001$. Also, Spanish /t/ has significantly higher VOT means in English to Spanish switches than in the reverse direction (38.77 vs. 29.67), $p = .002$. Both of these tendencies are suggestive of the beginning language effect. The

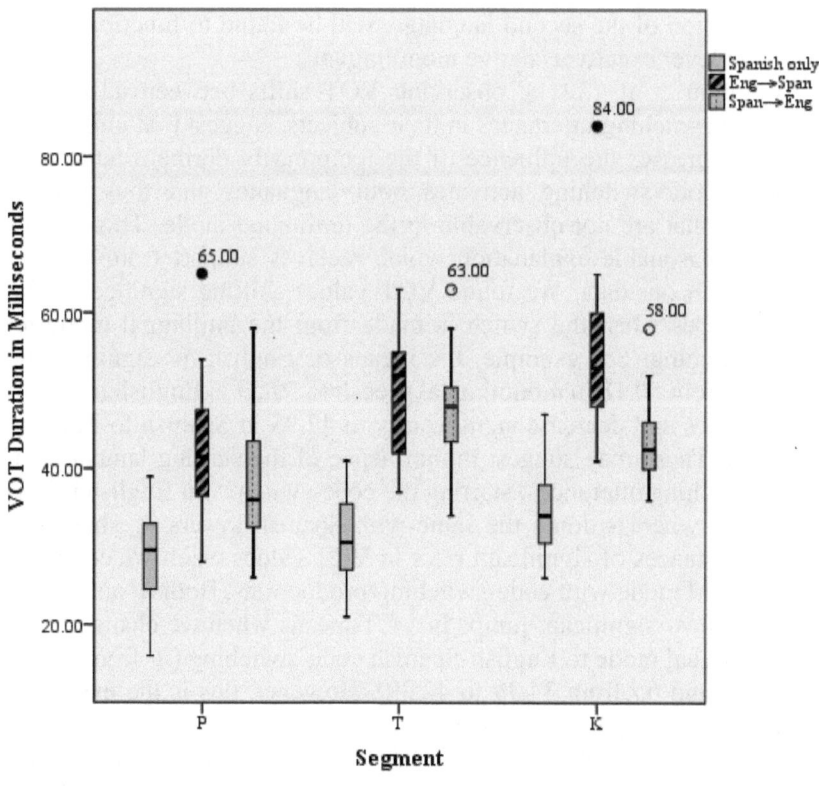

Figure 12.2 Bilinguals' Spanish VOTs in 'Spanish-only', 'English to Spanish switching', and 'Spanish to English switching' utterances.

measures of central tendency comparing Spanish VOTs are presented in Figure 12.2.

The data from our early sequential bilinguals demonstrate that subjects maintain two separate phonologies. Although not identical to those of monolingual norms, their representational systems remain independent. This is confirmed both in unilingual modes and in code-switched utterances. Such a picture is in accordance with the premise that the ability to create L2 phonetic categories may be inversely proportional to the time of first exposure to the L2 (Flege, 1992). Given that the average age of our subjects' exposure to English was 3;9, their formation of the L2 phonetic categories is understandable. At the same time, the VOT values we obtain are also supportive of Mack's (2003) suggestion that very few bilinguals, *if any* (our emphasis), regardless of age of acquisition of the second language, will be found to function at the phonetic level exactly as native monolinguals.

Antoniou et al. (2011), observing VOT shifts between unilingual and code-switching utterances in their subjects, suggest that unilingual mode suppresses the influence of the temporarily dormant language, whereas code-switching activates both languages and thus causes the shifts that are not observable in the unilingual mode. This is certainly a reasonable explanation which receives support from several instances in our data. We found VOT values shifting significantly in several cases when the switch is made from the unilingual mode to code-switching. For example, the means of English /p/ significantly increase from 50.18 in monolingual speech to 59.59 in English to Spanish switches and decrease significantly to 42.95 in Spanish to English switches. These may suggest the influence of the starting language in code-switching utterances; starting the code-switch with English raises the value, whereas doing the same with Spanish lowers it. There are further instances of significant rises in VOT values when we compare a unilingual mode with code-switching productions. Both /t/ and /k/ of Spanish show significant jumps in VOT means when we change from the unilingual mode to English-Spanish code-switching (/t/ from 29.69 to 38.77, and /k/ from 34.39 to 42.39). However, this is the extent of what we see as supporting evidence from our findings, as there are other cases where the significant shifts in VOT means point in the other direction. For example, Spanish /k/ is a case in point; while it, expectedly, jumps up in VOT significantly when we compare the monolingual productions with English to Spanish switches, /k/ also rises significantly in Spanish to English code-switches. Also worth mentioning are several cases where there were no significant shifts in the VOT means when the unilingual productions were compared to code-switchings (e.g., English and Spanish /t/ between unilingual mode and Spanish to English switches, and English /k/ and Spanish /p/ between unilingual mode and either code-switching mode). Thus, our results give only partial support to Antoniou et al.'s (2011) assertion.

There seems, however, to be a rather consistent pattern of significant changes in VOT means when we examine the direction of the switch between the two types of code-switching productions; in the three cases where this was observed, we saw the beginning language effect. The means for English /p/, which was 59.59 in English to Spanish constructions, drops significantly to 42.95 in Spanish to English code-switching. Similarly, English /k/, which has 71.75 in English to Spanish code-switching, is lowered significantly to 60.04 in Spanish to English switching. Finally, the means for Spanish /t/ goes down significantly from 38.77 to 29.67 when we change from English to Spanish switching to Spanish to English switching. These results are in conflict with the findings of Bullock et al. (2006), who finds the "precursor" language irrelevant. Our findings further conflict with Gonzalez-Lopez (2012), where the direction of switch did not appear to play a crucial role.

It might be argued that prosodic strengthening may cause VOT differences at switch sites in code-switching sentences. Since the beginning of a switch in a bilingual sentence could be considered as the beginning of a large prosodic unit, this would imply that an increase in VOT would occur in that site. Although our sentences are not perfectly controlled for this, there doesn't seem to be an effect of the switch site when we examine the available comparisons.

The commonly held view that phonetic influence occurs even in the speech of highly fluent early L2 dominant bilinguals when they switch languages has received confirmation with our findings. Antoniou et al. (2011), however, suggests that the L1 is less susceptible to phonetic interference than the L2, even for bilinguals who are L2 dominant. Bullock et al. (2006) makes a similar observation in that their subjects' Spanish values remained stable while English values dropped toward Spanish; that is, the shift affected only the L2, not the L1. Our results disagree with these. While the VOT means for English /p, t, k/ in our data were always within the established long-lag values (the lowest was 42.95, in Spanish to English switches), Spanish VOT means for /t/ and /k/ went beyond the norms (38.77 for /t/ and 42.39 for /k/ in English to Spanish switches). Since Spanish is affected more, it is reasonable to ask, "Why are more unmarked stops (Spanish unaspirated/short-lag stops) moving toward more marked (English aspirated/long-lag) stops?" The different markedness references we make between these two types of stops are phonetically grounded, as the more marked aspirated stops require keeping the glottis open long enough after the release of the oral closure to create a long interval of audible aspiration during the initial portion of the following vowel. In other words, any action of the larynx other than simple voicing or voicelessness co-occurring with oral articulation (breathy voice, aspiration, etc.) is a complicating factor (Maddieson, 2009). Further support for the more unmarked nature of unaspirated stops relative to aspirated ones also comes from child phonology (Macken & Barton, 1980; Pan, 1994; Davis, 1995), as well as data from languages of the world (Maddieson, 1984). The move from more unmarked short-lag to more marked long-lag productions that we observe in our subjects can be explained through language dominance. Having acquired their English rather early, coupled with greater daily use of English (self-reported), has resulted in L2 dominance, and this must have caused the increases in VOTs. Finally, in almost all types of sentences (monolingual and code-switching in either direction) and in both languages, overall results confirm the universal tendency that the lag is longer as the place of articulation moves from front to back.

A Note on Frequency

In considering VOT contrasts between participants' productions in Spanish and English, the following question is also posed: would L2 English speakers make closer approximations of English VOT productions for /p, t, k/ in words they hear and repeat more frequently? Asked more broadly, we can encapsulate this issue of frequency in the question: Are frequency effects correlated with language proficiency? Whaley (1978) establishes that the frequency of written words is predictive of the recognition times for a given set of targets. Whether or not word recognition time is predictive of more accurate L2 phonetic production is a question that is currently unanswered. Much of the prior research focusing on spoken word frequency is concerned with L1 language development in children, as quantified by the mean age of acquisition for a given word, rather than examining the relationship between frequency and L2 lexical or phonological acquisition (Brown, 1984).

Studies that have examined frequency and/or neighborhood density as predictive of the phonetic structure of speech have found that words existing in high frequency neighborhoods tend to be produced faster and more accurately (Vitevitch, 2002). Miller and Desterno (2009) claimed that VOT is robustly affected by contextual influences, including speaking rate and place of articulation. Van Dam and Port (2005) found that frequent words (e.g., talk, table) have a mean VOT roughly 10 milliseconds shorter than that of less frequent words (e.g., talc, taint) and that this effect was significantly stronger for words in a sentence (e.g., He will talk to his supervisor) than in list form. Baese-Berk and Goldrick (2009) examined specific types of neighborhood effects on VOT through the presence of a specific minimal pair lexical item. Their results showed productions with more extreme VOTs with the minimal pair neighbor (e.g., *cod-god*) than with words without a minimal pair neighbor (e.g., *cop-*gop*).

The hypothesis concerning frequency is that the likelihood of a word's occurrence may affect VOT values and that L2 English speakers may produce more English-like VOTs in highly frequently occurring words than in the less frequently occurring items. This hypothesis is derived from the assumption that L2 English speakers would have not only more examples of native-speaker input on frequently occurring words but also more practice shaping and refining their own acoustic output of frequently occurring words in the context of natural conversation. In other words, because of their high frequency these articulatory targets can be met faster than in low frequency words. While it is not reasonable to believe that every target word in this experiment receives an equal amount of real-world exposure for the L2 speaker, an attempt was made to construct the instrument in such as a way that frequently occurring items would be familiar to the particular demographics of the participants, whereas the infrequently occurring word set would be less likely to be encountered by these speakers.

In the current study each set of 12 targets consisted of 6 "frequently occurring" and 6 "less frequently occurring" tokens in each category, as delineated by the Brown corpus (1984).[2] English /p/ was selected as the target, as it showed the greatest variability in the VOT means in our data. A paired-sample *t*-test comparison of micro-sets of the target words was conducted whenever possible, as in the English-only sentences condition, where the words in the "frequent" column were *post*, *people*, and *pictures* compared with *pasta*, *potato*, and *pumpkin* in the infrequent category. The mean VOT duration for /p/ in frequently occurring words was 63 milliseconds, compared with 64 milliseconds for the infrequently occurring words. These comparisons were done in every instance where sufficient tokens were available to group words into frequent and infrequent categories, and we failed to find evidence that frequency skewed the direction of VOT in any of our targets for this study.

CONCLUSIONS

This chapter investigated the voiceless stop productions of English and Spanish in early sequential Spanish-English bilinguals. Our findings indicated that although bilinguals' productions were not identical to those of monolinguals of the two languages, the two language systems were clearly kept separate. Code-switching influenced the results and revealed the effects of the precursor language. As for the effects of markedness universals, we saw clear effects of the place of articulation and the amount of VOT in both languages and in all types of utterances. Spanish was the language that has been affected more than English with respect to VOT. The L2 English language dominance of the subjects was given as the explanation for this effect whereby the more unmarked (short-lag) stops have moved in the direction of the more marked longer-lag stops.

ACKNOWLEDGMENTS

We are grateful to the participants who gave their time generously to the study. Our thanks also go to Dr. Paulette Johnson for the statistical analysis.

NOTES

1　Antoniou et al. (2011) used carrier sentences as in the construction "say *target word* again."
2　However, because the research design had not included neighborhood density and phonetically similar pairs of words for each environment, it was impossible to do a comprehensive analysis of the effects of word frequency in these data.

REFERENCES

Antoniou, M., Best, C., Tyler, M., & Kroos, C. (2010). Language context elicits native-like stop voicing in early bilinguals' productions in both L1 and L2. *Journal of Phonetics* 38, 640–653.

Antoniou, M., Best, C., Tyler, M., & Kroos, C. (2011). Inter-language interference in VOT production by L2-dominant bilinguals: Asymmetries in phonetic code-switching. *Journal of Phonetics* 39, 558–570.

Baese-Berk, M., & Goldrick, M. (2009). Mechanisms of interaction in speech production. *Language and Cognitive Processes* 24, 527–554.

Bialystok, E., & Miller, B. (1998). The problem of age in second-language acquisition: Influences from language, structure, and task. *Bilingualism: Language and Cognition* 2, 127–145.

Brown, G. (1984). A frequency count of 190.000 words in the *London-Lund Corpus of English Conversation. Behavior, Research Methods, Instruments, and Computers* 16 (6), 502- 532.

Bullock, B., Toribio, A., Gonzalez, V., & Dalola, A. (2006). Language dominance and performance outcomes in bilingual pronunciation. *Proceedings of the 8th Generative Approaches to Second Language Acquisition Conference*, Cascadilla Proceedings Project, 9–16.

Davis, K. (1995). Phonetic and phonological contrast in the acquisition of voicing: Voice onset time in Hindi and English. *Journal of Child Language* 22, 275–305.

Flege, J. (1981). The phonological basis of foreign accent: A hypothesis. *TESOL Quarterly* 15, 443–455.

Flege, J. (1987). The production of "new" and "similar" phones in a foreign accent: Evidence for the effect of equivalence classification. *Journal of Phonetics* 15, 47–65.

Flege, J. (1991). Age of learning affects the authenticity of voice-onset time (VOT) in stop consonants produced in a second language. *Journal of the Acoustical Society of America* 89, 395–411.

Flege, J. (1992). Speech learning in a second language. In Ferguson, C., Menn, L., and Stoel-Gammon, C. (eds) *Phonological Development: Models, Research, and Application*, 565–604. Timonium, MD: York Press.

Flege, J. (1995). Second language speech learning: Theory, findings, and problems. In Strange, W. (ed) *Speech Perception and Linguistic Experience: Issues in Cross-language Research*, 233–277. Timonium, MD: York Press.

Flege, J., & Eefting, W. (1987). Production and perception of English stops by native Spanish speakers. *Journal of Phonetics* 15, 67–83.

Flege, J., & MacKay, I. (2004). Perceiving vowels in a second language. *Studies in Second Language Acquisition* 26, 1–34.

Flege, J., MacKay, I., & Piske, T. (2002). Assessing bilingual dominance. *Applied Psycholinguistics* 23, 567–598.

Flege, J., & Port, R. (1981). Cross-language phonetic interference: Arabic to English. *Language & Speech* 24, 125–146.

Fowler, C., Sramko, V., Ostry, D., Rowland, S., & Hallé, P. (2008). Cross language phonetic influences on the speech of French-English bilinguals. *Journal of Phonetics* 36 (4), 649–663.

Gonzalez-Lopez, V. (2012). Spanish and English word-initial voiceless stop production in code-switched vs. monolingual structures. *Second Language Research* 28 (2), 243–263.

Grosjean, F. (1982). *Life with Two Languages.* Cambridge, MA: Harvard University Press.

Grosjean, F. (2001). The bilingual's language modes. In Nicol, J. (ed) *One Mind, Two Languages: Bilingual Language Processing*, 1–22. Malden, MA: Blackwell.

Grosjean, F. (2008). *Studying Bilinguals.* Oxford: Oxford University Press.

Grosjean, F., & Miller, J. (1994). Going in and out of languages: An example of bilingual flexibility. *Psychological Science* 5, 201–209.

Guion, S., Flege, J., & Loftin, J. (2000). The effect of L1 use on pronunciation of Quechua-Spanish bilinguals. *Journal of Phonetics* 28, 27–42.

Hazan, V., & Boulakia, G. (1997). Perception and production of a voicing contrast by French-English bilinguals. *Language and Speech* 36, 17–38.

Hebblethwaite, B. (2010). Adverb code-switching among Miami's Haitian Creole-English second generation. *Bilingualism: Language and Cognition* 13 (4), 409–428.

Lisker, L., & Abramson, A. (1964). A cross-language study of voicing in initial stops: Acoustical measurements. *Word* 20, 384–422.

Lord, G. (2008). Second language acquisition and first language phonological modification. *Selected Proceedings of the 10th Hispanic Linguistics Symposium.* Somerville, MA: Cascadilla, 184–193.

Mack, M. (2003). The phonetic system of bilinguals. In Banich, M.T., & Mack, M. (eds) *Mind, Brain, and Language: Multidisciplinary Perspectives,* 309–351. Mahwah, NJ; Lawrence Erlbaum.

Mack, M., Bott, S., & Boronat, C. (1995). Mother, I'd rather do it myself, maybe: An analysis of voice onset time produced by early French-English bilinguals. *Idea* 8, 23–55.

Macken, M., & Barton, D. (1980). The acquisition of voicing contrast in English: A study of voice onset time in word-initial stop consonants. *Journal of Child Language* 7, 41–74.

MacLeod, A., & Stoel-Gammon, C. (2009). The use of voice onset time by early bilinguals to distinguish homorganic stops in Canadian English and Canadian French. *Applied Psycholinguistics* 30 (1), 53–77.

Maddieson, I. (1984). *Patterns of Sounds.* Cambridge: Cambridge University Press.

Maddieson, I. (2009). Calculating phonological complexity. In Pellegrino, F., Marsico, E., Chitoran, I., & Coupe, C. (eds) *Approaches to Phonological Complexity,* 85–109. New York: Mouton de Gruyter.

Magliore, J., & Green, K. (1999). A cross-language comparison of speaking rate effects on the production of voice onset time in English and Spanish. *Phonetica* 56, 158–185.

Miller, T., & Desterno, D. (2009). Individual talker differences in voice onset time: Contextual influences. *Journal of the Acoustical Society of America* 125 (6), 3974–3986.

Myers-Scotton, C. (1993). Common and uncommon ground: Social and structural factors in codeswitching. *Language in Society* 22 (4), 475–503.

Olson, D. (2013). Bilingual language switching and selection at the phonetic level: Asymmetrical transfer in VOT production. *Journal of Phonetics* 41, 407–420.

Pan, H.-H. (1994). *The voicing contrasts of Taiwanese (Amoy) initial stops: Data from adults and children.* Ph.D. thesis, Ohio State University.

Peterson, G., & Lehiste, I. (1960). Duration of syllable nuclei in English. *Journal of the Acoustical Society of America* 32, 693–703.

Piske, T., Flege, J., MacKay, I., & Meador, D. (2002). The production of English vowels by fluent early and late Italian-English bilinguals. *Phonetica* 59, 49–71.

Sancier, M., & Fowler, C. (1997). Gestural drift in a bilingual speaker of Brazilian Portuguese and English. *Journal of Phonetics* 25, 421–436.

Sebastian-Galles, N., Echeverria, S., & Bosch, L. (2005). The influence of initial exposure on lexical representation: Comparing early and simultaneous bilinguals. *Journal of Memory and Language* 37, 159–173.

Sundara, M., Polka, L., & Baum, S. (2006). Production of coronal stops by simultaneous bilingual adults. *Bilingualism: Language and Cognition* 9 (1), 97–114.

Thornburg, R., & Ryalls, J. (1998). Voice onset time in Spanish-English bilinguals: Early versus late learners. *Journal of Communication Disorders* 31, 215–229.

Toribio, A.J., Bullock, B., Botero, C., & Davis, K. (2005). Preservative phonetic effects in bilingual code-switching. In Gess, R., and Rubin, E. (eds) *Theoretical and Experimental Approaches to Romance Linguistics*, 291–306. London: John Benjamins.

Van Dam, M., & Port, R. (2005). Voice onset timing is shorter in high-frequency words. *Journal of the Acoustical Society of America* 117 (4), 2623–2628.

Vitevitch, M. (2002). The influence of phonological similarity neighborhoods on speech production. *Journal of Experimental Psychology: Learning, Memory, and Cognition* 28, 735–747.

Whaley, C. (1978). Word-nonword classification time. *Journal of Verbal Learning and Verbal Behavior* 17, 143–154.

INDEX